Assessing Intelligence in Children and Adolescents

The Guilford Practical Intervention in the Schools Series

Kenneth W. Merrell, Founding Editor
T. Chris Riley-Tillman, Series Editor

www.guilford.com/practical

This series presents the most reader-friendly resources available in key areas of evidence-based practice in school settings. Practitioners will find trustworthy guides on effective behavioral, mental health, and academic interventions, and assessment and measurement approaches. Covering all aspects of planning, implementing, and evaluating high-quality services for students, books in the series are carefully crafted for everyday utility. Features include ready-to-use reproducibles, lay-flat binding to facilitate photocopying, appealing visual elements, and an oversized format. Recent titles have Web pages where purchasers can download and print the reproducible materials.

RECENT VOLUMES

Assessing Intelligence in Children and Adolescents

A Practical Guide

JOHN H. KRANZLER
RANDY G. FLOYD

THE GUILFORD PRESS
New York   London

© 2013 The Guilford Press
A Division of Guilford Publications, Inc.
370 Seventh Avenue, Suite 1200, New York, NY 10001
www.guilford.com

Printed in Canada

This book is printed on acid-free paper.

Last digit is print number: 9 8 7 6 5 4 3 2

The authors have checked with sources believed to be reliable in their efforts to provide information that is complete and generally in accord with the standards and practice that are accepted at the time of publication. However, in view of the possibility of human error or changes in behavioral, mental health, or medical sciences, neither the authors, nor the editors and publisher, nor any other party who has been involved in the preparation or publication of this work warrants that the information contained herein is in every respect accurate or complete, and they are not responsible for any errors or omissions or the results obtained from the use of such information. Readers are encouraged to confirm the information contained in this book with other sources.

Library of Congress Cataloging-in-Publication Data

Kranzler, John H.
    Assessing intelligence in children and adolescents : a practical guide / John H. Kranzler, Randy G. Floyd.
        pages cm. — (The Guilford practical intervention in the schools series)
    Includes bibliographical references and index.
    ISBN 978-1-4625-1121-1 (pbk.)
    1. Children—Intelligence testing.   2. Teenagers—Intelligence testing.   3. Learning disabled children—Identification.   4. Learning disabled teenagers—Identification.   I. Floyd, Randy G., 1971–   II. Title.
    BF432.C48K73 2013
    153.9′3—dc23
                                                                2013025468

About the Authors

John H. Kranzler, PhD, is Professor and Program Director of School Psychology in the School of Special Education, School Psychology, and Early Childhood Studies at the University of Florida. He has received numerous awards for his research, including article-of-the-year awards in *School Psychology Quarterly* and *School Psychology Review*. Dr. Kranzler was Associate Editor of *School Psychology Quarterly* for 6 years and has served on the editorial boards of a number of other journals. His research focuses on the nature, development, and assessment of human cognitive abilities.

Randy G. Floyd, PhD, is Associate Professor of Psychology, Co-Director of the Child and Family Studies research area, and a member of the Institute of Intelligent Systems at the University of Memphis. Dr. Floyd is Editor of the *Journal of School Psychology* and has served on the editorial boards of several other journals. His research interests include the structure, measurement, and correlates of cognitive abilities, the technical properties of early numeracy measures, and the process of professional publication.

Preface

This book is a practical guide to the intellectual assessment of children and adolescents in the schools. Primarily intended for students of school psychology and for practicing school psychologists, it should also be useful for those counselors, teachers, administrators, and other school personnel involved in making decisions in schools based in part on the results of intelligence tests. In writing it, we have placed particular emphasis on empirically supported practices that will be useful within the response-to-intervention (RTI) model of school-psychological service delivery.

STATEMENT OF NEED

The assessment of intelligence has long been mandated by law for eligibility determination for special education and related services (e.g., intellectual disability [ID], specific learning disabilities [SLD], and intellectual giftedness). In the past, scores on standardized tests of intelligence (IQ tests) have been used in schools primarily as benchmarks against which to compare academic achievement or adaptive functioning. For example, central to most prior definitions of SLD is the concept of discrepancy in cognitive functioning. Children and youth have been identified with SLD when their academic performance or rate of skill acquisition falls substantially below what one would expect from their IQs, when that discrepancy is not attributable to certain exclusionary criteria (e.g., inadequate educational opportunity). However, the transition to the RTI model will have important implications for the use of intelligence tests in schools. To the best of our knowledge, at present no currently available textbook on intellectual assessment addresses the use of intelligence tests within an RTI context. One of our intentions in writing this book has been to fill that gap.

In addition to not addressing this need in the literature, many available books on intellectual assessment tend to be theoretically "agnostic" and present a range of theories and models of intelligence, thereby implying that readers should pick and choose any theory to meet their needs or personal predilections. Researchers in the field of intelligence, however, largely agree on the major substantive conclusions regarding the structure of cognitive abilities, the nature of individual differences, and other major emphases of research. Thus, another of our intentions in writing this book has been to emphasize the predominant theory of intelligence in the field today—the psychometric approach. Although there are various other theories of intelligence, the psychometric approach has by far the most empirical support in the literature.

Finally, the available books on intellectual assessment tend to describe approaches for interpreting test scores that, we believe, overstate the utility of intraindividual (ipsative) analysis for differential diagnosis and intervention planning. Although research on intelligence and its assessment may lead to breakthroughs, the empirical data at the present time do not clearly substantiate the validity of disordinal models (aptitude × treatment interactions) to inform decision making, although they do provide support for ordinal models (high vs. low general cognitive ability). Therefore, this book presents a method for interpreting test scores that emphasizes the interpretation of global composite scores rather than individual subtests, with implications for ordinal models of intervention when applied to conditions of incomplete instruction (Braden & Shaw, 2009). In sum, we have written this book to address the need for an updated, evidence-based, user-friendly resource to meet these needs.

DESCRIPTION OF THE CONTENT

This book is a practical guide for school personnel working at either the primary level (i.e., elementary schools) or the secondary level (i.e., middle and high schools). In particular, it should prove useful to school psychologists, school counselors, school social workers, teachers, administrators, and other school personnel. The book has 13 chapters, many of which include tables and figures, as well as checklists and assessment forms that school personnel can easily integrate into their practices.

Chapter 1 examines the definition and nature of intelligence from the psychometric perspective, as well as some of the criticisms of this model.

Chapter 2 discusses how and why individuals differ in intelligence. It includes an explanation of research in the differential model, or quantitative behavior genetics, as well as the implications of this model for modifying intelligence.

Chapter 3 highlights ethical principles and standards most relevant to testing children and adolescents. In particular, it reviews the most recent ethical guidelines from the American Psychological Association and the National Association of School Psychologists.

Chapter 4 addresses the reasons for assessment, typical assessment processes, and potential influences on test performance that can be controlled during standardized testing or acknowledged in the interpretation of test results. It also provides practical screening tools that will promote the most accurate assessment of cognitive abilities through standardized testing.

Chapter 5 first highlights the standards guiding the selection and use of tests. It continues with a review of the most critical characteristics of tests, including norming and item scaling, as well as the reliability and validity of their scores. This information will promote selection of the best intelligence tests by practitioners, based in part on the age, ability level, and backgrounds of the clients they serve.

Chapter 6 focuses on interpretation of examinee responses and resulting scores. It targets interpreting data from qualitative and quantitative perspectives, using interpretive strategies based on an understanding of the nature of cognitive abilities and relying on the scientific research base that illuminates empirically supported practices.

Chapter 7 provides a broad overview of the array of intelligence tests currently available. These include full-length multidimensional intelligence tests, which are the best known and most commonly used in research and practice, as well as nonverbal intelligence tests and brief and abbreviated intelligence tests.

Chapter 8 addresses two pathways by which assessment results are shared: psychological assessment reports and face-to-face contact with the parents or caregivers of the child or adolescent who has completed the assessment. It also addresses the process of sharing assessment results with supervisors during supervision meetings.

Chapter 9 highlights the evidence base describing the nature and correlates of psychometric g; advances in testing technology; and legal and practical constraints that warrant consideration of intelligence tests during use of the problem-solving model. It concludes that intelligence tests (1) will probably continue to play an important (though narrower) role in the schools than in the past and (2) should be included in modern problem-solving methods that seek answers to children's academic problems.

Chapter 10 describes the clinical condition known as ID and offers practical guidelines for assessing children suspected of having this condition. It addresses varying diagnostic and eligibility criteria for ID, offers recommendations for best practices in assessment, and discusses best practices in interpreting test results.

Chapter 11 discusses the use of intelligence tests in the identification of giftedness. We first review contemporary theories of giftedness. Following this, we address the definition of giftedness and issues in its identification.

Chapter 12 examines the different conceptualizations of SLD and the implications of these definitions for its identification. The use of intelligence tests in the identification of SLD has long been surrounded by controversy, which continues to this day. We address best practices in assessment that apply regardless of the SLD criteria used for identification.

Chapter 13 discusses best practices in the use of intelligence tests with children and youth from diverse backgrounds. After briefly reviewing research on test bias, we address the pros and cons of the most widely recommended best practices with this population.

Acknowledgments

We thank the many people who supported us during our writing of this book. In particular, we thank our wives and children—Theresa, Zachary, and Justin (JHK) and Carrie and Sophie (RGF)—for their enthusiasm about this book and their patience across the 3 years we devoted to developing it.

We also thank doctoral students in our school psychology programs who contributed literature reviews, retrieved articles, and helped with formatting and proofing. In particular, Ryan Farmer contributed substantially to two chapters in this book. In addition, Tera Bradley, Rachel Haley, Haley Hawkins, Sarah Irby, Jennifer Maynard, Phil Norfolk, Kate Price, Triche Roberson, Colby Taylor, and Isaac Woods deserve specific recognition. Furthermore, students enrolled in the 2010, 2011, 2012, and 2013 assessment practica at the University of Memphis were the sources of many of the examples we used, and they helped to refine our thinking about central issues and the resources we provided.

We are also appreciative of our colleagues and collaborators who provided source material for and feedback about our chapters; they include Dr. Thomas Fagan, Dr. Kevin McGrew, and Dr. Matthew Reynolds. In addition, Dr. Matthew Reynolds and Dr. Joel Schneider provided thorough and generous recommendations to us after reviewing a complete draft of this book. Finally, several professionals provided guidance to us as we developed and refined the screening tools described in Chapter 4. They include Courtney Farmer and Dr. David Damari. Overall, we benefited greatly from the support and assistance of these individuals.

We missed the opportunity to work with the late Dr. Kenneth W. Merrell throughout the development of this book, but we are grateful for his recruiting us to write it and for his support and feedback as we developed the book proposal. We would also like to express thanks to Acquisitions Editor Natalie Graham, Senior Production Editor Jeannie Tang, and Copyeditor Marie Sprayberry, all at The Guilford Press, for their guidance (and patience) as we developed and fine-tuned each chapter.

Contents

CHAPTER 1

What Is Intelligence?

A basic assumption underlying the "American dream" is that all people are created equal. Many Americans see success in life as resulting primarily from ambition, hard work, and good character, regardless of the circumstances into which one was born (e.g., gender, race/ethnicity, and socioeconomic status). This commitment to the concept of equality underlies much of the controversy that has long surrounded research and theory on intelligence and its assessment (e.g., Cronbach, 1975; Gould, 1996). Despite these well-intentioned egalitarian ideals, today's society is heavily oriented toward intelligence and intellectual achievement (e.g., Browne-Miller, 1995; Gifford, 1989). Ambition, hard work, and good character will not guarantee success in life; intelligence is also required (e.g., Gottfredson, 2011; Nisbett et al., 2012).

In schools, the assessment of intelligence is mandated by current federal special education law—the Individuals with Disabilities Education Improvement Act of 2004 (IDEA, 2004)—for the identification of intellectual disability (ID). In addition, IDEA allows, but does not require, the use of intelligence tests for the identification of specific learning disability (SLD). Finally, although gifted students are not protected under IDEA in its current form, exceptionally high intelligence (IQ) is a key component used in most states to identify intellectual giftedness (McClain & Pfeiffer, 2012). In these instances, the overall score on standardized IQ tests is primarily used as the benchmark against which to compare students' current academic achievement or adaptive behavior (i.e., age-appropriate ability to act independently, interact socially with others, care for oneself, etc.). For example, ID is identified when an individual has significantly below-average IQ and comparable deficits in adaptive functioning, among other criteria. In contrast, SLD has traditionally been identified when there is a significant discrepancy between an individual's level of academic performance and IQ, and when that discrepancy cannot be explained by certain exclusionary criteria (e.g., inadequate educational opportunities and sensory disorders). For identification of giftedness, high scores on intelligence tests are seen as necessary but not sufficient for high accomplishment. In addition to a sufficiently high level of general intelligence, other factors are required, such as motivation, creativity, and task commitment (e.g., Reis & Renzulli, 2011). Chapters 10–12 provide more detailed information on the use of intelligence tests in schools for the determination of eligibility for special education and related services.

The purpose of this chapter is to define *intelligence* and to describe how people differ in terms of their intellectual abilities. We begin by addressing two common objections to intelligence research and assessment. The first objection asserts that because intelligence is not a real thing, how can we measure something that does not exist? The second objection contends that since there is no consensus definition of intelligence, how can we measure something we cannot define?

DOES INTELLIGENCE EXIST?

The great American psychologist E. L. Thorndike (1874–1949) stated that "whatever exists at all exists in some amount" (Thorndike, 1918, p. 16, as quoted in Eysenck, 1973). Many laypersons also believe that intelligence exists as a "real thing" that underlies intelligent behavior (Berg & Sternberg, 1992). Treating an abstract concept as a concrete, physical entity, however, is a common mistake in reasoning known as *reification*. Intelligence, like gravity, is nothing more than an idea, or construct, that exists in the minds of scientists. Scientific constructs are hypothetical variables that are not directly observable.

Individuals exist, of course, and their behavior can be observed and measured. Careful examination of these measurements leads to the development of constructs that attempt to explain these factual observations. The appropriateness and usefulness of these constructs depends upon the degree to which they help us to understand, describe, and predict behavior. Thorndike, therefore, was wrong: Intelligence is not a "real thing" that exists in some amount. It is a hypothetical construct that scientists have posited to explain certain types of behavior. *Intelligence*, then, exists, but only as a scientific construct.

HOW CAN WE MEASURE SOMETHING WE CANNOT DEFINE?

Despite over 100 years of theory and research, the field of psychology has never reached a consensus on a definition of *intelligence* (e.g., see Sternberg & Kaufman, 2011). No other psychological phenomenon has proven harder to define than intelligence. In 1921, the *Journal of Educational Psychology* published a symposium titled "Intelligence and Its Measurement" (Buckingham, 1921). In

> Despite over 100 years of theory and research, the field of psychology has never reached a consensus definition of *intelligence*.

this symposium the editor asked 14 leading experts to define intelligence, among other questions. He received 14 different replies. Sample responses from selected experts included the following:

- "The power of good responses from the point of view of fact." (Thorndike)
- "The ability to carry on abstract thinking." (Terman)
- "Intelligence involves the capacity to acquire capacity." (Woodrow)
- "The ability of the individual to adapt himself adequately to relatively new situations in life." (Pintner)
- "Intelligence is what the tests test." (Boring)

The main source of disagreement in this symposium concerned whether intelligence is one single general ability or a number of different abilities. The only point on which the respondents tended to agree was that intelligence is related to "higher mental processes," such as abstract reasoning or problem solving.

In 1986, Sternberg and Detterman published a book titled *What Is Intelligence?* They were interested in determining whether there was greater consensus among contemporary researchers than there had been 65 years earlier. They asked 24 prominent experts in the field of intelligence to respond to the same questions that the participants answered in the 1921 symposium. Here are a few sample definitions of intelligence from these experts:

- "Intelligence is a quality of adaptive behavior." (Anastasi)
- "Intelligence is the repertoire of knowledge and skills available to a person at a particular point in time." (Humphreys)
- "Intelligence is defined as the general factor . . . of psychological tests." (Jensen)
- "Intelligence is the reification of an entity that does not exist; it is a number of somewhat independent broad abilities." (Horn)

As Sternberg and Detterman (1986) noted, "striking diversity" was apparent among the respondents' definitions, despite over half a century of research on the nature and measurement of intelligence since the 1921 symposium. Nonetheless, consistent with the earlier findings, most of the participants mentioned that intelligence is related to higher-order cognitive functions. Differences among experts were also prevalent on the "one versus many" question of the generality of intelligence.

Conceptions of Intelligence

One reason for this lack of consensus stems from the fact that one can view intelligence from different perspectives (see Eysenck, 1998). Figure 1.1 shows the relationship among three different conceptions of intelligence. The first concerns the biological substrate that underlies all intelligent

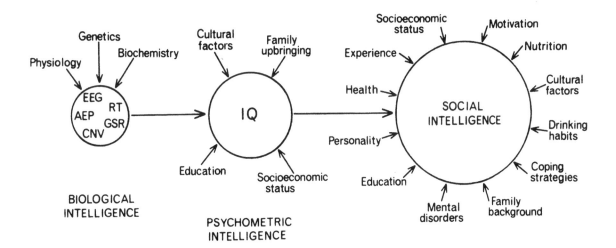

FIGURE 1.1. Relations among biological, psychometric, and social (or practical) intelligence. From Eysenck (1998, p. 62). Copyright 1998 by Transaction Publishers. Reprinted by permission.

thought and action. *Biological intelligence* sets the limits of intellectual development. Intelligence is influenced by genetics, because genes determine the neurological structures and the physiological and biochemical functioning of the brain. As shown within the circle for biological intelligence, brain functioning can be measured in a number of different ways, including the electroencephalograph (EEG), averaged evoked potentials (AEP), galvanic skin response (GSR), central nerve conduction velocity (CNV), and reaction time (RT) on elementary cognitive tasks, among other methods (e.g., see Colom & Thompson, 2011; Deary, Penke, & Johnson, 2010; Haier, 2011; Nisbett et al., 2012).

The second conception of intelligence is psychometric intelligence. *Psychometric intelligence* refers to the "intelligent" behavior that is sampled on standardized tests of intelligence ("IQ tests"). Individual differences in biological intelligence can be measured only indirectly by psychometric intelligence tests. The behaviors measured on these tests are related to biological functioning, but they are also influenced by one's background and experience. Cultural factors, family upbringing, level and quality of education, and socioeconomic status are all importantly related to intelligence test performance (e.g., Gottfredson, 2008; Jensen, 1998).

The third and final conception of intelligence is social (or practical) intelligence. *Social intelligence* refers to the overt behavior that is considered "intelligent" in specific contexts, cultures, or both. Examples include academic achievement in school and performance at work. What is considered intelligent behavior may differ to some degree across contexts and cultures, even though the basic cognitive and biological processes underlying such behavior may be the same. Intelligent behavior in the "real world" is determined in part by biological intelligence and in part by background and experience, but also by a host of other noncognitive factors (e.g., personality, healthy lifestyle, and mental health).

Thus, although these three meanings of the term *intelligence* overlap to a considerable degree, they differ in their breadth or inclusiveness. Given that there are different ways in which to view intelligence, it is perhaps not surprising that a consensus definition has eluded the field. It is important to note that this lack of consensus worries scientists much less than it appears to worry journalists, the mass media, and other laypersons. This is because scientists are more aware that consensus definitions come at the end of a line of investigation, not near the beginning when inquiry is still in the formative stages.

In any case, the key point to keep in mind is not whether tests of intelligence measure something that we all agree upon, but whether we have discovered something that is worth measuring. As we shall see in Chapter 2, despite the absence of a consensus definition of intelligence, the vast amount of research that has been conducted over the past century clearly supports its meaningfulness as a scientific construct that can be assessed with considerable accuracy. The bottom line is this: We use intelligence tests because they predict important social outcomes better than anything else that we can currently measure independently of IQ (e.g., Gottfredson, 2011).

THEORIES OF INTELLIGENCE

Scientific knowledge consists of the gradual accumulation of information by different researchers, from different types of research, and in different domains. Scientific theories are essentially "bold conjectures" that attempt to explain the known evidence in a field of study. According to philosopher of science Karl Popper (1968), "good" scientific theories make important and useful predictions that can be subjected to empirical tests. Theories that are not potentially falsifiable are known as *pseudoscientific* theories (e.g., Freud's psychoanalytic theory). Theories of *intelligence* are scientific theories that attempt to explain differences among individuals in their ability to solve the myriad problems people confront almost daily, to learn from those experiences, and to adapt to a changing environment (e.g., Neisser et al., 1996). Theories of intelligence, however, vary in the degree to which they have been substantiated and, as a result, the extent to which they are accepted in the scientific community.

The Psychometric Paradigm

At present, the scientific theory that has by far the most empirical support is the psychometric approach to the study of intelligence. Although there are various competing theories of intelligence in the literature (e.g., see Ceci, 1990; Gardner, 1983; Das, Naglieri, & Kirby, 1994; Sternberg, 1985), the psychometric paradigm "has not only inspired the most research and attracted the most attention (up to this time) but is by far the most widely used in practical settings" (Neisser et al., 1996, p. 77).

Psychometrics is the scientific field of inquiry that is concerned with the measurement of psychological constructs. Although psychometricians study other psychological phenomena (e.g., personality, attitudes, and beliefs), the definition and measurement of intelligence have been a primary focus. According to the psychometric paradigm, intelligence involves the ability to reason abstractly, solve complex problems, and acquire new knowledge (e.g., Neisser et al., 1996). The construct of intelligence, therefore, reflects more than

> According to the psychometric paradigm, intelligence involves the ability to reason abstractly, solve complex problems, and acquire new knowledge.

"book learning" or "test-taking skill" (e.g., Eysenck, 1998; Gottfredson, 2002; Neisser et al., 1996). Contrary to the view of expert opinion often reported by the mass media, most scholars with expertise in the field of intelligence agree with this working definition of intelligence (Snyderman & Rothman, 1987).

Psychometric g

Two facts of nature must be explained by any theory of intelligence—and both are adequately addressed in the psychometric paradigm. The first is known as the *positive manifold* (Spearman, 1904). The positive manifold refers to the fact that all tests of cognitive ability (i.e., objectively scored tests on which individual differences are not due to sensory acuity or motor deftness) are positively intercorrelated. This means that, on average, individuals who score high on one kind of cognitive test will tend to score high on *every* other kind of cognitive test, and vice versa. The existence of the positive manifold indicates that all tests of cognitive ability share something in common that is related to differences in performance (i.e., an underlying source of individual differences, or variance).

The second fact of nature that must be explained pertains to the description of the underlying structure of these positive intercorrelations. Specifically, the central question here is whether these correlations are related to a single cognitive ability or to a number of different abilities. Charles Spearman (1904) hypothesized that the positive correlations observed among all tests of cognitive ability result from a single underlying general ability that is shared by all tests. In other words, he asserted that all cognitive tests correlate positively because they measure the same thing to some degree. He invented factor analysis to estimate this underlying source of variance, which he called the *general factor*, or simply psychometric g. The purpose of factor analysis is to determine whether the correlations among a number of cognitive tests can be explained by some smaller number of inferred hypothetical constructs (i.e., factors; Carroll, 1993). Specifically, Spearman hypothesized that every test measures g and one other ability that is unique to that specific test (or highly similar tests).

Figure 1.2 displays Spearman's original two-factor theory. This figure shows the relationship among nine tests of cognitive ability and psychometric g. As can be seen, each of these tests overlaps to some degree with g (as expected, given the positive manifold), but not with each other. Also note that some tests are more closely related to g than others. S_1, for example, overlaps to a considerable extent with psychometric g, whereas S_2 is related to g to a much lesser degree. The portions of S_1 and S_2 that do not overlap with psychometric g reflect the portion of individual differences that are specific to each respective test.

What is psychometric g? Perhaps the most undisputed fact about g is that it is related to information-processing complexity (e.g., see Jensen, 1998). Spearman discovered that the tests correlating most highly with g—or the most g-loaded tests—are those that involve what he called *abstractness* and the *eduction of relations and correlates* (Spearman & Jones, 1950). Abstractness refers to ideas and concepts that cannot be perceived directly by the senses. The eduction of relations and correlates pertains to the perception of relations through inductive or deductive reasoning, as opposed to the simple reproduction of known rules. For example, take tests of cognitive ability that involve mathematics. Tests that correlate the most highly with psychometric g are those that involve solving problems, such as word problems in which the requisite arithmetic operations are not made explicit. The test taker must deduce from the description of the problem which arithmetic operations are required and then apply them. In contrast, tests that involve the

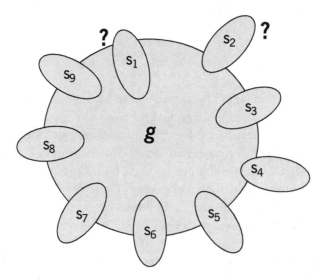

FIGURE 1.2. Spearman's two-factor theory of intelligence.

perfunctory application of explicit arithmetic operations, such as addition and subtraction work-sheets, tend to be much less *g*-loaded. In other words, the relative *g*-loadedness of these kinds of tests is not related to the fact that they concern mathematics, but to the complexity of information processing required.

In addition to tasks that require inferring relations about abstract concepts, tests that correlate highly with psychometric *g* are those that require more conscious mental manipulation. A straightforward illustration of this phenomenon can be found by comparing the *g*-loadings of the Forward and Backward Digit Span tests of the Wechsler Intelligence Scale for Children—Fourth Edition (WISC-IV; Wechsler, 2003). On both tests, one must repeat a string of digits presented once at a rate of one digit per second. One repeats the digits in Forward Digit Span in the same order as presented, and in Backward Digit Span in the opposite order as presented. Thus, on Backward Digit Span, one must retain the string of digits that have been presented in short-term memory and then repeat them, just as in Forward Digit Span, but with the added requirement of reversing the digits. Because it involves more conscious mental manipulation, Backward Digit Span is more highly correlated with *g* than is Forward Digit Span (Jensen, 1998).

> **A test's correlation with *g* is related to the complexity of information processing required, rather than to its requisite specific skills or knowledge content.**

Another noteworthy characteristic of *g* is that it cannot be described in terms of the surface characteristics of the different cognitive ability tests used in factor analysis. Spearman referred to this phenomenon as the *indifference of the indicator* (Spearman & Jones, 1950). For example, take the Block Design and Vocabulary subtests of the WISC-IV. On Block Design one must arrange colored blocks to match a pattern, and on Vocabulary one must define the meaning of different words. With their entirely different information content and response requirements, these two subtests would seem to call for quite different thought processes; yet they are two of the most highly *g*-loaded subtests on the WISC-IV (Jensen, 1998). A test's correlation with *g*, therefore, is related to the complexity of information processing required, rather than to its requisite specific skills or knowledge content.

Although it is now well established that psychometric *g* is related to processing complexity on cognitive tasks and not their surface characteristics, it is important to note that this is merely a description of *g*. Like all factors, *g* is not, strictly speaking, an explanatory construct. Factor analysis can be used to explain how various cognitive ability tests are related to each other, but it does not provide a causal explanation of the abilities or how they are organized. Therefore, the construct of *g* itself calls for an explanation. As Eysenck (1998) stated, "It is one thing to postulate a general factor of intelligence as the central conception in the theoretical framework which explains the observed phenomena in the field of mental testing; it is a different thing to postulate the nature of this factor" (p. 10).

The underlying causal mechanism of *g* is still largely unknown. Over the past 30 years, however, research at the interface between brain and behavior suggests that individual differences in intelligence are integrally related to a property of the brain known as *neural efficiency*, which is related to speed and efficiency of cognitive processing. This idea has received increased attention (e.g., Jensen, 2006; Nettelbeck, 2011). In Chapter 2, we further discuss how and why individuals differ in intelligence.

Group Factors

Not long after Spearman (1927) introduced the two-factor theory, he and other pioneers in factor analysis discovered group factors in addition to *g*. Unlike *g*, which enters into all cognitive tests, group factors are common only to certain groups of tests that require the same kinds of item content (e.g., verbal, numerical, or spatial) or cognitive processes (e.g., oral fluency, short-term memory, perceptual speed).

Thurstone's (1938) theory of *primary mental abilities* (PMAs) was the first theory of intelligence that did not include a general factor. His theory was based on the results of a new statistical technique that he developed, called *multiple factor analysis*. Multiple factor analysis initially allowed for the identification of a number of mental abilities, but no general factor. Thurstone's methodology also allowed for the identification of different kinds of cognitive abilities that were related to the factors discovered. Like Spearman's, his methodology was a product of his assumptions. Whereas Spearman's method of factor analysis was based on the assumption that only one factor is present in the correlation matrix, Thurstone's method was predicated on the notion of multiple abilities and no general ability.

Thurstone originally believed that the positive manifold is not the result of a general factor that underlies all tests of cognitive abilities, but stems from a number of fundamental abilities or PMAs. He identified seven PMAs: Verbal Comprehension, Perceptual Speed, Space Visualization, Inductive Reasoning, Deductive Reasoning, Rote Memory, and Number Facility. These factors were seen to be related to a variety of tests that shared common features. He believed that performance on any particular test, however, did not involve all the PMAs. Thurstone developed a special set of tests, called the PMA tests, to measure each of these factors.

For Thurstone's theory to be correct, each of the PMA tests had to correlate with only one factor. Furthermore, there would be no general factor with which every test correlated (representing psychometric *g*). This pattern of results in factor analysis is known as *simple structure*. Table 1.1 presents an idealized version of the results of a factor analysis showing simple structure. As can be seen here, there are six tests of cognitive ability and three factors. Each of the tests correlates perfectly with one factor and not at all with the other factors. In this case, each test represents a single group factor, uncontaminated by any other PMA. The factors are interpreted in terms of the characteristics of the tests on which they load. Thurstone's goal was to develop a battery of "factor-pure" tests such as these to measure each of the PMAs.

Results of factor analyses of Thurstone's PMA tests, however, do not contradict the existence of a general factor (e.g., see Cattell, 1971). Because all tests correlate with psychometric *g* to some

TABLE 1.1. Idealized Version of Simple Structure

Test	Factor		
	I	II	III
A	1.00	—	—
B	1.00	—	—
C	—	1.00	—
D	—	1.00	—
E	—	—	1.00
F	—	—	1.00

extent, it is only possible to approximate simple structure by allowing the factors themselves to be correlated. However, when this is done, the resulting correlations between factors can also be factor-analyzed. When these correlations are factor-analyzed, psychometric g emerges as a second-order factor. When factor analyses are conducted at different levels, this is known as *higher-order factor analysis*. Thus the finding that there is a psychometric g as well as group factors among the PMA tests indicates that Spearman and Thurstone were both correct in what they initially believed, but wrong about what they denied.

Agreement was finally reached on a general psychometric paradigm that has lasted to this day (see Carroll, 1993). According to this paradigm, individuals have a number of different abilities for solving intellectual problems and for adapting to the environment. Among these abilities, psychometric g is particularly important. In addition to g, there are specific abilities to deal with various types of problems under specific circumstances, such as those involving visual–spatial, numerical, or memory abilities. During this early period of research, a number of theories postulated by such factor-analytic luminaries as Vernon, Cattell, and Guilford attempted to describe the structure of cognitive abilities (see Carroll, 1982). Nonetheless, because opinions differed about the most appropriate method of factor analysis, consensus as to the best model of the structure of cognitive ability was not reached.

The Structure of Intelligence

One of the main reasons for this lack of consensus with regard to the structure of intelligence had to do with the fact that the early theorists were limited to a type of factor analysis called *exploratory factor analysis* (EFA). EFA is most useful in the early stages of research, when initial hypotheses about the underlying factors are generated. EFA does not test the fit between competing theories and the data within a statistical modeling framework. In the 1980s, however, use of a new statistical procedure known as *confirmatory factor analysis* (CFA) provided a way out of this theoretical dead end. CFA is a general model of factor analysis that contains all earlier models as special cases. CFA is a "sharper" factor-analytic tool than earlier models and can be used both to estimate and to test alternative factor models. In CFA, specific theories are used to construct models of the underlying structure of a battery of tests to determine how well they "fit" or explain the data. Furthermore, the "goodness-of-fit" provided by the models based on competing theories can be examined to determine which one provides the best description of the data. The results of more recent analyses using this new approach show that a hierarchical model of cognitive ability best fits the data (Keith & Reynolds, 2012; Gustafsson, 1984). In these models, both g and a number of group factors are represented as independent dimensions of cognitive ability (e.g., Johnson, te Nijenhuis, & Bouchard, 2008).

At the current time, the most widely accepted theory of the structure of human cognitive abilities is Carroll's (1993) three-stratum theory (e.g., Brody, 1994; Eysenck, 1994; Sternberg, 1994). Carroll's theory is based on the re-analysis of 467 data sets. It is largely an extension and expansion of the earlier theories of cognitive abilities, such as the Horn–Cattell theory of fluid and crystallized abilities (Gf-Gc; Horn, 1994; Horn & Noll, 1997). According to Carroll, "there is abundant evidence for a factor of general intelligence" (1993, p. 624), but also for a number of group factors. As shown in Figure 1.3, in the three-stratum theory psychometric g and group factors are arranged in a hierarchy based on their generality. *Generality* refers to the number of other factors with which a particular factor is correlated. The most general factor, psychometric g, is located at the

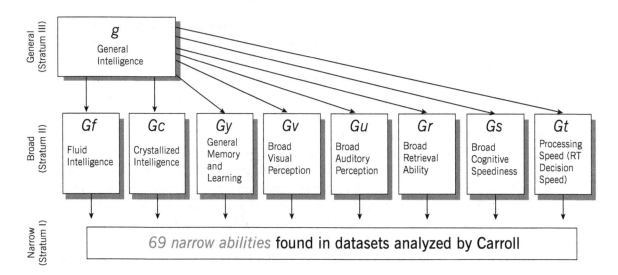

FIGURE 1.3. Carroll's three-stratum theory of the structure of human cognitive abilities. Adapted from McGrew and Flanagan (1998). Copyright 1998 by Allyn & Bacon. Reprinted by permission of Pearson Education, Inc.

top of this hierarchical structure at stratum III. Eight broad cognitive abilities (e.g., Fluid Intelligence and Crystallized Intelligence) that are similar to Thurstone's PMAs constitute stratum II; and stratum I consists of many narrow cognitive abilities (e.g., Visual Memory, Spelling Ability, and Word Fluency). *Intelligence*, therefore, is multidimensional, and consists of many different cognitive abilities (Sternberg, 1996).

In recent years, Carroll's (1993) three-stratum theory and Horn and Cattell's Gf-Gc theory have been integrated into what is referred to as the *Cattell–Horn–Carroll* (CHC) theory of cognitive abilities. This model has the same factor structure as the three-stratum theory, with a prominent psychometric g, but with several relatively small differences among the broad abilities posited at stratum II (e.g., Schneider & McGrew, 2012). CHC theory is increasingly being used by test developers to create theoretically driven tests that measure the general and broad factors of human intelligence.

CHC Theory and IQ Testing

How well do current intelligence tests measure the factors in the CHC theory? Given that psychometric g is related to the complexity of cognitive processing, all of the most widely used intelligence tests are excellent measures of g (see Carroll, 1993). Due to the practical limitations of psychological assessment, the battery of subtests on intelligence tests tends to be fairly small. This precludes the measurement of all factors in the CHC theory. Typically, in addition to g, intelligence tests measure no more than three to five broad abilities at stratum II (Keith & Reynolds, 2012). The WISC-IV, for example, measures five broad abilities (viz., Fluid Intelligence, Crystallized Intelligence, General Memory and Learning, Broad Visual Perception, and Broad Cognitive Speediness), and psychometric g (Keith, Fine, Taub, Reynolds, & Kranzler, 2006). Moreover, none of the intelligence tests currently in use measures all of the abilities at stratum II. At the present time, a thorough assessment of the broad stratum II abilities requires either (1) administration of multiple intelligence tests measuring different abilities or (2) adoption of the *cross-battery approach* to intellectual assessment (e.g., Flanagan, Alfonso, & Ortiz, 2013).

What do intelligence tests measure? The global composite score on virtually every intelligence test is an excellent measure of *g*. Psychometric *g* is the largest factor on intelligence tests (e.g., Canivez & Watkins, 2010a, 2010b; Jensen, 1998; Nelson & Canivez, 2012). Psychometric *g* usually explains more variance than all group factors combined (Canivez, 2011; Kranzler & Weng, 1995), even when intelligence tests are not developed within the framework of CHC theory (e.g., Kranzler & Keith, 1999). Furthermore, the predictive validity of intelligence tests is largely a function of psychometric *g* (e.g., Gottfredson, 2002; Hunter, 1986; Jensen, 1998; Ree & Earles, 1991, 1992). On most educational and occupational criteria, the general factor usually explains from 70% to 90% of the predictable variance, depending on the criterion (e.g., Kaufman, Reynolds, Kaufman, Liu, & McGrew, 2012; Thorndike, 1985, 1986). In addition, the more complex the criterion, the more predictive psychometric *g* tends to be. Nelson and Canivez (2012), for example, found that psychometric *g* accounted for approximately 80% of the variance explained by the Reynolds Intellectual Assessment Scales (RIAS; Reynolds & Kamphaus, 2003) on a variety of academic achievement outcomes. Psychometric *g* is predictive of many important social outcomes beyond tests, such as years of education and socioeconomic status (Gottfredson, 2008). The general factor is also related (negatively) to such problem behavior as dropping out of high school, living in poverty, and incarceration (e.g., Herrnstein & Murray, 1994).

Despite the predictiveness of psychometric *g*, the predictiveness of intelligence tests is far from perfect. For example, in schools, the average correlation between measures of *g* and reading comprehension is approximately +.70. Thus the overall score on intelligence tests explains about 50% of the differences between children in the ability to comprehend text—at best. This means that up to 50% of the remaining variance must be explained by other cognitive and noncognitive variables beyond *g*, such as conscientiousness and ambition. Predictive validity coefficients between *g* and outcomes in the workplace are typically lower. As Gottfredson (1997) has stated, this implies that "the effects of intelligence—like other psychological traits—are probabilistic, not deterministic. Higher intelligence improves the *odds* of success in school and work. It is an advantage, not a guarantee. Many other things matter" (p. 116; emphasis in original).

> **The effects of intelligence are probabilistic, not deterministic. Higher intelligence is an advantage, not a guarantee.**

Criticism of the Psychometric Paradigm

The main criticism of the psychometric paradigm is not that it is incorrect, as it has substantial empirical support, but that it is incomplete. According to Sternberg (1988a, 1988b), this approach focuses on only one (or, at most, two) of the essential aspects of intelligence, and thus cannot lead to a complete understanding of intelligence. Others, such as Ceci (1990), have argued that the syllogism implied in this line of investigation (*g* = IQ = real-world success) obscures the complex link between micro-level processing and intelligent behavior. Ceci has also contended that alternative interpretations of the data are possible. In any case, as mentioned previously, at the present time the psychometric approach—with its vast empirical support—is clearly the predominant theory of intelligence.

It is also important to note that although the three-stratum and CHC theories are now widely accepted as working models of the structure of intelligence, "the consensus is by no means unanimous, and in any case, scientific truth is not decided by plurality (or even majority) vote" (Sternberg, 1996, p. 11). While virtually every researcher within the psychometric paradigm agrees that the structure of human cognitive abilities is hierarchical, at least some question the appropriateness of an overarching psychometric g at stratum III of the factor hierarchy. In fact, several theories of intelligence outside the psychometric approach do not include a general ability—such as Sternberg's (1985) triarchic theory and Gardner's (1983, 1993, 1999, 2006) theory of multiple intelligences, as well as more recent theories such as the Planning, Attention, Simultaneous, and Successive (PASS) processes theory (e.g., Naglieri & Otero, 2012; Das, Naglieri, & Kirby, 1994), and Ceci's bioecological framework (e.g., Ceci, 1990). Although these contemporary theories have contributed significantly to the study of intelligence, the psychometric paradigm has been the most thoroughly researched and has by far the most empirical support.

SUMMARY

What, then, is intelligence? Most experts agree that intelligence involves the ability to reasoning and think abstractly, acquire new knowledge, and solve complex problems (Snyderman & Rothman, 1987). The vast literature on the structure of human cognitive abilities clearly indicates that it is multidimensional. This means that any single score on intelligence tests will not explain the full range of these dimensions (Sternberg, 1996). In the psychometric paradigm, however, g plays a particularly important role. Not only is g the largest factor in batteries of cognitive tests, but it is also the "active ingredient" in cognitive tests' predictiveness. Psychometric g is not merely linked to the surface characteristics of cognitive ability tests; rather, g is *directly* related to the complexity of information processing. Finally, psychometric g is measured quite well by most, if not all, of the most widely used intelligence tests. Certain group factors are also measured on most of these tests, but typically no more than a few are measured on any one test.

CHAPTER 2

How and Why Do People Differ in Intelligence?

It is a truism that no two people are exactly the same. Even identical twins are not *exactly* alike. Indeed, individuals differ on virtually every biological and psychological attribute that can be measured. Individual differences are observed in physical characteristics such as height, weight, blood type and pressure, visual acuity, and eye coloration; they are also observed in psychological characteristics such as personality, values, interests, and academic achievement, among others. Individuals also differ in intelligence—that is, in their general, broad, and specific cognitive abilities (e.g., see Carroll, 1993).

The scientific study of how and why people differ in terms of their psychological characteristics is known as *differential psychology* (e.g., Revelle, Wilt, & Condon, 2011). In contrast to *experimental psychology*, where differences among people are seen as a source of error to be controlled, in differential psychology those differences are the focus of research. For school psychologists and other professionals working with children and youth who have learning problems, understanding individual differences in intelligence is particularly important—not only for the identification of school-related difficulties, but also for the effective planning and evaluation of school-based interventions (e.g., Fiorello, Hale, & Snyder, 2006).

The purpose of this chapter is to explain how and why individuals differ in intelligence. We begin by discussing how individuals of the same age differ in intelligence. We then discuss developmental differences. Finally, we address why individuals differ in intelligence; we consider both the heritability and the malleability of intelligence.

THE DISTRIBUTION OF INTELLIGENCE

Around 1870, the Belgium astronomer Adolphe Quetelet (1796–1874) made a discovery about individual differences that impressed him greatly. His method was to select a physical characteristic, such as height; obtain measurements on a large number of individuals; and then arrange the results in a frequency distribution. He found the same pattern of results over and over again, for all sorts of different things. Quetelet discovered that the distribution of these characteristics closely approximated a bell-shaped curve. The symmetrical, bell-shaped curve that results from plotting human characteristics on frequency polygons is known as the *normal* (or *Gaussian*) *distribution*. The normal curve is bell-shaped, is perfectly symmetrical, and has a certain degree of "peakedness."

Sir Francis Galton (1822–1911) was the first to discover that individual differences in intelligence closely approximate the normal distribution. Figure 2.1 shows an idealized normal distribution of intelligence test scores (IQs). As can be seen here, the average (or mean) of the distribution is 100. Most individuals have scores that are near the average, with increasingly fewer scores near the extremes of each tail. The figure shows the percentage of cases in the distribution that can be found in the different areas of the normal curve when it is divided into standard deviation units. The same proportion of scores fall within the different areas of all normal curves when standard scores are used (e.g., *z* scores, *T* scores, or deviation IQ scores). This is very important from a practical standpoint, because it allows us to determine the percentage of cases in the distribution that fall below or above any particular score, or the percentage of cases falling between any two scores.

Given that the percentage of scores in a normal distribution always equals 100%, a person's IQ can be understood in terms of its *percentile rank*. Percentile ranks are frequently used to describe standardized test scores, and for good reason: They are the easiest kind of score to understand. The percentile rank of a score is simply the percentage of the whole distribution falling below that score on the test. An individual whose score is at the 75th percentile scored higher than about 75% of the

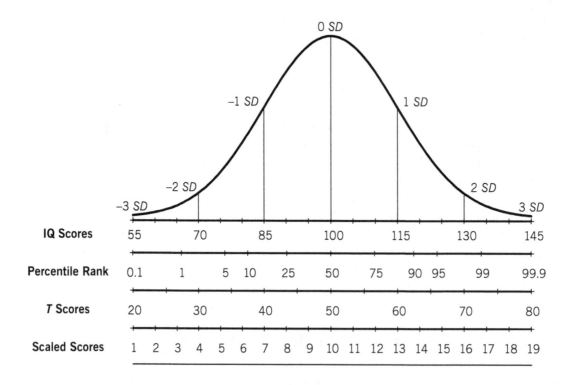

FIGURE 2.1. Theoretical normal distribution.

persons in the norm group; someone whose score is at the 50th percentile scored higher than about 50%; and so on. Most intelligence tests are developed to have a mean standard score of 100 and standard deviation of 15. Therefore, an IQ of 115, for example, has a percentile rank of 84, meaning that it surpasses 84% of all scores in the normative sample. Roughly 68% of the population has IQs that fall between 85 and 115.

The normal distribution serves as a reasonably accurate model of the frequency distribution of intelligence test scores. For individuals with IQs falling between 70 and 130, which accounts for approximately 95% of the population, the normal curve is a very good model of the distribution of scores. Nevertheless, when the 5% of scores at the extreme tails of the distribution are included, the normal distribution is not perfectly accurate. Much of the deviation from the normal curve for intelligence is due to the fact that there is a greater proportion of individuals with IQs at the very low end of the distribution (i.e., below 50 or so) than predicted by the normal curve.

> **The normal distribution serves as a reasonably accurate model of the frequency distribution of intelligence test scores.**

Intellectual disability (ID) is typically defined by IQs below 70 or 75 (among other criteria; see Chapter 10). Individuals with mild ID (i.e., with IQs between 55 and 70) represent the lower tail of normal variability in intelligence. Severe and profound ID (corresponding to IQs below 50), however, does not tend to result from normal variability (e.g., Percy, 2007), but from either accidents of nature (i.e., single-gene defects or chromosomal abnormalities) or brain damage (e.g., birth complications, extreme nutritional deficiency, or head injury). These anomalous conditions tend to have such dramatic effects that they completely outweigh the usual genetic and environmental factors that determine a person's intelligence. Nevertheless, for most practical purposes, the normal curve provides a reasonable approximation to the distribution of intelligence—particularly when we are dealing with individuals within two standard deviations of the mean of the distribution.

DEVELOPMENTAL DIFFERENCES IN INTELLIGENCE

Alfred Binet (1857–1911) is widely regarded as the father of modern intelligence tests. The French Ministry of Education commissioned Binet and Théophile Simon (1873-1961) to find a way to identify children and youth who were at risk for educational failure. Binet and Simon began with the assumption that children become more intelligent with age, because older children are capable of doing things that younger children cannot. They developed a set of short questions and simple tasks that most children were capable of successfully completing at different ages. They then administered these items to representative samples of children at 1-year intervals from the ages of 3 to 15 years. Binet and Simon grouped items based on the percentage of children in each age group who got each item correct. For example, if a particular test item could be solved by the average child at the age of 6 years, then the age level of the problem was 6 years. Any child who passed this item was said to have a *mental age* (MA) of 6 years. They identified five items at each age level, so that they could measure MA in months as well as years. By comparing MA to *chronological age* (CA), Binet and Simon were able to determine whether a child was above or below average in relation to same-age peers. They found that at each age level, the distribution of scores on their intelligence test was approximately normal.

Wilhelm Stern (1871–1938) was the first to describe intelligence by the ratio of MA to CA to derive a *mental quotient*, which was later changed to the *intelligence quotient*, or IQ. IQ was obtained by multiplying by 100 to remove the decimal point; that is, IQ = MA/CA × 100. Thus an 8-year-old child with a MA equivalent to the average 10-year-old would have an IQ of 125 (10/8 × 100); an 8-year-old child with a MA equivalent to the average 8-year-old would have an IQ of 100 (8/8 × 100); and an 8-year-old with a MA equivalent to the average 6-year-old would have an IQ of 75 (6/8 × 100). Despite its appeal, it quickly became apparent that the new IQ scale was not useful after about 16 years of age, given that intellectual skills do not continue to develop steadily after that age. For adults this method is clearly inappropriate, because their MA would remain relatively constant, while their CA would constantly increase with time. Although many teenagers would perhaps believe in the veracity of the consistently decreasing IQ of their parents, this is clearly inappropriate. For this reason, all current intelligence tests use a point scale in which an individual's score is compared to a normative sample of same-age peers.

Figure 2.2 shows the theoretical growth curve of intelligence, based on repeated testing of the same individuals over time. As shown in the figure, between the ages of 4 and 12 years or so, the rate of cognitive growth is fairly linear. After that age, the rate of gain begins to decrease gradually as the individual reaches maturity, between 16 and 20 years of age. The development of intelligence, therefore, is similar to that of height. Although scores on IQ tests are relatively unstable during infancy and the preschool years, they stabilize rather quickly during the early school years and remain that way throughout adulthood (e.g., Humphreys, 1989). This means that the rank order of intelligence test scores will tend to remain relatively the same as individuals move from childhood to adulthood. Prior to age 4 or 5, however, the long-term stability and predictive power of intelligence tests are of less value (Goodman, 1990). In addition, the stability of test scores decreases with time. More recent test results will be a better indicator of a person's current cognitive ability than tests administered in the distant past.

Figure 2.3 shows the growth curves for fluid general intelligence for three hypothetical individuals. Although the cognitive ability of all three increases over time, plateauing at about the age of 15 years, the relative ranking of each person remains the same. Because children's IQs are

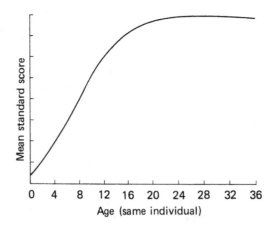

FIGURE 2.2. Theoretical growth curve based on repeated testing of the same individual. From Eysenck (1979, p. 59). Copyright 1979 by Springer-Verlag. Reprinted by permission.

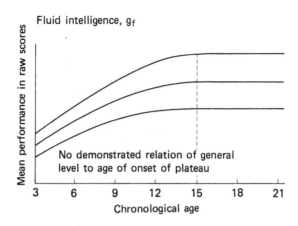

FIGURE 2.3. Growth curve of fluid ability (Gf) with age. From Eysenck (1979, p. 75). Copyright 1979 by Springer-Verlag. Reprinted by permission.

derived from comparison to same-age peers, this means that children's scores on intelligence tests will remain relatively the same, despite the fact that their cognitive ability is steadily developing. An 8-year-old and a 16-year-old with IQs of 100 are not the same in terms of their general reasoning abilities. On the contrary, it simply means that they are average for their respective age groups. Students who obtain the same IQ from one age to another have simply maintained their relative standing in relation to same-age peers, while their cognitive abilities may have developed considerably. It is also important to note that although IQ scores are generally quite stable over time, the consistency of scores is not perfect. Just like height, many individuals' level of intelligence may remain roughly constant in relation to that of same-age peers over time, but others' may not. The average change in IQs for individuals between 12 and 17 years of age, for example, is about 7 points, but for some people it can be as much as 18 points (e.g., Neisser et al., 1996).

> **Although intelligence test scores are generally quite stable over time, the consistency of scores is not perfect.**

Although much is known about the development of intelligence through childhood, research on change in cognitive abilities in adulthood and old age is less clear—largely due to methodological issues surrounding the use of cross-sectional research designs, cohort effects, and which cognitive abilities are to be measured and how (e.g., see Salthouse, 2010). Nevertheless, examination of the age norms for widely used intelligence tests among adults, such as the Wechsler Adult Intelligence Scale—Fourth Edition (WAIS-IV; Wechsler, 2008), are fairly straightforward (Deary, 2001). For some subtests on the WAIS-IV, there is little change across age among adults; for other subtests, age-related decrements in ability are apparent. The subtests on which older and younger people tend to compare well are vocabulary, general information, and verbal reasoning. These subtests draw upon one's knowledge base that has been accumulated through experience over time (i.e., Crystallized Intelligence, or Gc).

The cognitive subtests on which marked differences between older and younger people are observed are those that tend to be speeded or involve abstract or spatial reasoning. These subtests measure current cognitive functioning, because they involve solving problems here and now, often with novel content and under speeded conditions (i.e., Fluid Intelligence or Gf). For example, results from Schaie's (1996) Seattle Longitudinal Study for verbal ability (Gc) and inductive reasoning indicated that average scores on verbal ability remained fairly constant across age. On inductive reasoning, in contrast, average scores decreased considerably across age. It is important to note that these were average changes in inducting reasoning. For some people, performance on Gf tasks such as inductive reasoning does not change or improves with age. What does age affect? One theory proposed by Salthouse (1996) is that age-related changes in cognitive abilities are caused by slowing in the speed of information processing in the brain. Salthouse found that the effects of age on the brain were primarily on the general factor of intelligence (psychometric g). Changes observed in the measures of Gf and Gc across the lifespan are due to their relationship to g, not something specific to each broad ability at stratum II of the three-stratum theory (see Carroll, 1993, and Chapter 1, this volume). Further research on the study of cognitive aging is needed, however—particularly given that life expectancy is increasing dramatically, and thus the proportion of older people in the population is growing.

WHY DO PEOPLE DIFFER IN INTELLIGENCE?

Given the controversy that has surrounded research on the so-called "nature–nurture" issue in intelligence over the years, it may come as a surprise to learn that the main focus of research in this area no longer involves the question of whether individual differences in intelligence are related to genes or the environment (Nisbett et al., 2012). Results of surveys indicate that most psychologists believe that *both* genetic and environmental factors are at least partly related to variability in intelligence (Snyderman & Rothman, 1987). As Ceci (1990) has put it, "there are so many reports in the behavior-genetics literature of substantial heritability coefficients, calculated from an enormous variety of sources, that it is unlikely they could all be wrong" (p. 130). Rather, the focus of much contemporary research is on the identification of specific genes responsible for the heritability of intelligence, and on specific pathways between genes and behavior (e.g., Plomin & Spinath, 2004). Before we discuss research on the heritability of intelligence, it is important to describe how researchers investigate the relative contributions of nature and nurture to individual differences in behavioral traits such as intelligence.

> **Most psychologists believe that both genetic and environmental factors are at least partly related to variability in intelligence.**

Quantitative Behavior Genetics

Quantitative behavior genetics, or the *differential model*, is used to examine the contributions of genetics and the environment to individual differences in behavioral traits. Research in behavior genetics is best understood as an attempt to partition *variance*. Variance is the average of the squared deviations of every score from the mean of the distribution:

$$SD^2 = \frac{\sum \left(X - \overline{X} \right)^2}{N}$$

where Σ is "the sum of," X refers to each obtained score, $\overline{X}$ is the mean of X, and N refers to the total number of scores. The variance is interpreted as the "amount of information" in a distribution (Cronbach, 1990).

In quantitative behavior genetics, variance in an observable, measurable characteristic of an individual—the phenotype *(VP)*—is partitioned into components of variance related to the genotype *(VG)* and the environment *(VE)*. Thus $VP = VG + VE$. The proportion of variance in the phenotype that is attributable to variance in the genotype is known as *heritability* (h^2) of a particular trait $(h^2 = VG/VP)$. *Environmentality* reflects differences in the phenotype that are associated with the environment and with measurement error (i.e., $1 - h^2$). The environmental component of variance can be further partitioned into two subcomponents, *shared* and *nonshared*. Shared environmental influences reflect common experiences that make individuals in the same family similar to each other and different from those in other families (e.g., socioeconomic status, parenting style). Nonshared environmental influences reflect unique life experiences that make members of the same family different from one another (e.g., peer groups). In addition, phenotypic variance may also be influenced by combined genetic and environmental influences, such as genotype–environment correlations. Genotype–environment correlations occur when people's genetic propensities are related to the environments they experience. A common example in the schools is the identification and placement of children in special classes for the intellectually gifted.

All procedures for estimating the relative contributions of heredity and environment in quantitative behavior genetics involve correlating measurements taken from groups of people who are and are not biologically related, and then comparing these correlations with those expected from a purely genetic hypothesis. The genetic correlation for identical, or *monozygotic* (MZ), twins is 1.00, because they share 100% of their genetic makeup. Since non-twin offspring (i.e., full siblings) receive 50% of their genes from each parent, the parent–child genetic correlation is .50. The genetic correlation for fraternal, or *dizygotic* (DZ), twins is also .50, because they too share 50% of their genes. Persons who are not biologically related have no genes in common, so the genetic correlation between these individuals is .00. When the correlations for a particular kinship (e.g., MZ twins) differ substantially from the predicted genetic correlation, results do not substantiate a purely genetic hypothesis. If there is no resemblance between family members, then the genetic hypothesis is disconfirmed for that particular trait.

Family, twin, and adoption studies are the three basic research designs used in the differential model. These designs essentially exploit different combinations of genotypes and environments that occur naturally in the population. In family studies, estimates of h^2 are based on comparisons of parents with their offspring and of siblings with each other. Because members of the same family share both common genes and environment, evidence of familial similarity is consistent with the genetic hypothesis, but cannot confirm it. Twin and adoption studies must be used to separate the relative contributions of genetics and the environment to phenotypic variance, because they essentially control for the effects of genes or the environment.

Twin studies are one of the most powerful designs in the differential model. If a particular trait is influenced by genetics, then the correlation between MZ twins should be greater than the correlation between DZ twins, because MZ twins share 100% of their genes and DZ twins share only 50%. Correlations for MZ and DZ twins reared together reflect the phenotypic variance accounted for by the combined effects of genes and common environment. Adoption studies are another invaluable source of information on the relative contributions of genetics and the environment to phenotypic variance, because they too separate the effects of common genes and common environment. In adoption studies, adoptive parents are compared to their adopted children, to whom they are completely genetically dissimilar, and biological parents are compared to their adopted-away children, with whom they have no environmental experiences in common. Any resemblance between adopted children and their adoptive parents, therefore, can be attributed to the effects of shared environment; conversely, any resemblance between adopted-away children and their biological parents can be attributed to genetics. Pairs of adopted and unadopted children reared together can also be compared in adoption studies to estimate the effects of common environment. Particularly noteworthy are studies in which the adoption and twin methods are combined. In these studies, of which there are relatively few, MZ and DZ twins who have been separated at birth and reared apart are compared.

Heritability of Intelligence across the Lifespan

Bouchard and McGue (1981) reviewed the literature of familial studies of the heritability of intelligence. They reviewed over 100 independent studies, summarizing over 500 correlations among more than 100,000 family members. Taken as a whole, results of these studies were consistent with a genetic hypothesis, but provided support for the influence of the environment on individual differences on intelligence (see Table 2.1). Not only were the correlations between MZ twins greater than those between family members with less genetic overlap, even when MZ twins were reared apart, but the obtained correlations across kinships did not deviate substantially from the expected genetic correlations. Evidence for the role of environment was reflected in the fact that correla-

TABLE 2.1. Average IQ Correlations among Family Members

Relationship	Average r	Number of pairs
Reared-together biological relatives		
MZ twins	.86	4,671
DZ twins	.60	5,533
Siblings	.47	26,473
Parent–offspring	.42	8,433
Half-siblings	.35	200
Cousins	.15	1,176
Reared-apart biological relatives		
MZ twins	.72	65
Siblings	.24	203
Parent–offspring	.24	720
Reared-together nonbiological relatives		
Siblings	.32	714
Parent–offspring	.24	720

Note. MZ, monozygotic; DZ, dizygotic. Adapted from McGue, Bouchard, Iacono, and Lykken (1993). Copyright 1993 by the American Psychological Association. Adapted by permission.

tions between biological relatives reared together were greater than those between individuals of the same degree of kinship reared apart; and correlations between biologically unrelated persons reared together were substantially greater than zero. Neither of these findings can be explained by genetics alone. For these data, h^2 for general intelligence was estimated to be .51 (Chipeur, Rovine, & Plomin, 1990), indicating that slightly more than half the phenotypic variance was accounted for by genetic factors. Shared environmental influences accounted for 11–35% of the variance, depending on kinship data used in the estimation. Nonshared environmental variance was found to explain 14–38% of the variance. Therefore, the results of this review indicated that environment and genetics contribute roughly equally to variability in psychometric g.

A later review of the literature by McGue, Bouchard, Iacono, and Lykken (1993), however, reached a somewhat different conclusion regarding the relative contributions of heritability and environmentality to individual differences in general intelligence across the lifespan. They found that the correlation between the IQs of MZ twins increased across the lifespan. The correlation between DZ twins, in contrast, although fairly stable between 4 and 20 years of age, decreased dramatically after late adolescence. Interestingly, subsequent research has shown that shared environmental influences account for between 30% and 40% of the variance in IQ until the age of about 20 years, after which the amount of variance explained drops to zero (Loehlin, 2007). Nonshared environmental effects, in comparison, remain fairly constant across the lifespan, explaining somewhere between 10% and 20% of the variance from 4–6 years of age into adulthood.

Further substantiation that the underlying genetic and environmental determinants of IQ variability change over the lifespan comes from adoption studies. Among persons who were not biologically related, but reared together, research indicates that average correlation between siblings during childhood is rather substantial, accounting for approximately 25% of the variance in IQ (e.g., Bouchard, 2009; Nisbett et al., 2012). During adulthood, however, this correlation again decreases to zero. Taken together, these results indicate that the environmental effects influencing variability in intelligence are *nonshared*. Neisser et al. (1996) have stated:

> No one doubts that normal child development requires a certain minimum level of responsible care. Severely deprived, neglectful, or abusive environments must have negative effects on a great many aspects—including intellectual—of development. Beyond that minimum, however, the role of family experience is in serious dispute. (p. 88)

Interpreting Heritability Coefficients

Several important points must be kept in mind when we are interpreting h^2 estimates, however. First, h^2 is a statistic that describes the ratio of genotypic variance to phenotypic variance in a population. Although it does indicate that physiological functioning is related to individual differences in the trait, it provides no information on the specific areas of the brain responsible for that variation or how they operate. Second, estimates of h^2 refer to populations, not to individuals. An h^2 of .50 does not indicate that half of an individual's measured trait is attributable to genes and half to the environment. Third, estimates of h^2 that are greater than zero do not imply biological determinism. Genotypes do not directly cause phenotypic expression. As Rushton (1995) has stated, "they code for enzymes, which, under the influence of the environment, lay down tracts in the brains and nervous systems of individuals, thus differentially affecting people's minds and the choices they make about behavioral alternatives" (p. 61).

Malleability of Intelligence

The effects that genes have on individual differences in intelligence are better described as genetic influence than as genetic determinism. Being born with a particular set of genes does *not* predetermine behavioral traits. Particular genotypes do not correlate perfectly with expressed phenotypes. This is clearly seen in the correlations for identical twins reared together that are less than perfect. Despite the fact that identical twins share the same genotype, their expressed level of intelligence is highly correlated, but not exactly the same. These differences can only be explained by the environment. "Gene action always involves an environment—at least a biochemical environment, and often an ecological one" (Neisser et al., 1996, p. 84). Thus, traits with substantial heritable components, such as intelligence, are susceptible to environmental intervention.

Behavior geneticists use the concept of *reaction range* (RR) to explain variability in phenotypes for a particular genotype. Figure 2.4 shows the hypothetical effects of three different environments (viz., restricted, natural, and enriched) upon four different genotypes for the expression of intelligence. For all genotypes, the level of intelligence that is expressed is lower when individuals are raised in a deprived environment and higher when they are brought up in an enriched environment. The RR for any genotype is limited, however, as is reflected in the vertical lines on the right of the figure. As can be seen here, within any particular environment there will be differences among individuals, depending upon their genotypes. Also, the RR is larger for some genotypes than for others. More specifically, there is a wider RR for those with more advantaged genotypes. Genes, therefore, do not determine behavior; instead, they determine a range of responses to the environment.

Over the course of development, environmental effects can give rise to considerable variation in the phenotypic expression of any single genotype. Nevertheless, as Jensen (1981) has asserted, "there are probabilistic limits to the reaction range, and one of the tasks of genetic analysis is to explore the extent of those limits in the natural environment and to discover the environmental

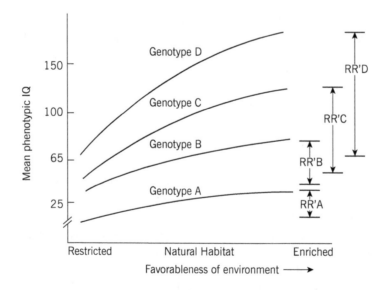

FIGURE 2.4. Hypothetical reaction range (RR) for four genotypes. Adapted from Platt and Sanislow (1988). Copyright 1988 by the American Psychological Association. Adapted by permission.

agents that affect them" (p. 485). At the current time, despite numerous efforts to discover ways to increase children's intelligence, the empirical evidence indicates that there are indeed limits to the malleability of IQ (e.g., Spitz, 1999). Results of early intervention programs for preschoolers, such as Project Head Start, have consistently shown that there is a "fade-out" of any gains in IQ points within 3 years of program termination (for reviews, see Clarke & Clarke, 1989; Locurto, 1991; Spitz, 1986).

In addition, those intervention programs that have resulted in substantial and durable gains in IQs often fail to evince comparable improvement on tasks that are highly correlated with IQ. On the Milwaukee Project (e.g., Garber, 1988), for example, large differences of about 30 IQ points were observed between the experimental and control groups, but no significant differences were observed on measures of academic achievement that are closely related to intelligence, such as reading comprehension. These results suggest that these gains in IQ resulted from "teaching to the test" and did not reflect real increases in IQ (e.g., Jensen, 1989a). Results of adoption studies—which are arguably the most intensive "interventions" imaginable—suggest that gains or losses of about 10–12 IQ points are the most that can be expected from dramatic environmental interventions (e.g., Locurto, 1990, 1991; Nisbett et al., 2012; Rowe, 1994). Last, although certain cognitive skills definitely can be taught "at least to some of the people, some of the time" (Sternberg, 1996, p. 13), research has shown that such learning tends to be quite context-bound and does not transfer to other cognitive domains (e.g., Detterman & Sternberg, 1993).

Taken as a whole, research indicates that IQ is *imperfectly malleable*. With the exception of instances of extreme social isolation and neglect, most environments are functionally equivalent for the development of intelligence. Of course, the failure of most intervention programs over the past 50 years to dramatically increase IQ does not preclude novel interventions from doing so in the future. Nonetheless, "if environmental interventions are to succeed, they must be truly novel ones, representing kinds of treatments that will be new to most populations" (Rowe, 1994, p. 223).

> **Research indicates that IQ is *imperfectly malleable*. Most environments are functionally equivalent for the development of intelligence.**

SUMMARY

Much of the research and theory on individual differences in intelligence can be summed up as follows: (1) The distribution of general intelligence is approximately normal among people of the same age; (2) intelligence develops from childhood to maturity, plateauing at about 16 years of age; (3) changes in cognitive abilities occur across the lifespan, with cognitive abilities related to Gc being the least affected and those related to Gf being the most affected; (4) both genetic and environmental factors are importantly related to individual differences in intelligence, but the relative contribution of each changes over the lifespan; and (5) IQ is somewhat, but not completely, malleable.

CHAPTER 3

Ethics in Assessment

It is important that students in training and professionals engaged in the practice of psychology read and frequently review the most recent ethical guidelines from the American Psychological Association (APA; go to *www.apa.org/ethics/code/index.aspx*). For those engaged in the practice of school psychology (especially in school settings), we also recommend referencing similar guidelines from the National Association of School Psychologists (NASP; go to *www.nasponline.org/ standards/2010standards.aspx*). This chapter highlights the ethical principles and standards from these two professional groups that are most relevant to testing children and adolescents. In many ways, this chapter forms one segment of the foundation for the remainder of the chapters in this book that focus on professional practices. For broader coverage of ethical standards and principles, as well as coverage of laws and court decisions relevant to testing children and adolescents, please consider the following texts: Jacob, Decker, and Hartshorne (2011) and Sattler (2008, Chapter 3). Content from the *Standards for Educational and Psychological Testing* (American Educational Research Association [AERA], APA, & National Council on Measurement in Education [NCME], 1999) is discussed in Chapter 5.

THE AMERICAN PSYCHOLOGICAL ASSOCIATION

In its Ethical Principles of Psychologists and Code of Conduct, including the 2010 Amendments, the APA (2002, 2010a) addresses five general principles that should serve as aspirations for professional practice: beneficence and nonmaleficence; fidelity and responsibility; integrity; justice; and respect for people's rights and dignity. Table 3.1 presents descriptions of these general principles. The APA's Ethical Principles of Psychologists and Code of Conduct also includes 10 specific ethical standards. Table 3.2 lists each of these standards and highlights some components that are most relevant to the practice of testing. In particular, Standard 9 comprises 11 components related to assessment. These components address four themes: high-quality assessments; control of information; interpretation of assessment results; and competence.

TABLE 3.1. General Ethical Principles from the American Psychological Association's Ethical Principles of Psychologists and Code of Conduct, and Their Descriptions

Beneficence and Nonmaleficence

Psychologists strive to benefit those with whom they work and take care to do no harm. . . .

Fidelity and Responsibility

Psychologists . . . uphold professional standards of conduct, clarify their professional roles and obligations, accept appropriate responsibility for their behavior, and seek to manage conflicts of interest that could lead to exploitation or harm. . . .

Integrity

Psychologists seek to promote accuracy, honesty, and truthfulness in the science, teaching, and practice of psychology. . . .

Justice

Psychologists . . . take precautions to ensure that their potential biases, the boundaries of their competence, and the limitations of their expertise do not lead to or condone unjust practices.

Respect for People's Rights and Dignity

Psychologists respect the dignity and worth of all people, and the rights of individuals to privacy, confidentiality, and self-determination. . . . Psychologists are aware of and respect cultural, individual, and role differences, including those based on age, gender, gender identity, race, ethnicity, culture, national origin, religion, sexual orientation, disability, language, and socioeconomic status and consider these factors when working with members of such groups. Psychologists try to eliminate the effect on their work of biases based on those factors . . .

Note. Copyright © 2010 by the American Psychological Association. Adapted with permission. The official citations that should be used in referencing this material are as follows:

American Psychological Association. (2002). Ethical principles of psychologists and code of conduct. *American Psychologist,* 57, 1060–1073.

American Psychological Association. (2010a). Amendments to the 2002 ethical principles of psychologists and code of conduct. *American Psychologist,* 65, 493.

No further reproduction or distribution is permitted without written permission from the American Psychological Association.

High-quality assessments are supported by three components of Standard 9. Component 9.01 states that psychologists should base their conclusions and recommendations offered in oral and written reports on evidence from the most appropriate methods of assessment. Opinions about a person's psychosocial functioning should be based on the results of a formal assessment, not on hearsay, rumors, or other sources of unverifiable information. In the same vein, Component 9.02 conveys that psychologists should rely on sound evidence when selecting which assessment techniques to use, modify, and interpret. More specifically, they should consider reliability and validity evidence (see Chapter 5) relevant to their assessment techniques and the clients they serve, and when this evidence is not strong or plentiful, they should articulate the limitations of their assessment results. Thus psychologists should work diligently in selecting,

> **Psychologists should consider reliability and validity evidence relevant to their assessment techniques and the clients they serve, and when this evidence is not strong or plentiful, they should articulate the limitations of their assessment results.**

TABLE 3.2. Ethical Standards from the American Psychological Association's Ethical Principles of Psychologists and Code of Conduct (Including the 2010 Amendments)

Standard 1: Resolving Ethical Issues

Standard 2: Competence

2.01 Boundaries of Competence

(b) Where scientific or professional knowledge in the discipline of psychology establishes that an understanding of factors associated with age, gender, gender identity, race, ethnicity, culture, national origin, religion, sexual orientation, disability, language, or socioeconomic status is essential for effective implementation of their services or research, psychologists have or obtain the training, experience, consultation, or supervision necessary to ensure the competence of their services, or they make appropriate referrals . . .

2.03 Maintaining Competence

Psychologists undertake ongoing efforts to develop and maintain their competence.

2.04 Bases for Scientific and Professional Judgments

Psychologists' work is based upon established scientific and professional knowledge of the discipline.

Standard 3: Human Relations

3.09 Cooperation with Other Professionals

When indicated and professionally appropriate, psychologists cooperate with other professionals in order to serve their clients/patients effectively and appropriately.

3.10 Informed Consent

(a) When psychologists conduct research or provide assessment, they obtain the informed consent of the individual or individuals using language that is reasonably understandable to that person or persons [in most circumstances].

(b) For persons who are legally incapable of giving informed consent, psychologists nevertheless (1) provide an appropriate explanation, (2) seek the individual's assent, (3) consider such persons' preferences and best interests, and (4) obtain appropriate permission from a legally authorized person, if such substitute consent is permitted or required by law.

Standard 4: Privacy and Confidentiality

4.01 Maintaining Confidentiality

Psychologists have a primary obligation and take reasonable precautions to protect confidential information obtained through or stored in any medium . . .

4.02 Discussing the Limits of Confidentiality

(a) Psychologists discuss with persons and organizations with whom they establish a scientific or professional relationship (1) the relevant limits of confidentiality and (2) the foreseeable uses of the information generated through their psychological activities.

Standard 5: Advertising and Other Public Statements

Standard 6: Record Keeping and Fees

6.01 Documentation of Professional and Scientific Work and Maintenance of Records

Psychologists create, and to the extent the records are under their control, maintain, disseminate, store, retain, and dispose of records and data relating to their professional and scientific work . . .

(continued)

TABLE 3.2. *(continued)*

Standard 7: Education and Training

Standard 8: Research and Publication

Standard 9: Assessment

Standard 10: Therapy

Note. Copyright © 2010 by the American Psychological Association. Adapted with permission. The official citations that should be used in referencing this material are as follows:

American Psychological Association. (2002). Ethical principles of psychologists and code of conduct. *American Psychologist, 57,* 1060–1073.

American Psychological Association. (2010a). Amendments to the 2002 ethical principles of psychologists and code of conduct. *American Psychologist, 65,* 493.

No further reproduction or distribution is permitted without written permission from the American Psychological Association.

administering, scoring, or interpreting the results of their assessment instruments, to ensure that they facilitate the most accurate assessments and produce the best outcomes for their clients. Finally, in Component 9.08, psychologists are implored to avoid old and obsolete tests as a basis for current assessments, decisions about interventions, or recommendations. In reference to intelligence testing, tests normed more than 10 years ago should be avoided, if possible (see Chapter 5). We also assert that there is about a 2-year window in which psychologists should make the transition from an older version of a test to a more recently published version of that test, but we recognize that professional judgment must be applied in considering this transition (see Dombrowski, 2003; Lichtenstein, 2010; Oakland, 2003). Psychologists, however, must clearly stay up to date in their assessment knowledge.

Control of information is addressed in three components. Two focus on informed consent and confidentiality. Component 9.03 states that psychologists should ensure both (1) that their clients are informed about the nature and purpose of the assessment, what other parties (if any) are privy to the information yielded by the assessment, and confidentiality and its limits; and (2) that they (or, in the case of minors, their parents) consent to the assessment. Psychologists always inform clients about the kind of assessment they are about to conduct, and tell them why they are assessing them, in a language they can understand. Psychologists also obtain informed consent before conducting assessments, except when (1) the assessment is required by law or government regulations; (2) informed consent is implied as part of a customary educational, institutional, or organizational activity; or (3) one purpose of the testing is to evaluate a client's ability to make decisions independently of a guardian.

Component 9.04 targets release of assessment results and conveys that psychologists release these results to only their clients, others to whom their clients have released the results, and others as required by law or court order. Assessment results include the following: an examinee's raw and standardized scores; the examinee's actual responses to test questions and stimuli; and the psychologist's notations and records about the examinee's statements and behavior during the assessment. In addition, in Component 9.11 psychologists are implored to maintain *test security* by avoiding release of test manuals, test items, test pages, other testing materials, and test protocols, consistent with law and contractual obligations. Because well-developed assessment instruments are the products of years of effort to develop and refine them, it is important for test users to honor these efforts. More specifically, users are prohibited not only from duplicating these resources in hard copy and digital forms without permission, but also from sharing specific test content—and

> **Psychologists are implored to maintain *test security* by avoiding release of test manuals, test items, test pages, other testing materials, and test protocols.**

even response strategies—that might inflate test scores due to invalidity in assessment (see Chapter 4). Essentially, revealing such information spoils the test's ability to differentiate those who possess the underlying knowledge or skills from those who do not; in other words, validity is undermined. Consistent with this theme, in practice administrations during training, answers to items should not be provided upon an examinee's request, and at no point should others not in training be allowed to peruse the testing materials or be advised regarding how to improve performance on such tests. It is important to note that completed test protocols are "educational records" in school settings. So, despite psychologists' being held to high standards for maintaining privacy and confidentiality of records as well as intellectual property rights, copyright interests, and test security standards, parents' rights to examine their children's records may supersede them. Thus, they may examine test protocols, including specific items, but this review is typically conducted with guidance by a competent professional. Parents, however, do not have a legal right to review the personal notes of psychologists.

Interpretation of results is addressed in three components. Component 9.06 implores psychologists to consider any attribute of the person being assessed that might undermine the accuracy of test interpretations. These attributes include external and internal influences that are not relevant to the construct targeted by the assessment, such as the client's test-taking abilities and any situational, personal, linguistic, and cultural differences (see Chapters 4 and 13). Component 9.09 reminds psychologists that they are responsible for drawing valid conclusions from the assessment instruments that they employ as part of their assessments, regardless of who administers and scores these instruments and in cases of electronic administration and scoring. In addition, Component 9.10 implores psychologists to convey assessment results clearly to clients.

Finally, competence is addressed not only in Standard 2 in general (see Table 3.2), but also in Component 9.07 of Standard 9. In it, psychologists are encouraged to ensure that psychological techniques are employed by only qualified individuals or, in the case of training, under the supervision of those who are qualified.

THE NATIONAL ASSOCIATION OF SCHOOL PSYCHOLOGISTS

In its Principles for Professional Ethics, the NASP (2010a) addresses many of the same themes, principles, and specific ethical standards as addressed in the APA's (2002, 2010a) Ethical Principles of Psychologists and Code of Conduct, but it uses slightly different terms to describe them. In this section of the chapter, the NASP's broad ethical themes I, III, and IV are discussed first, and then emphasis is placed on the broad ethical theme II because of its focus on assessment. Again, full access to the NASP's Principles for Professional Ethics (2010a) is available at *www.nasponline. org/standards/2010standards.aspx.*

General Principles

Theme I addresses three principles related to respecting the dignity and rights of all individuals to whom school psychologists provide services. These principles are most similar to the five general ones offered by the APA (see Table 3.1). They implore school psychologists to honor the rights of others to participate and to decline participation in the services they provide. For example, school psychologists should ensure that parents provide informed consent (typically, written consent) for the provision of extensive or ongoing psychological or special education services (including assessment) for their children before these services begin. Although administration of all intelligence tests (and other psychological tests) requires consent, because the tests could be seen as intrusions on privacy beyond what might be expected in the course of ordinary school activities, other assessment practices (such as review of records, classroom observations, academic screening, and progress monitoring) do not typically require parental consent, if those conducting them are employees of the district in which they practice. School psychologists should also consider seeking and obtaining children's assent (i.e., their affirmative agreement) to participate in assessment or intervention activities; such assent is not required legally or ethically, but it is best practice (Jacob et al., 2010). Furthermore, these principles guarantee the rights to privacy and confidentiality to those who participate in school psychology services, while promoting information about the limits of confidentiality. Finally, school psychologists should promote fairness and justice for all.

> **School psychologists should collaborate and engage in respective interactions with other professionals to promote the well-being of students and families with whom they work.**

Theme III addresses honesty and integrity in interactions with parents, children, and other professionals. Its principles urge school psychologists to accurately present their competencies and to clearly convey the nature and scope of their services. School psychologists should collaborate and engage in respectful interactions with other professionals to promote the well-being of students and families with whom they work. In addition, they should strive to avoid relationships in which they may lose objectivity and diminish their effectiveness because of prior and ongoing personal relationships or their service in multiple professional roles (as evidenced through financial or other conflicts of interest).

Theme IV addresses responsibilities to society as a whole and to more specific institutions within it. Its five principles encourage school psychologists to apply their knowledge and skills to promote healthy environments for children. School psychologists should be aware of federal, state, and local laws governing educational and psychological practices. They should contribute to the instruction, mentoring, and supervision of those joining the field or desiring to expand their skills, as well as to conducting and disseminating research. Finally, they should be self-aware of ethical conflicts they may experience and act accordingly, and should also provide peer monitoring to promote public trust in school psychology services.

Competence in Assessment

Theme II, of all the general ethical themes highlighted by the NASP, most directly addresses competence and responsibilities in assessment practices. Its first principle addresses competence. School psychologists are implored to reflect on their training experiences and to engage in only those practices stemming from these experiences. They are also encouraged to participate in exercises to enhance their understanding and skills in working with students and families from diverse backgrounds, as well as to engage in professional development activities (such as attending professional conferences and self-study) to remain current in their knowledge and practices. In the same vein, the second principle encourages conscientious professional behavior and acceptance of the responsibilities that come with being a school psychologist. Specific reference is made to ensuring the accuracy of written reports, clearly communicating assessment results and other information, and monitoring the effects of recommendations and interventions. (See Chapter 8 for more information about preparing psychological reports and presenting information to parents and other caregivers.)

The third principle directly addresses assessment and intervention practices, and we highlight specific recommendations addressing assessment practices. One series of recommendations addresses measurement integrity and the fidelity of interpretations. For instance, school psychologists should rely on scientific evidence to select the optimal assessment instruments. In particular,

> **School psychologists should rely on scientific evidence to select the optimal assessment instruments.**

they should select those with the strongest body of reliability and validity evidence supporting their use for the intended purposes (see Chapter 5). They should not violate the rules for uniform administration of standardized assessment instruments (see Chapter 4); if they do so, by error or by design through the use of test accommodations, they should report this in their oral and written descriptions of assessment results (see Chapter 8). Furthermore, they should use the most recently published and up-to-date normative data available (see Chapter 5) and exercise sound professional judgment in evaluating the results of computer-generated summaries of results and interpretive narratives.

Theme II includes recommendations addressing general ideals of assessment practices. These ideals include broad and comprehensive assessments: (1) those that stem from multiple sources of information, including informants (e.g., teachers, parents, and students) and assessment instruments; and (2) those that represent all areas of suspected disability, such as health, vision, hearing, social–emotional functioning, motor abilities, and communicative status. When these assessments are complete, results should be presented in a clear and meaningful way (see Chapter 8). In addition, several recommendations for assessing children from culturally and linguistically diverse backgrounds are provided. For example, school psychologists are implored to conduct assessments that are fair for all those assessed. Thus, the process of selecting assessment instruments should

> **The process of selecting assessment instruments should include consideration of the potential examinee's disabilities and other limitations, as well as the examinee's cultural, linguistic, and experiential background.**

include consideration of the potential examinee's disabilities and other limitations, as well as the examinee's cultural, linguistic, and experiential background (see Chapters 5 and 13). In addition, administration of assessment instruments and interpretation of their results should also take into account these characteristics of the examinee, to ensure that the results accurately represent the targeted constructs being measured. For example, school psychologists should promote quality control in the training and use of interpreters during testing practices (see Chapter 13).

The next principle under Theme II addresses record keeping. In particular, school psychologists are implored to include only documented and relevant information from reliable sources in their records, which include psychological reports (see Chapter 8). Consideration of this standard should ensure that school psychologists report only information that is directly relevant to the referral concerns or eligibility decisions. For example, they should reflect on whether personal information about a child's immediate and extended family (e.g., histories of substance use or mental health problems) is relevant. In addition, they should ensure that they report the source of such information to support its truth value. The final principle under Theme II addresses intellectual property and copyright law, as well as record keeping, test security, and parents' and guardians' access to testing material (as previously discussed). It is particularly important to make sure that access to assessment results on computers and computer networks is restricted to authorized professionals. If this is not possible, then it is best to avoid the use of networked computers altogether and use the best personal computer security available. Psychologists should also assume that email is permanent and potentially public.

SUMMARY

Assessments should be grounded in the ethics of psychology. We find that with each additional reading of the APA's (2002, 2010a) Ethical Principles of Psychologists and Code of Conduct and the NASP's (2010a) Principles for Professional Ethics, we are inspired to do more than is commonplace and to be stronger advocates for children, families, and schools. We are also reminded of general and specific standards that we meet only partially or inconsistently.

On the one hand, we should aspire to ideals such as beneficence, justice, and integrity; strive for excellence in all aspects of our practices; and engage in lifelong learning to achieve and maintain expertise in professional ethics. On the other hand, we should be practical in applying day-to-day ethical practices involving assessment. We should remember that parents and children have the right to know the services we provide and the right to privacy; that assessment results are privileged and sensitive information; that our test content should remain secure to ensure its validity in assessment; and that we should strive to use the best assessment instruments and promote optimal testing environments to produce the most meaningful test results. We hope that the following chapters provide the information that will allow you, our readers, to reach these goals most effectively.

CHAPTER 4

The Assessment Process
with Children and Adolescents

with Ryan L. Farmer

It is important to have a strong knowledge of the reasons for assessment, the typical steps in the assessment process, and the potential influences on test performance that can be controlled during standardized testing or acknowledged when interpreting test results. This chapter addresses these issues and provides practical tools that will promote the most accurate assessment of cognitive abilities through standardized testing.

THE COMPREHENSIVE ASSESSMENT PROCESS—
AND HOW INTELLIGENCE TESTS FIT IN

Assessment is a broad term that refers to the process of collecting data to make informed decisions. Psychological and educational assessments are typically conducted for one of five reasons (and sometimes for multiple reasons). First, they are conducted for *screening* purposes—to rapidly identify those with specified characteristics, so that more in-depth assessment may be conducted. Screening children for hearing or vision deficiencies, for reading problems (via oral reading fluency probes), and for internalizing problems such as depressive disorders (via self-report rating scales) is relatively common. Intelligence tests (including brief or abbreviated intelligence tests; see Chapter 7) are often used to screen for intellectual disabil-

> **Assessment is a broad term that refers to the process of collecting data to make informed decisions.**

Ryan L. Farmer, MA, is a doctoral candidate at the University of Memphis. His research interests include intelligence assessment, threat assessment, and psychometric considerations in test selection.

ity (ID) and intellectual giftedness. Second, assessments may be conducted for *diagnosis* or *eligibility determination*. Assessment data may be used to determine whether a child or adolescent meets one of the criteria for a mental disorder as outlined in the *Diagnostic and Statistical Manual of Mental Disorders* (American Psychiatric Association, 2000, 2013), or such assessment may be prescribed by legislation (currently the Individuals with Disabilities Education Improvement Act of 2004 [IDEA, 2004]) to determine eligibility for special education services. Third, assessment may be conducted for *problem solving*—to identify problems, validate them, and develop interventions to address a concern. Fourth, assessments may be completed for *evaluation* purposes. For example, repeated assessments may be completed to determine the effectiveness of interventions (via progress monitoring) through the administration of fluency-based academic tasks. Finally, assessments may be completed as *indirect interventions*—because of their direct effects on the person being assessed—so that the process of completing the assessment leads to changes in the person and his or her behavior.

It is important to understand that *testing* is a more specific term than *assessment*, and that testing is typically only one component of an assessment. *Testing* refers to the process of collecting data via standardized procedures for obtaining samples of behavior, to draw conclusions about the constructs underlying these behaviors. A *construct* is an "attribute of people, assumed to be reflected in test performance" (Cronbach & Meehl, 1955, p. 283). In the case of intelligence tests, these constructs are cognitive abilities. When considering testing, most psychologists think of individualized standardized testing (i.e., tests administered by an examiner on a one-to-one basis with the examinee for screening, diagnostic, or eligibility purposes), and this book focuses on such tests. In contrast, most educators think about group-administered tests—those administered to a class or to all students in a school (as in end-of-the-year, high-stakes tests) for evaluation purposes.

Just as tests are only one component of the assessment process, there are many other components: reviews of records (e.g., report cards, prior reports and test scores, and incident reports); reviews of permanent products (e.g., completed class assignments); interviews conducted with parents, teachers, and other caregivers; systematic direct observations in classroom, home, or clinic settings; behavior rating scales completed by parents, teachers, and other caregivers; and interviews with and self-report rating scales completed by children and adolescents. Given the high degree of comorbidity (i.e., overlap) of academic and behavior problems displayed by children and adolescents, comprehensive assessments are often necessary to ensure that all relevant problems are evaluated (Frick, Barry, & Kamphaus, 2009). Best practice in assessment is to complete a multimethod, multisource, and multisetting assessment of children and adolescents' learning, as well as their behavioral and emotional functioning (American Educational Research Association [AERA], American Psychological Association [APA], & National Council on Measurement in Education [NCME], 1999; Whitcomb & Merrell, 2012), and such assessments are largely mandated for determining eligibility for special education. Thus the best assessments draw data from many different assessment techniques, from the child or adolescent being assessed as well as multiple knowledgeable persons who observe the child or adolescent, and from behaviors displayed across more than one setting (e.g., the testing session alone).

Intelligence tests are only one component—and sometimes an unessential component—of comprehensive assessments. Because intelligence tests produce measures of one of the most explanatory variables in all of the social sciences, psychometric g, we believe that they should be considered in seeking answers to children's academic problems. We do not claim, however, (1) that they should always be included in a comprehensive assessment or (2) that hours and hours of intelligence testing and days of poring over its results are necessary in most cases. In fact, we recommend the following texts, which target other assessment instruments and methods that may be more useful in identifying the central problems underlying academic problems and developing effective interventions: Kamphaus and Campbell (2006); Chafouleas, Riley-Tillman, and Sugai (2007); Frick et al. (2009); Mash and Barkley (2007); Whitcomb and Merrell (2012); Sattler and Hoge (2006); and Steege and Watson (2009).

> **Because intelligence tests produce measures of one of the most explanatory variables in all of the social sciences, psychometric g, we believe that they should be considered in seeking answers to children's academic problems.**

PRELIMINARY ASSESSMENT

Gathering Background Information

A thorough history of the child or adolescent being assessed should be obtained prior to administering intelligence tests. Background information is often needed to determine age of onset of the presenting problem (i.e., during which developmental period the problem surfaced); the course or prognosis of the problem (i.e., whether the presenting problem is becoming worse over time); etiology (e.g., whether the problem runs in the family), and the results of previous assessments or interventions. In particular, the following types of information should be obtained: referral information; demographic information (including age, grade, and race/ethnicity); family structure and history; the child or adolescent's medical history (including prenatal and perinatal history, genetic conditions, ear infections, head injuries, and surgeries and hospitalizations); developmental history (including speech–language milestones and motor milestones); social history (including major life stressors and traumatic events); and educational history (including grades, prior test scores, academic problems, behavior problems, and prior interventions). Although this information could be obtained by using a response form (a.k.a. paper-and-pencil format—e.g., the Behavior Assessment System for Children, Second Edition [BASC-2] Structured Developmental History Form; Reynolds & Kamphaus, 2004), this information should be obtained in an interview if possible. Interviews provide the opportunity to follow up on issues raised by informants, and they also facilitate rapport building. (The working relationship between an assessment professional and a client during assessment is often called *rapport* in the professional training literature.) Your rapport with informants will promote their engagement in the assessment process and facilitate your clear communication of results after the assessment is complete.

Screening

In addition, a thorough screening for possible impediments to testing should be conducted. Throughout this chapter, we consistently address methods to identify and prevent or minimize *construct-irrelevant* influences on test scores (AERA et al., 1999). These confounds as they apply to validity evidence are described in more detail in Chapter 5, but in this chapter we address them as relevant to individual testing cases. According to Bracken (2000),

> An assumption made about the psychoeducational assessment process is that examiners have made every effort to eliminate all identifiable construct-irrelevant influences on the child or ado-

lescent's performance and the resultant test scores. That is, the goal in assessment is to limit assessment to only construct-relevant attributes (e.g., intelligence), while limiting the influence of construct-irrelevant sources of variation (e.g., fatigue, lack of cooperation, emotional lability). Before important decisions can be made with confidence about a child or adolescent's future educational plans, possible treatments, or medications, examiners must be comfortable with the validity of assessment results. Only when all construct-irrelevant sources of variation have been eliminated or optimally controlled can examiners attest to the validity of the assessment results. (p. 33)

Basic methods can be used to screen for problems with sensory acuity, speech and language, motor control, and behavior as potential confounds. Based on our review of the literature and consultation with professionals in such fields as optometry, audiology, speech–language pathology, and physical therapy, we have identified items that parents, teachers, or both should complete as part of the initial stage of assessment (American Speech–Language–Hearing Association, n.d.; Centers for Disease Control and Prevention, n.d.; Gordon-Brannan, 1994; Colour Blind Awareness, n.d.; Teller, McDonald, Preston, Sebris, & Dobson, 2008; Mathers, Keyes, & Wright, 2010; Suttle, 2001). For this book, we have created several assessment tools that are collectively called the Screening Tool for Assessment (STA).

Form 4.1 is the STA Parent and Caregiver Screening Form, and Form 4.2 is the STA Teacher Screening Form.[*] These forms include items addressing visual acuity problems (items 1–6), color blindness (items 7–10), auditory acuity problems (items 11–16), speech and articulation problems (items 17–22), fine motor problems (items 23–29), and noncompliance (items 30–32). If the patterns of item-level responses indicate serious concerns (e.g., if more than half of the items are marked "Yes"), you should delay testing and inquire about the extent of these apparent problems, discuss whether prior screenings have indicated problems, or consider whether more thorough screening should be conducted. If problems in these areas cannot be corrected before an assessment (e.g., vision problems corrected with glasses), you should (1) select tests so that they are not influenced by them or (2) develop test accommodations to implement during testing. Overall, it is important to consider these influences and eliminate them, because they are potential confounds that will undermine the accuracy and meaningfulness of your test results.

THE TESTING PROCESS

In this section, we address how to prepare yourself and the testing environment for testing, how to establish rules and expectations for the testing session, how to build rapport and interact with children and adolescents during test administration, how to observe test session behaviors, and how to judge the "validity" of the test results.

Preparing for Testing

As you prepare for the testing session, you should be physically and mentally ready to test; appropriately arrange the testing materials and adjust the testing environment to maximize efficiency

---

[*] All forms appear at the ends of the respective chapters.

and eliminate potential confounds; and have a thorough grasp of the test's administration procedures (e.g., rules for subtest stopping points and querying).

Dress, Accessories, and Equipment

Because most testing sessions last approximately 2 hours, you should dress comfortably yet professionally. Although most sessions will be completed at a table with you sitting in a chair, you may need to sit on and crawl about on the floor when you are testing young children. Dressing in comfortable slacks and loose-fitting clothes is important (see Bracken, 2000, for more information about testing young children). In addition, you should be mindful of how your accessories may interfere with testing. For example, decorative rings and bracelets should be avoided, and discretion should be used in selecting ties, necklaces, and earrings. These personal items should not become distractions during testing.

In the same vein, we discourage use of cell phones during testing. Although we know psychologists who use their cell phones for timing during testing, the risk is too great for cell phones (especially smart phones) to cause distractions by vibrating, ringing, beeping, or otherwise providing audible notifications. In addition, it is common for children to use their parents' cell phones for games and other activities, so they may see your phone as a game console rather than a part of the testing equipment. We also occasionally have seen psychologists using digital wrist watches for timing. Unless such a watch is removed from the wrist, using it will be cumbersome; furthermore, wrist watches are often somewhat difficult to manipulate because of their small buttons. We recommend using "old-school" athletic digital stopwatches or digital kitchen timers. These devices should fit in the palm of the hand, should count up (and not only down, as some timers do), and should have beepers removed so that they operate silently.

It is becoming increasingly common for both intelligence and achievement tests to require tape players or CD players for administration. One example is the Woodcock–Johnson III (WJ III) battery (Woodcock, McGrew, & Mather, 2001). In general, you should (1) select the highest-quality equipment (e.g., a tape player with good speakers and a counter), and (2) test this equipment before initiating testing. Headphones (a.k.a. ear buds) are also a necessity, especially with tapes that require items to be queued up. Using CDs and CD players is far easier than using audiotapes and tape players, because you can move across items without using headphones or a counter.

Finally, you should have other materials at your disposal. Of course, numerous pencils are needed, and you will need to consider variations in the types of pencils required across tests. For example, erasers are prohibited during administration of some tests; they should be removed before testing. In addition, #2 lead pencils are typically called for, but sometimes red pencils are required. You should also maintain a collection of tangible incentives. For example, small stickers may be useful to reinforce attentive and compliant behaviors during testing. For young children, small food items (e.g., M&Ms and raisins) may also be helpful for the same purpose. Issues pertaining to the use of such incentives are addressed later in this chapter.

Selecting and Arranging the Testing Environment

You should select a testing environment that has minimal distractions and is otherwise ideal for testing (Bracken, 2000). The room should be well lighted, be kept at a comfortable temperature, and have adequate ventilation. It should contain furniture that is appropriately sized for the child or adolescent being tested. Chairs should be short enough so that a child's feet can touch the floor, and if they cannot, consider placing a box or large books under the child's feet (Kamphaus, 2001). Tabletops should have smooth surfaces, and children should be able to reach them without straining.

You should also consider where you and the child or adolescent being tested should sit. Although the pattern of seating (e.g., sitting across from examinees or beside them) is dictated by the test's standardized procedures, you should strive to seat yourself at the long end of a rectangular table (if possible), in order to arrange your materials more easily and to allow for more writing space. Circular tables are not ideal for testing when (1) they are so wide that you cannot comfortably reach across the table, or (2) it is difficult to space testing material appropriately from the edge and to judge the correctness of some responses when there is no straight edge. Also, seat the child or adolescent so that he or she is not facing distractions (e.g., a window with a view of the playground), and consider arranging the seating so that you are between the child or adolescent and the testing room door.

You should consider the time of day for testing. In elementary school settings, it may be that testing in the morning is ideal; in high school settings, the opposite may be true for adolescents, who may be groggy in the morning. In clinic settings, weigh the costs and benefits of testing at the end of the school day or in the early evening versus having the child or adolescent miss school to complete testing.

Finally, you should reserve enough time to complete each test in its entirety for two reasons. First, most tests were normed that way (see Chapter 5). Second, completing a test in one session prevents you from having to use different norms to score subtests if the delay is extremely lengthy. (In general, if the delay between sessions is no more than 2 weeks, use the child or adolescent's age at the time of the first session unless other recommendations appear in the test's scoring guidelines.)

Knowing the Test and Preparing Testing Materials

We cannot stress enough the importance of your being prepared for testing. It is vital not only to prepare yourself for testing, bring the right support materials, and select and arrange the testing environment, but also to know the administration and scoring procedures well and to prepare the testing materials for an efficient administration. Sattler (2008) has conveyed the importance of preparation for testing—especially for psychologists in training:

> Your goal is to know your tasks well enough that the test administration flows nicely, leaving you time to observe and record the child or adolescent's behavior. To do this you will need to have learned how to apply the administration and scoring rules, how to find test materials quickly, and how to introduce and remove the test materials without breaking the interaction and flow between you and the child or adolescent. Do not study a test manual as you give the test, because doing so will prolong the testing, may increase the child or adolescent's anxiety, and may lead to mistakes in administration. However, in most cases you must refer to the directions and scoring guidelines in the test manual as you administer the test. Most individually administered tests do not require you to memorize test directions. Use highlighters, adhesive flags, index tabs, and other aids to facilitate swift and efficient use of the test manual. (p. 201)

When you are first learning to administer a test, it can be daunting to remember all the rules of standardized administration while maintaining rapport, administering and scoring items, and observing test behavior. To help you reach these goals, you should mark up your test records in advance of testing. Start points can be circled; varied rules for discontinuing can be highlighted; and unique queries, pronunciations of items, and reminders to prevent common errors can be written on sticky notes or in blank spaces on test records. These markings will lessen the amount of information you need to juggle in your mind during testing.

In addition to knowing the intricacies of the tests, it is also useful to prepare your test materials (opening manuals to the first page, setting up easels, setting out pencils, organizing manipulatives for presentation, cueing up tapes for auditory administration, etc.) before initiating the testing session. Of course, if you are pressed for time, these activities can be completed while building rapport; however, this dual tasking is not ideal, because it does not allow you to exert optimal attending skills during the early stage of rapport building.

What should you do if parents request that they be able to observe your testing session by sitting in the testing room with you? It is not a good idea to allow parents to do so if the child or adolescent is age 4 or older (see Bracken, 2000). We have found that most parents understand and respond appropriately when it is explained that the tests were not developed to be completed with a parent in the room, and that their being in the room may be disruptive to the child or adolescent and lead to lower scores. Kamphaus (2001) has suggested that parents should also be told that they should consider how stressful it may be (for them!) to observe the assessment: "Parents want their child to do well, and when they do not, it can be extremely punishing to a parent, especially when they know that their child is taking an intelligence test" (p. 98). If a parent insists on being in the room, or if the child will not separate from the parent despite coaxing, the parent can sit in the testing room outside the child's line of vision (i.e., behind the child). The parent should be instructed (1) to stay silent during testing and (2) not to reveal the content of test items after the session is complete (in order to maintain test security).

Beginning Testing

First Contact and Initial Rapport Building

Because most intelligence tests require one-on-one administration, you will need to retrieve the child or adolescent from a classroom or other school setting (for a school-based assessment) or from a waiting room (for a clinic-based assessment) to initiate testing. It is important to begin developing rapport from the initial contact and to maintain rapport throughout the testing sessions. This rapport is likely to be relatively short-term—across fewer than four sessions and perhaps an additional meeting to describe the results. Your goal in fostering rapport is to obtain information about the child or adolescent, versus to facilitate verbal discussion, reflection, and initiation of therapeutic techniques and strategies for addressing psychological problems (as in counseling and psychotherapy). Thus, the goal of rapport building and rapport maintenance during testing is to ensure enough of a bond with the child or adolescent so that he or she (1) does not feel negative emotions (e.g., fear or worry) that might undermine the assessment, and (2) is motivated to respond to test items and questions in a manner that represents the targeted areas well. In doing so, you want to consider the child or adolescent's age and find the appropriate balance between being approachable (fun, interesting, and humorous) and being more formal and businesslike (Bracken, 2000).

Before you meet the child or adolescent for the first time, consider information you may already possess that may aid you in generating topics of conversation. For example, you may have already gathered information from parents (via their completion of initial interviews or developmental history forms) and from direct observations of the child or adolescent. In addition, you may have scanned materials posted outside the classroom and learned something about the child or adolescent. From these sources, you may have learned about topics or people on which recent classroom projects have focused. In addition, for school-based assessments, it is wise to consult briefly with the child or adolescent's teacher to ensure that you are retrieving the child or adolescent during a segment of the day that does not cause major disruption of important activities in the classroom or during activities that the child or adolescent finds most enjoyable, such as those during support classes. If the timing is not right, you can return to your testing room, engage in other activities (such as scoring protocols or emailing colleagues), and then return later to retrieve the child or adolescent.

When you first meet the child or adolescent, smile, greet the child or adolescent in a friendly manner, and use his or her name. We suggest offering your hand to shake, and, with young children, squatting to be roughly at their eye level when you first meet them. Also, keep the greeting brief; you will have more time to chat and explain your goals soon afterward. You might say, "Hi, Erica. My name is Ms. Barker. I am here to work with you today and talk about school. Please walk with me to my room." We admit to falling prey to a strategy that, on occasion, backfires. Consistent with guidelines for securing a child or adolescent's assent during research projects, we often ask, "Would you like to come with me?" at the end of our greetings. The occasional problem is that children or adolescents may respond negatively, saying that they would rather not do so. When such a response occurs, it lengthens the greeting process, but it may also allow the child or adolescent to express reasons for hesitations that you can address.

As you begin to converse with the child or adolescent while you walk toward the testing room, continue your rapport building by asking open-ended questions about "easy" topics (hobbies, how the day is going, any fun activities the child or adolescent has completed recently, etc.). We find discussion of favorite colors or favorite letters (for young children), pets, and sports to be particularly easy for many children. As you facilitate conversation, strive to be engaging and enthusiastic about the child or adolescent's responses and experiences. Use extenders (e.g., "Oh" and "Umm") and brief positive feedback (e.g., "That's cool" and "I like that, too") in response to the child or adolescent's statements, so that you do not monopolize the conversation. Most children and adolescents appreciate this focused attention from an adult.

Addressing the Purpose of Assessment and Confidentiality

Once the child or adolescent is in the testing room, and you have silenced your cell phone and placed a "Do Not Disturb" sign on the door, you can provide more details about your goals for the testing session. Although excellent scripts are offered in Sattler (2008) and Kamphaus (2001), use a script like this one that is appropriately modified to address important issues related to the assessment. You might begin this way:

"I met your mother/father and your teacher, and now I want to get to know you. They tell me that you have been having a hard time at school. I want to know more about what you have already learned at school and how you go about learning new things, and I want to talk about what we can do to make school better for you. Our work today should last about 2 hours. Is this a good plan to you?"

Most children and adolescents will nod their heads. Then you might ask the child or adolescent to repeat to you what you have said. Say, "So tell me what we're going to do today," and accept any reasonable summary.

    Consistent with the legal and ethical guidelines discussed in Chapter 3, it is important to explain confidentiality and its limits. Although we do not believe that these issues are commonly addressed with children or adolescents before testing sessions, it is best practice to do so. You might say,

> "We need to follow certain rules when we work together today. I want you to feel that you can talk to me, so I'll keep what you tell me between you and me [or private]. That means that I won't go telling your friends, anyone outside of school, or anyone else besides your parents and teacher[s] about our work together. What I share with your parents and teacher[s] will be things to make school better for you. How does that sound?"

Then you can explain the limits of confidentiality and its limits:

> "Again, I will keep our work together private unless several things happen: (1) You tell me that someone (like an adult) has hurt you or someone you know; (2) you tell me that you are going to hurt someone; (3) you tell me that you are going to hurt yourself; or (4) if a police officer or court judge requires me to share the information. When these things happen, you and I would need to talk more about them and share them with your parents, teacher[s], and other adults who care about you. What do you think about this part?"

    You can close the introduction to the testing session by summarizing, adding other rules, encouraging communication with you, and perhaps inserting humor as a bridge to introducing the test. You might say,

> "Other than these things, what we talk about stays between you and me, because I want to help make school better for you. It is very important that you try your best and that you are honest with me because we need to figure things out together."

You may want to add other rules, depending on the child or adolescent's age. For example, for young children you may add rules about staying in the room and asking your permission before touching objects in the room. For others, you may also encourage them to communicate their discomfort at any point during the testing session. Finally, you can consider lightening the mood by telling a joke or by saying something obviously incorrect. For example, some of our favorite strategies in this vein are calling a child by the wrong name (e.g., "OK, are you ready to move on, Esmeralda-ina?" and "So I've forgotten. Your name is Eli . . . Manning, right?") and indicating that the child is much older than his or her actual age (e.g., "I have it written here that you are 10 years old. Is that right?" and "So is it correct that you are in the ninth grade?"). Almost all children will correct your errors. If these questions are asked with a wry smile, we have found that children tend to find them a bit silly; when you say, "Oh, that's right!" and shake your head, throw up your arms, and look exasperated by your error, this technique aids in rapport building. You should develop your own strategies like these to lighten the mood.

Introduction to Testing and Screening for Confounds

Before you begin testing, it is important to describe your expectations for testing and to screen for potential sensory deficits and other personal influences on test performance, in order to rule out potential construct-irrelevant influences on performance on the day of the testing.

Most intelligence tests have incorporated introductions to testing in their standardized procedures, but we encourage you to review them carefully and enhance them with some additional content to promote clear expectations. Essentially, you want to ensure that the children and adolescents understand at least four different components of the testing: (1) that they will complete various tasks; (2)

> Before you begin testing, it is important to describe your expectations for testing and to screen for potential sensory deficits and other personal influences on test performance.

that some of these tasks' items will be easy and others difficult; (3) that they should exert effort and persistence to do their best; and (4) that is it acceptable to report that they do not know answers. We tend to read introductory directions for most intelligence tests and supplement these with "It's OK to ask questions, guess, or say, 'I don't know.'"

Ice Breakers and Screening

From our experience and review of the literature, we understand that it has historically been very common for psychologists to administer simple tasks as "ice breakers" before beginning testing. Drawing tasks, such as the Bender–Gestalt (Bender, 1938) and the House–Tree–Person (Buck & Warren, 1992), were often administered prior to intelligence tests in years gone by. One goal of their administration appears to have been engaging a child or adolescent in some low-stress, paper-and-pencil task before beginning to administer the intelligence test items, which are often orally administered. These tasks provided another buffer between entering the testing room and beginning testing. In some cases, these tasks also allowed examiners to screen directly for potential problems that may undermine the validity of the test scores. However, in our review of the literature, we found no ice-breaking activity that accomplished all of these goals—especially effectively screening for the variety of problems that may undermine accurate testing. To accomplish these goals, we developed the STA Direct Screening Form to accomplish this goal (see Forms 4.3 and 4.4).

The STA Direct Screening Form begins with general questions targeting emotional states and preparedness for testing. The first section covers global impressions of health and mental state, the prior night's sleep, feelings of confidence, and motivation. The next section includes sections devoted to screening for sensory deficits and fine motor control problems. These questions are not intended to be administered in a rigid fashion; instead, they should guide your brief screening interview. Be sure to follow up responses with appropriate extenders, paraphrasing, more specific questions ("What do you mean?"), and "soft" commands (e.g., "Tell me more about it"). There is no reason to complete additional screening if all evidence converges on the absence of sensory deficits and fine motor control problems, but direct assessment of these issues may be useful. The remainder of the STA Direct Screening Form contains assessment items targeting sensory deficits, fine motor control problems, as well as articulation problems and intelligibility.

First, the STA Direct Screening Form includes items targeting visual acuity. Children and adolescents are asked to name letters printed on a page to screen for potential vision problems that may interfere with the test administration (see Form 4.3 for instructions and Form 4.4 for items). The letters printed on the top line should be large and distinct enough for every examinee to see, and corrective feedback can be used to train young or low-functioning examinees. It is essentially a practice trial. After the completion of this trial, you should ask examinees to read the rows below it. Because no intelligence test uses type smaller than the second row of letters (from the top) in Form 4.4 (i.e., 12-point type), vision screening is passed if the examinee accurately reads seven of the nine items in any row below the top row. Do not administer the vision screening items to those (especially young children) who have not yet mastered the names of all letters of the alphabet.

Second, direct assessment items target color blindness. Examinees are asked to identify the colors of six squares (see Form 4.3 for instructions and Form 4.4 for items). They should be able to identify all six colors, and errors in identifying the red and green squares will be especially diagnostic for color blindness in those old enough and high-functioning enough to know color names. Do not administer the color blindness items to those who have not yet mastered the names of the basic colors. Third, direct assessment items target fine motor skills (see Form 4.3 for instructions and Form 4.4 for items). Examinees are asked to trace a horizontal line, a star, and a circle, and to write a simple sentence. Do not administer the item requiring writing to those (especially young children) who have not yet mastered letter printing. Consider deviations from the lines and malformed letters, as well as unsteady pencil grips, hand tremors and jerky movements, impulsive and messy responding, and signs of frustration when an examinee is completing these items, as these may be associated with fine motor control problems. Responses are judged qualitatively; the screening is passed if the examinee responds with reasonable accuracy in tracing or the writing is legible to a stranger who would not know what the sentence in the last item should say.

The remaining direct assessment items from the STA Direct Screening Form do not require visual stimuli (as those included in Form 4.4 do). The next items target auditory acuity (see Form 4.3). These screening items require the examinee to play a listening game, where you give brief commands and the examinee points to parts of his or her face and body (Howard, 1992). During Part A, administer all the items in a slightly louder voice than typical to establish a baseline understanding of the commands, but during Part B, ask the examinee to close his or her eyes while you readminister the items in a whisper. During Part B, observe behavioral signs of hearing problems, such as turning the head to favor one ear and delayed or vague responding (e.g., hovering of the hand near their head). The screening is passed if the examinee responds accurately to at least five of the seven items in Part B.

Finally, direct assessment items target articulation and intelligibility (see Form 4.3). The child or adolescent is asked to close his or her eyes and to repeat words you have stated at a normal volume. These items were developed for the STA on the basis of Shriberg's (1993) findings regarding the development of more challenging phonemes in children. Phonemes included in each word represent the so-called "Late 8" sounds (i.e., the last eight sounds that children are expected to acquire in speech). Phonemes are represented in three positions (initial, medial, and final) across the words (when possible), because these phonemes present different levels of difficulty at each position. For our purposes, we have used the International Phonetic Alphabet when sounds match the English alphabet letters (e.g., /l/). However, when appropriate phonetic symbols would not be commonly recognized (e.g. ʃ representing the *sh* sound), a representation of that phoneme appears in quotation marks. When you are considering patterns of responses, keep in mind that 75% of children should acquire the phonemes /l/, /z/, /s/, *sh*, and *zh* by age 5. The phonemes *th* (voiced, as in the word *although*, and voiceless, as in the word *think*) and /r/ should be acquired by age 6 (Shriberg, 1993). On the form, circle incorrect phonemes; the screening is passed if the examinee provides at least 20 of the 23 correct phonemes.

In addition, a brief rating of intelligibility is available that coincides with items on the STA Parent/Caregiver and Teacher Screening Forms (Forms 4.1 and 4.2). *Intelligibility* is best defined by Bowen (1998) as the percentage of an individual's spoken language that can be readily understood by an unfamiliar listener. Flipsen's (2006) intelligibility formula is as follows:

$$\frac{\text{Age in years}}{4} \times 100 = \% \text{ understood by an unfamiliar listener}$$

As such, a child's intelligibility should increase by 25% for each year after birth. A 1-year-old is expected to be 25% intelligible to strangers, whereas a 3-year-old is expected to be 75% intelligible to strangers. Taking comparable ratings from familiar listeners (e.g., parents) and unfamiliar listeners (e.g., you as the examiner) results in a clinical, albeit subjective, accounting of intelligibility in children. For the purposes of assessment, low intelligibility can affect a child's ability to respond verbally to items. As such, low intelligibility ratings should be considered potentially invalidating when your examiner rating is below 75%. In these cases, it may be wise to consider using language-reduced composite scores or multidimensional nonverbal intelligence tests.

Interacting with Children and Adolescents during Testing

Once you are reasonably confident that the examinee has no sensory acuity, fine motor, speech, or other personal problems that will undermine testing, introduce the first test items. In general, begin testing when the child or adolescent appears ready—and sooner rather than later.

> **In general, begin testing when the child or adolescent appears ready—and sooner rather than later.**

Standardized Procedures

Following standardized administration procedures, once these are studied and practiced repeatedly, should allow for a brisk administration. In addition, we cannot stress enough the importance of following standardized procedures with almost rigid adherence. Kamphaus's (2001) point about this is spot on: "If an examiner does not use standardized procedures, then he or she should not use the norms tables" (p. 106). Although it is possible to interpret intelligence tests from a qualitative and idiographic perspective (see Chapter 7), the best-validated findings come from interpretation of norm-referenced scores. We agree with Kamphaus's point that psychologists in training should think about their own experience of taking group-based standardized tests, such as the ACT, the SAT, and the GRE. You should consider all the rules and decorum (the proctors, the reading of scripts, and the strict time limits) that are central to the standardized testing enterprise, and strive to replicate such strict adherence. You should read instructions, item introductions, and feedback after errors exactly as they are written—even if you are motivated to improve the examinee's understanding. For example, Sattler (2008) has implored examiners to "never ad lib, add extraneous words, leave out words from instructions or the test questions, or change any test directions because you think that the altered wording would improve the child's performance (unless the test manual permits changes)" (p. 203).

Accurate timing of items on intelligence tests is vital to measuring individual differences in cognitive abilities, and we have five points to offer about timing. First, there is no reason to hide your stopwatch or otherwise be surreptitious in timing. We agree with Kamphaus (2001) that you should be natural about timing and use of the stopwatch. Now, perhaps more than ever, children and adolescents are accustomed to completing timed (and fluency-based) tests; it is unlikely that they will be unnerved by your using it. Second, timing should begin once you have completed the instructions. Once timing for an item or subtest has been initiated, you should not stop timing until the item is complete or the time limit has ended. Do not stop timing when children or adolescents ask questions, when they make errors in response to individual items, or when you must prompt to maintain standardization. Third, discontinue the items or subtests when the time limit has expired, or record the exact completion time (typically rounding down to the nearest second vs. recording minutes, seconds, and milliseconds). Fourth, score the last response provided within the time limit. Most subtests have you award no credit for items completed after the time limit, although there are a few exceptions in which partial credit is given for incomplete performance. Finally, do not share the time limit or the time remaining with the child or adolescent, even if asked. If you are asked a question during a timed trial, you might make eye contact and calmly say, "Just keep working," and then break eye contact so as to not engage in conversation.

We are seeing a trend toward more explicit description of "soft time limits" targeting test items—especially items requiring expression of knowledge and oral expression. In general, you should present the next test item after allowing a child or adolescent an appropriate amount of time to respond to a difficult question. However, some tests require that a response to an item be given in about 20 or 30 seconds, to enhance the efficiency of testing. Other tests, as noted previously, apply an absolute time limit to item-level responses. You should find the right balance between (1) allowing examinees to continue working on responses after the time limit has expired, and (2) stopping them in development of a response and ushering them to the next item. It is important, however, to score the response that was available before the time limit expired.

Extending and Clarifying Responses

During testing, you may need to encourage the examinee to extend or clarify an initial response. Typically, you should offer *queries*, such as "What do you mean?" and "Tell me more about it." Although these queries are very similar across intelligence tests, you should always use the queries prescribed by each test. We recommend using sticky notes or the like in the test record to remind you of these queries when you are administering several different tests as part of an assessment. For most intelligence tests, the administration manual provides sample responses that must be queried, but you should also query vague responses, regionalisms, or slang responses that are not clearly incorrect. However, you should be careful not to query any clear-cut responses that contain enough information to score without a query. Furthermore, you should record on your protocol the points when you queried (using Q to represent a query).

In general, you should consider all parts of a response—those parts that are offered before the query is issued, and those offered after the query is issued. In other words, score the whole of the response. For example, when asked about the meaning of the word *colander*, the child offers "You use it in the kitchen with water," and after you query the response, he or she offers, "It keeps you from pouring hot pasta down the drain," you would consider both parts of the response, and the child would earn as many points as if he or she had combined both parts into one sentence. However, it gets tricky when the response after the query is mediocre or outright flawed. If you issue a query, and the child offers a weak response or otherwise fails to improve the initial response (e.g., "Colanders are plastic and white"), score the quality of the initial response. However, if the query reveals a fundamental misconception—a totally flawed understanding—about the content of the item (e.g., "Colanders chop up food into pieces"), the initial response, regardless of its quality, is spoiled, and the item is scored 0.

Dealing with Audio Players

Using an audiotape player or CD player introduces challenges into the testing session that were not commonly experienced by those administering intelligence tests in the past. In addition to needing one more piece of equipment, if you are using an audiotape player, it is important to use a player that has a counter so that you can link your subtest start points to items on the tape. Doing so requires preparation, a set of headphones (if adjustments must be made during testing), and a good deal of rewinding and fast-forwarding. A CD player largely eliminates these problems, because most start points can easily be located.

When you are using any type of audio player, it is important to look away from the examinee (e.g., at your test record) when the item is being played, and then look expectantly at the examinee once the item has been completed. In addition, it is important to stop the CD or pause the tape (when allowed) to allow examinees who are slow to respond more time to formulate a response. Although there should be enough time between items for most children and adolescents to respond, we recommend (1) being conscious that the next item may be presented before a response can been offered, and (2) stopping or pausing before such incidents occur.

Scoring and Recording Responses

You should strive for a brisk administration, while also taking your time to score responses concurrently with the administration. If you cannot decide on a score for an item, leave it blank, mark it with a question mark, continue to complete the last item, or meet the discontinue rule while not including this item; score the item in question at a later time. When you are scoring, both example responses and general scoring criteria should be consulted, but keep in mind that the examples listed in the test manuals are guides to scoring and that some professional judgment (a.k.a. "real thinking" on your part) may be required. If you are a beginning tester or are learning a new test, we strongly encourage you to have a second party review your item scoring and raw score calculation. We are also strong advocates of using scoring software to prevent errors when the norm tables presented in manuals are consulted.

It is important to score all items according to the examples, general criteria, and scoring guides provided in test manuals, and to avoid applying subjective judgments that "bend the rules" for examinees. However, as just noted, professional judgment is needed—especially in cases where the examinee responds in a manner that is more sophisticated than the sample responses. For example, an adolescent may respond to a picture vocabulary item by reporting the genus and species of a beetle, rather than referring to it as an "insect" in general or a "beetle" more specifically. Some children may calculate the exact number of weeks in a year (yielding a decimal fraction), versus telling you that there are 52 full weeks in the year. In such cases, it is incumbent on you to search books or the Internet, or to do the calculations yourself, to determine whether the response is correct or incorrect. In the same vein, you should not penalize the child or adolescent for mispronunciations due to articulation problems or to regional or dialect differences.

It is difficult to know how to score initial responses that include both correct and incorrect components. Although you should always consult the test manuals for specific guidelines, here are two commonalities across them. First, if several responses to an item are given, ask which one the child or adolescent wants you to score. You can say, "You said *X*, and you said *Y*. Which one is it?" or the like. (Note that some intelligence test manuals encourage you to score the last response given.) Second, for many tests, if the child or adolescent provides numerous correct responses of varying quality and the item is scored on a scale, score the best response.

When administering the tests, you should record verbatim responses to the degree possible. Record them in the lines on the test record or beside the item. However, exercise some discretion in selecting only the core of the responses to record. For instance, you need not record the initial stem of a response (e.g., "I think that an encyclopedia is a . . . "), interjections (e.g., "Darn!"), or idiosyncratic responses (e.g., "I think we learned that in third grade" or "That is a tough one") that are not clinically meaningful. Thus, extraneous content need not be recorded. It is also important to be able to use abbreviations when appropriate, but never place them in the item-scoring column.

Breaks, Check-Ins, and Encouragement

It is important to monitor the child or adolescent's motivation and persistence during testing, and to encourage full responses to all items. Throughout the testing session, you should "read" the child or adolescent's behavior, including facial expressions, posture, and verbalizations, to determine his or her level of motivation and fatigue (Kamphaus, 2001). Although you typically want to keep small talk to a minimum during subtests, we recommend "checking in" between subtests with questions like "How are you feeling?" and "Ready for the next one?" to gauge motivation and fatigue. We encourage energetic, brisk administrations of the tests, but for some children and adolescents, you may call for breaks every 30 minutes or so. You must consider, though, that (1) some children and adolescents have a difficult time readjusting to the testing session after a break; and (2) in a school setting, breaks lengthen the assessment session and potentially prevent exposure to valuable instructional content in the classroom setting.

Engaging in strategies to encourage full expression of knowledge and skills during testing is vital. Although you are able to provide encouraging feedback after correct responses to sample items—and some tests do, in fact, allow for such feedback after responses to test items—you should generally strive to give no indication of whether responses to test items are correct or incorrect. In particular, you should not indicate the quality of the examinee's responses through your facial expression or your verbalizations. We encourage our students in training to practice their "stone face with a smile" expressions throughout testing, and to develop nonevaluative verbalizations that can be consistently used. For example, we believe that saying "OK" or "That's fine," and nodding after responses, are both acceptable behaviors—as long as examiners are diligent about using them for both correct and incorrect responses. Others may assert that presenting the next item signals clearly that the last response has been accepted, but we find that, with preschool- and elementary-school-age children, some other way of accepting their response seems warmer and more responsive.

We recommend two types of feedback designed to praise a child or adolescent's effort during testing. First, use various comments to recognize effort. Examples include "Thanks for your hard work," "I like how you thought through that one," "Excellent effort! Keep it up!" and "Keep giving it your all." We also encourage well-timed general comments, such as "You are doing a great job," and "Good work," that cannot be linked to correct responses and that are intermingled with comments about effort. Second, we encourage physical gestures and brief physical contact, such as fist bumps. We admit to engaging in some seemingly hokey behaviors, such as prompting children to give us "high fives" and offering "thumbs-up" gestures paired with phrases like "Good job" and a smile. Of course, these behaviors must be moderated in keeping with the child or adolescent's age. For example, preschoolers tend to enjoy silliness from adults, but the same cannot be said for many adolescents. In particular, adolescents may be particularly sensitive to insinuation of false praise or to repetitions of platitudes.

The use of tangible and edible incentives during testing is a topic of frequent debate (see Fish, 1988). We agree with Sattler (2008) that such incentives should not be used under normal circumstances; they may introduce unnecessary complexity and potential hazards into the testing situation (e.g., activating food allergies and choking, in the case of food items). However, we have seen benefits of the use of incentives with preschool-age children, children with ID, and children with attention-deficit/hyperactivity disorder (ADHD) when they are used to reinforce compliance and responding to items. We offer these recommendations. First, if you plan to use food items, obtain the parent or caregiver's permission to do so. Many food items, such as M&M candies or marshmallows, may be prohibited by the family. Obtaining such permission in school settings is often impractical. Second, food items often interfere with testing because they have the potential to make a mess (e.g., tortilla chip remnants on the testing table or chocolaty saliva running down a child's mouth). Food items are probably best reserved for preschoolers, but for older children and adolescents, we recommend that a token economy or point system be implemented so that they earn rewards for compliance (e.g., sitting in the chair and attempting as many questions as possible) that can be traded in at the end of the testing session for valued items (e.g., trading cards, stickers, and colorful pencils).

Monitoring the motivation and persistence of children and adolescents, and encouraging them to respond fully requires guiding them to work though the most difficult test items. Although you may have already shared with them that they can report that they do not know some answers (and that no one is expected to be able to answer all items), you should encourage them to guess by reminding them with "It's OK to guess" or "It's OK to answer even if you are not sure," and encouraging them to "Give it a try" or "Give it a shot." After using these techniques (and driving home the point that guessing is not a problem) and reading their behaviors as the testing progresses, you may also ask, "Want to give it a try or move to the next one?" or "Want to pass on this one?" Furthermore, you should be sensitive to their perceptions of failures, and remind them that effort is more important to you than correct responses. There seems to be some benefit of reminding children and adolescents that some items were developed for older adults. You may say, "Remember I told you that some of these items would be hard; they must be for moms and dads, huh?" or "That was a tough one, wasn't it? I like how well you worked on it, though."

Responding to Questions

Some anxious or inquisitive children and adolescents may barrage you with questions. Others, due to some of their limitations, may require you to respond to pleas for assistance. For example, some may ask you for feedback on items, asking "Was I right?" or "How am I doing?"; others may ask you for the answers to questions that they could not produce. Your standard responses to these issues should be to say, kindly, that you cannot tell them how well they are doing or what the correct answers are. Comments such as "You're doing fine, and I appreciate your hard work," and "Your answer sounds good to me," work well. We often refer to our testing rules to justify our inability to share the correct answers. We say, "I'm sorry that I can't tell you; it's one of the rules I must follow in doing my job."

Unless the test item targets an ability that would be enhanced by repeating the item (e.g., sub-tests targeting Short-Term Memory or Listening Ability), you can repeat questions or items upon request, but when you do so, it is important that you repeat it in its entirety so that you do not parse its components for them. For example, on a subtest targeting quantitative reasoning that requires children to calculate the difference in miles between two cities, a child might ask, "Did you say in miles?" Rather than replying in the affirmative, you should repeat the whole item to require the child to parse the important information from it. You may also repeat items when a response suggests that the child misheard or misunderstood words used in the item.

Observing Behaviors during the Test Session

As we have noted earlier in this chapter, you should observe test session behaviors to judge how these behaviors might undermine the validity of your score results. Even if you have gone through all the efforts to eliminate or to control optimally for construct-irrelevant sources of variation in test scores, it is possible that some of the child or adolescent's characteristics may exert their influences and produce biased results. In particular, behaviors that produce downwardly biased results, such as those associated with anxiety, fatigue, inattention, extreme disappointment, and noncompliance, should be monitored closely.

Commonplace Practices

Two practices for recording and summarizing test session behaviors have become commonplace. The first practice is writing descriptions of behaviors of interest in the margins of the test record. These narrative "behavior observations" may be used to enhance memory when examiners are summarizing test results and writing reports, as well as to contribute to a better understanding of low norm-referenced scores yielded after testing has been completed. These behavior observations are often written concisely. Examples include such notes as "Seems anxious: fidgety, picks at skin around fingernails," "Says hates math," or "Is a live wire: bouncing in chair, grabbing testing materials, out of seat." Although some of these behaviors may be a reaction to test content (e.g., the one about hating math), these behaviors sometimes represent our failures to eliminate or optimally control for construct-irrelevant influences. Because behavior in one-on-one testing environment does not accurately represent behaviors in other environments, you should be more concerned about producing valid test scores than about observing the child or adolescent's reaction to the testing session. You should not sit passively and record behaviors that confound your results; you should intervene. For example, with an adolescent who appears to lack motivation, you could ask, "Is everything OK? You are looking a bit tired," problem-solve based on the response, and terminate the testing session if needed (Kamphaus, 2001). The second practice is summarizing (after testing is complete) noteworthy behaviors displayed during the testing session. Almost every intelligence test record includes a brief checklist or prompts addressing language usage, attention, activity level, attitude, cooperativeness, mood, and self-confidence. Both methods may assist you in describing the testing environment in your report after detailed memories of the session have decayed.

Innovative Practices

Two innovative practices cast light on our understanding of test session behaviors and their potential influences on the validity of assessment. First, A. S. Kaufman, N. L. Kaufman, and their collaborators (see Kaufman & Kaufman, 2004a) have developed a brilliant way to monitor and record potential construct-irrelevant influences on item-level performance: having the examiner review and complete a brief checklist of common influences associated with each subtest. Their *qualitative indicators* include *disrupting indicators*, including not monitoring accuracy, failing to sustain attention, impulsively responding incorrectly, perseverating despite feedback, refusing to engage in a task, being reluctant to commit to a response, being reluctant to respond when uncertain, and worrying about time limits. Conversely, they include *enhancing indicators*, including closing eyes to concentrate, asking for repetition of items, persevering after initial struggles, trying out options, being unusually focused, verbalizing related knowledge, verbalizing a strategy for recall, and working quickly but carefully. Reviewing a checklist of such items during or after the administration of each subtest allows examiners to identify and document potentially confounding influences. Second, rating scales have been developed to assess behavioral excesses that may interfere with test performance. Two of the most well-developed and psychometrically sound instruments of this kind are the Guide to Assessment of Test Session Behavior (Glutting & Oakland, 1993) and the Achenbach System for Empirically Based Assessment Test Observation Form (TOF; McConaughy & Achenbach, 2004). The completion of postassessment rating scales such as the TOF may be especially useful for students in training, because it sensitizes them to unusual and perhaps meaningful behaviors during the testing session. For discussion of these methods, see McConaughy (2005).

Meaningfulness of Behavior Observations

Examiners' narrative descriptions and ratings of observations completed after the testing session are likely to be negatively affected by errors in memory (Lilienfeld, Ammirati, & David, 2012; Watkins, 2009), so we encourage recording behaviors of interest immediately after they occur during testing. The most accurate summaries of behaviors during the test session would probably stem from review of such notes recorded in the protocol. There is no doubt that these varying types of behavior observations can be completed in concert, but we encourage relying first on direct observation and immediate recording of them. We should perhaps conclude, upon reflection, that specific behaviors were not undermining test scores unless notes indicated such throughout protocol.

Posttesting Considerations

Debriefing

We admit to frequently making the mistake of not conducting some sort of debriefing after completing a test session (and not teaching our students to do so!). After a full testing session, it is tempting to say, "We're done today. Thanks for working so hard with me. Let's go back to your classroom," or the like, but it is an ideal practice to spend a bit more time debriefing. First, it may help to maintain rapport with the child or adolescent—especially if multiple testing sessions will be completed. Kamphaus (2001) has suggested honestly acknowledging challenges the child or adolescent faced during testing. Statements like "I realize that you were a little unhappy about being here today, but you tried hard to do what I asked and I really appreciate that" (Kamphaus, 2001, p. 111) may go a long way in building and maintaining your relationship with the child or adolescent. In addition, it may allow you to answer questions or allay fears the child or adolescent may have. Second, if you inquire about the child or adolescent's experience of the test, as well as what he or she liked and did not like, you may identify probable construct-irrelevant influences on test results. Third, debriefing is consistent with the goal of keeping the child or adolescent informed about the outcomes of the testing. Sattler (2008) has suggested repeating some of your introductory statements regarding these outcomes, such as your sharing that you will summarize the results in a report and meet with parents and teachers to discuss the results so that the examinee's experience at school will be improved. We strongly encourage taking additional time at the end of each testing session to debrief the child or adolescent.

Validity of Results

After testing is complete, you must make two decisions. One decision is to determine whether the results are "valid." This validity is not exactly the same type as that discussed in Chapter 5, but the concepts are similar. Essentially, you need to judge whether the intelligence test subtests were administered in a way—and the child or adolescent reacted to them in a way—that permits you to say with confidence that the resulting scores well represent the ability or abilities you targeted. In other words, you must judge whether the inference made about the child or adolescent's cognitive abilities are reasonably accurate, based on his or her test behavior.

> **You must judge whether the inference made about the child or adolescent's cognitive abilities are reasonably accurate, based on his or her test behavior.**

Although statements about the validity of testing results are often made at a global level when printed in reports (see Chapter 8 for examples), we encourage consideration of the meaningfulness of subtest scores, which are the foundation of all other scores for intelligence tests. It is possible that the results from one subtest are invalid and all other results are valid. We encourage you to specify which scores are likely to be invalid and describe what led you to conclude this. Perhaps there is a continuum of validity of assessment. On one end is an ideal testing environment and a perfect standardized administration. There were no interruptions; the child or adolescent was optimally motivated to respond and displayed no behavior problems; and there was consistent performance across items, with no apparent guessing or failure to answer the easiest items. Such sessions are not uncommon. On the other end is a testing session that goes awry. You are testing in a broom closet near a noisy hallway and a train track; you are not at your best due to caffeine withdrawal; you fumble through the testing materials; and the child or adolescent is unruly and unmotivated. In cases such as the latter, you may conclude that all of the data collected as part of the assessment are meaningless in representing the child or adolescent's cognitive abilities. If so, you should not report the scores in your report or discuss them. You should promptly schedule another testing session and develop a plan for improving it. Furthermore, you should briefly summarize this event in your report, justify your decision not to report your initial results, and describe your rationale for administrating a second intelligence test.

The most difficult validity decisions are those between the extremes on the continuum—those cases in which there was probably some interference in measurement during testing. We have found that these instances are rarely addressed by examiners and included in reports, but we urge giving more attention to them and their influence on test scores. They may stem from influences generally associated with the testing environment. For example, some children and adolescents may be less engaged in the testing late in the session, and the results are lower scores on the last few subtests administered. Others may struggle in completing items from one subtest and seem to be dejected afterward. Still others will react in an unexpected way to standard test directions, test items, and prompts and queries. For example, some will simply not understand the requirements of the task as a whole, despite completing practice items satisfactorily. Others may adopt the strategy of providing you more information than you required—going on and on when defining words or providing the correct answer and also five variants of it. Still others will offer a new response— effectively changing their answer—when queried for more information. These external influences and idiosyncratic reactions almost certainly have an impact on test scores, but it is admittedly difficult to determine when they reflect true ability deficits versus construct-irrelevant influences.

Testing of Limits and Follow-Up Assessment

There are at least two methods for addressing potential construct-irrelevant influences and the validity of test results: (1) testing of limits and (2) follow-up testing using similar measures. *Testing of limits* refers to readministration of subtest items after completion of a test, during which additional cues are given, modeling of correct responses is completed, items are presented in a different fashion, responses are allowed in another modality (e.g., spoken vs. written), time limits are eliminated, and probing questions are asked. The goal is to test hypotheses about why a child or adolescent missed an item or series of items. For example, in cases in which the child or adolescent quickly missed all items on a subtest requiring him or her to repeat orally presented numbers backward, you could use concrete objects (e.g., tiles or blocks with numbers on them) to demonstrate how to reverse numbers presented orally to ensure that the child or adolescent understands what is required. Alternately, you could request that they teach you how to complete an easy item. Afterward, you could administer the items again to determine whether the intervention has yielded dividends. Regardless of the outcome, you should never change raw scores obtained from a standardized test administration, but you should consider explaining the reason for a low score and eliminating the affected score from your report.

Testing of limits has been formalized in some published tests, such as the Wechsler Intelligence Scale for Children—Fourth Edition Integrated (WISC-IV Integrated; Kaplan et al., 2004). It contains 16 "process tests" that reflect changes in the task requirements of subtests through adaptations to their stimuli, to response requirements, and to the nature of the subtests themselves. Some of these adaptations are minor, such as laying a grid over an image to facilitate reconstruction of that design with blocks; others are substantial, such as requiring children to point to images of numbers in sequence rather than repeat orally presented numbers. Performance on most of these process tests yields norm-referenced scores that can be compared to those stemming from the original standardized administration of subtests from the Wechsler scales. Higher scores on the process tests than on the original subtests are thought to indicate that the process targeted by the adaptation must have interfered with performance on the original subtest. For example, an examiner might conclude that a child or adolescent who performed notably better on the subtest requiring recall of number factors, calendar facts, geography, science, and history when provided with multiple-choice options than when provided with no external cue experienced memory retrieval problems that interfered with his or her initial performance on the subtest without the cues. We worry, though, that repeated exposure to the same items during testing of limits has unknown but probably facilitative effects on the responses of the child or adolescent.

In addition, when we develop hypotheses regarding construct-irrelevant influences on test scores, we often engage in some additional testing employing related measures. If we believe that some distraction during testing, some misunderstanding on the child or adolescent's part, or some other influence unduly affected test scores, we usually turn to resources offered as part of the cross-battery approach (Flanagan, Ortiz, & Alfonso, 2013) to find an alternative subtest purported to measure the same specific ability to test our hypothesis. Often we identify alternative subtests that go about measuring the ability in a different way—somewhat like those included in the WISC-IV Integrated (Kaplan et al., 2004), but from another test. For example, if a child scored poorly on a subtest that requires repeating orally presented numbers in reverse, we might follow up with a related subtest that requires him or her to order orally presented numbers and letters in ascending order. Alternately, we might follow up with a subtest that more closely matches the content and response processes of the one in question. Although we are not certain that the extra effort to examine all of our hypotheses in this vein is always warranted, judicious use of this technique may allow you to distinguish more clearly between low scores indicating ability deficits and low scores due to construct-irrelevant influences.

SUMMARY

It is important to have a strong knowledge of the reasons for assessment, typical assessment processes, and potential influences on test performance that can be controlled during testing or acknowledged when interpreting test results. In this chapter, we have offered detailed descriptions of these processes and equipped you with tools and resources to facilitate and evaluate the validity of your test scores for each child or adolescent you assess.

Screening Tool for Assessment (STA)— Parent and Caregiver Screening Form

Child's name: _____   Glasses/contact lenses: Y/N

Parent or caregiver's name: _____   Hearing aid/cochlear implant: Y/N

Please read each item carefully and circle Yes or No.

1	My child closes or covers one eye when looking at some things.	Yes	No
2	My child frequently squints his or her eyes.	Yes	No
3	My child complains that some images are blurry or hard to see.	Yes	No
4	My child holds objects unusually close to his or her face when looking at them.	Yes	No
5	My child seems to blink a lot.	Yes	No
6	My child becomes frustrated or upset when doing close-up work such as reading, math, and puzzles.	Yes	No
7	My child uses the wrong color names for objects, such as saying that there are purple leaves on trees.	Yes	No
8	My child has a short attention span when coloring or drawing with colors or colored markers.	Yes	No
9	My child has difficulty identifying red or green.	Yes	No
10	My child has difficulty reading when the words are on colored pages.	Yes	No
11	My child does not respond to loud noises sometimes.	Yes	No
12	My child's listening skills are behind what I expect.	Yes	No
13	My child turns up the volume too loud on electronic equipment.	Yes	No
14	My child does not follow spoken directions well.	Yes	No
15	My child often says, "Huh?" or asks you to repeat something you have said.	Yes	No
16	My child does not respond when called.	Yes	No
17	My child's speech is behind what I expect.	Yes	No
18	My child has difficulty pronouncing some words.	Yes	No
19	My child substitutes sounds in words (e.g., *wed* for *red*).	Yes	No
20	My child leaves sounds out of words (e.g., *root* for *fruit*).	Yes	No

21	How much of your child's speech do you understand?	25%	50%	75%	100%
22	How much of your child's speech would a stranger understand?	25%	50%	75%	100%

(continued)

23	My child has difficulty stacking blocks.	Yes	No
24	My child has difficulty fitting puzzle pieces together.	Yes	No
25	My child has difficulty drawing a straight line.	Yes	No
26	My child has difficulty drawing a circle.	Yes	No
27	My child has difficulty printing his or her first name.	Yes	No
28	I can usually read my child's handwriting.	Yes	No
29	A stranger would usually be able to read my child's handwriting.	Yes	No
30	My child is often defiant.	Yes	No
31	My child often refuses to do what I ask.	Yes	No
32	My child breaks a lot of rules at home.	Yes	No

Are there any other issues that might affect how well your child performs during the upcoming testing sessions? Please describe them below.

FORM 4.2

Screening Tool for Assessment (STA)—Teacher Screening Form

Student's name: _____   Glasses/contact lenses: Y/N

Teacher's name: _____   Hearing aid/cochlear implant: Y/N

Please read each item carefully and circle Yes or No.

1 The student closes or covers one eye when looking at some things.   Yes   No

2 The student frequently squints his or her eyes.   Yes   No

3 The student complains that some images are blurry or hard to see.   Yes   No

4 The student holds objects unusually close to his or her face when looking at them.   Yes   No

5 The student seems to blink a lot.   Yes   No

6 The student becomes frustrated or upset when doing close-up work such as reading, math, and puzzles.   Yes   No

7 The student uses the wrong color names for objects, such as saying that there are purple leaves on trees.   Yes   No

8 The student has a short attention span when coloring or drawing with colors or colored markers.   Yes   No

9 The student has difficulty identifying red or green.   Yes   No

10 The student has difficulty reading when the words are on colored pages.   Yes   No

11 The student does not respond to loud noises sometimes.   Yes   No

12 The student's listening skills are behind what I expect.   Yes   No

13 The student turns up the volume too loud on electronic equipment.   Yes   No

14 The student does not follow spoken directions well.   Yes   No

15 The student often says, "Huh?" or asks you to repeat something you have said.   Yes   No

16 The student does not respond when called.   Yes   No

17 The student's speech is behind what I expect.   Yes   No

18 The student has difficulty pronouncing some words.   Yes   No

19 The student substitutes sounds in words (e.g., *wed* for *red*).   Yes   No

20 The student leaves sounds out of words (e.g., *root* for *fruit*).   Yes   No

21 How much of the student's speech do you understand?   25%   50%   75%   100%

22 How much of the student's speech would a stranger understand?   25%   50%   75%   100%

(continued)

23	The student has difficulty stacking blocks.	Yes	No
24	The student has difficulty fitting puzzle pieces together.	Yes	No
25	The student has difficulty drawing a straight line.	Yes	No
26	The student has difficulty drawing a circle.	Yes	No
27	The student has difficulty printing his or her first name.	Yes	No
28	I can usually read the student's handwriting.	Yes	No
29	A stranger would usually be able to read the student's handwriting.	Yes	No
30	The student is often defiant.	Yes	No
31	The student often refuses to do what I ask.	Yes	No
32	The student breaks a lot of rules at school.	Yes	No

Are there any other issues that might affect how well the student performs during the upcoming testing sessions? Please describe them below.

FORM 4.3

Screening Tool for Assessment (STA)—Direct Screening Test Record

Student's name: _____   Glasses/contact lenses: Y/N

Date: _____   Hearing aid/cochlear implant: Y/N

GENERAL SCREENING QUESTIONS

I want to ask you a few questions before we start today.

How are you feeling today?

Did you sleep well last night?

How confident (or nervous) are you feeling about our work together today?

How ready are you to do your best on every task today?
or How motivated are you to do well on these tasks today?

Do you wear glasses or contacts or have trouble seeing?

Do you have any trouble telling colors apart?
or Are you color-blind?

Do you wear a hearing aid or have trouble hearing?

Do you have any trouble writing with a pencil?
or How neat is your handwriting?

Do you have any trouble picking up and moving items such as coins?

Note. Paraphrase and follow up with more specific questions if needed. Use the child or adolescent's oral language during interview to estimate intelligibility of speech.

(continued)

VISION SCREENING

Present Vision Screening items from the STA Direct Screening Response Form.

Look at these letters on this sheet of paper. Please tell me the letters in the top row.

Stimuli	Number incorrect	Total correct
E O P Z T L C D F		/9

Correct errors if necessary, and repeat until all items are correct in sequence.

Without picking up the sheet, tell me the letters in the other rows. There is no reason to go fast. Slow and careful reading is best.

Mark those items missed.

Stimuli	Number incorrect	Total correct
T D P C F Z O E L		/9
D Z E L C F O T P		/9
F E P C T L O Z D		/9

COLOR BLIND SCREENING

Present Color items from the STA Direct Screening Response Form.

See these squares. Name these colors for me. (Alternatively, **What is this color?**)

Stimuli	Correct response	
Black	Yes	No
Blue	Yes	No
Red	Yes	No
Green	Yes	No
Yellow	Yes	No
Purple	Yes	No

Total correct: /6

FINE MOTOR SCREENING

Present items from the Fine Motor page of the STA Direct Screening Response Form. Administer items in sequence as age and developmental level dictates.

If the examinee attempts to rotate the paper, say, **Don't move the paper; keep it in one place.**

1. **Take this pencil and trace this dotted line. Follow on the line, and make one smooth line.**
2. **Now trace this star. Follow on the lines.**
3. **Now trace this circle. Follow on the line.**
4. **Write this sentence, "The dog ran," on this line.**

(continued)

Stimuli	Successful		Stimuli	Successful			
Line	Yes	No	**Circle**	Yes	No	**Total Yes:**	/4
Star	Yes	No	**Sentence**	Yes	No		

HEARING SCREENING

Part A: **Let's play a game about listening. I want you to point to parts of your body. Ready? Listen carefully. I will tell you where to point.**

Administer the initial items slightly louder than normal.

Item	Correct response	
Point to your nose.	Yes	No
Point to your hair.	Yes	No
Point to your face.	Yes	No
Point to your ear.	Yes	No
Point to your chin.	Yes	No
Point to your shoulder.	Yes	No
Point to your mouth.	Yes	No

Total correct, Part A: _____

Part B: **Now I want you to point to the same parts of your body, but this time I want you to close your eyes while I tell you where to point. Ready? Listen carefully.**

Administer these items at a low volume that is above that of a whisper, but still able to be heard by the examinee. Put your hand a few inches in front of your mouth during administration.

Item	Correct response	
Point to your face.	Yes	No
Point to your nose.	Yes	No
Point to your ear.	Yes	No
Point to your hair.	Yes	No
Point to your shoulder.	Yes	No
Point to your mouth.	Yes	No
Point to your chin.	Yes	No

Total correct Part B: _____

(continued)

ARTICULATION SCREENING

Please close your eyes, listen carefully, and say what I say.

Carefully articulate each word at a normal volume. Carefully watch the lips of the child or adolescent while he or she is responding.

If you cannot determine how to score a response, say "Please, say (item) again" as often as needed.

Circle the phonemes in the Sounds column that were incorrectly pronounced. Subtract number of incorrect phonemes from 23 to determine the percentage correct, using the table provided.

Item	Sounds		#Correct	%Correct	#Correct	%Correct
Lizard	/l/	/z/	0	0%	19	83%
This	th	/s/	1	4%	20	87%
Wreath	/r/	th	2	9%	21	91%
Shoes	sh	/z/	3	13%	22	96%
Seal	/s/	/l/	4	17%	23	100%
Think	th	—	5	22%		
Mouthwash	th	sh	6	26%		
Garage	/r/	zh	7	30%		
Feather	th	/r/	8	35%		
Pillow	/l/		9	39%		
Zebra	/z/		10	43%		
Soothe	th		11	48%		
Television	zh		12	52%		
Listen	/s/		13	57%		
Washer	sh		14	61%		
			15	65%		
Total sounds:	**23**		16	70%		
Number of incorrect sounds: _____			17	74%		
Number of correct sounds: _____			18	78%		

INTELLIGIBILITY

After completing the STA Direct Screening Test, rate the proportion of the child or adolescent's speech you were able to understand.

	Some	Most	Almost all	All
How much of the child or adolescent's speech did you understand?	25%	50%	75%	100%

Screening Tool for Assessment (STA)—
Direct Screening Response Form

Examinee's name: _____   Date: _____

E O P Z T L C D F

T D P C F Z O E L

D Z E L C F O T P

F E P C T L O Z D

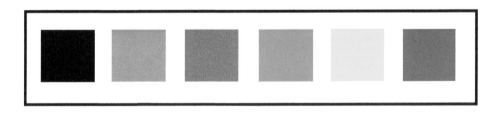

(continued)

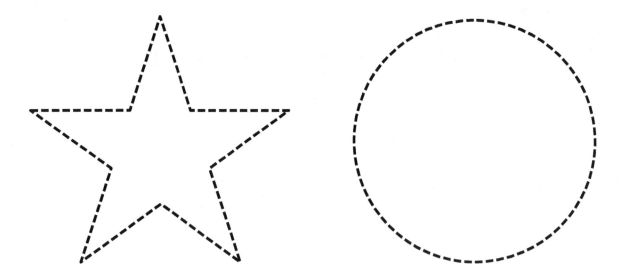

The dog ran.

_____

CHAPTER 5

Selecting the Best Intelligence Tests

Before you can begin to make sense of the meaningful scores from intelligence tests, you should ensure that you fully understand the measurement properties of the tests you are using and their resultant scores. With this information, you can select the best intelligence test for your needs, based in part on the age, ability level, and backgrounds of the clients you serve. This chapter highlights standards guiding the selection and use of tests, and it continues with a review of the most critical characteristics of tests—including norming and item scaling, as well as the reliability and validity of scores.

THE JOINT TEST STANDARDS

In addition to the American Psychological Association's (APA's) Ethical Principles of Psychologists and Code of Conduct and the National Association of School Psychologists' (NASP's) Principles for Professional Ethics (APA, 20002, 2010a; NASP, 2010a; see Chapter 3), you should be familiar with the *Standards for Educational and Psychological Testing* (American Educational Research Association [AERA], APA, & National Council on Measurement in Education [NCME], 1999). This document was last published in 1999, but at the time of our writing this chapter, a new edition was slated for publication in late 2013. We briefly describe its organization and key components, and then discuss how these components can be applied to selecting the best test for your assessment needs.

The *Standards* document was developed to facilitate scientifically sound and ethical testing practices, as well as to promote evaluation of such practices, and it has traditionally been organized into three sections. The first section addresses test construction, evaluation, and documentation, and its chapters have targeted validity; reliability and errors of measurement; test development and revision; scales, norms, and score comparability; test administration, scoring, and reporting; and sup-

> **The *Standards* document was developed to facilitate scientifically sound and ethical testing practices, as well as to promote evaluation of such practices.**

porting documentation. The second section addresses fairness in testing, and its chapters have targeted the rights and responsibilities of test takers, as well as testing of individuals with diverse linguistic backgrounds and disabilities. The third section addresses testing applications, and its chapters have targeted responsibilities of test users; psychological and educational assessment; testing in employment and credentialing; and testing in program evaluation and public policy.

In this chapter, we focus on general standards and guidelines for test use and general guidelines for psychological testing. Chapter 4 has addressed issues in the assessment process; Chapters 6 and 8 address interpretation and reporting of scores; and Chapter 13 highlights issue related to fairness and nondiscriminatory assessment. As conveyed in the *Standards* (AERA et al., 1999), evaluation of the acceptability of tests and their measurement characteristics involves, at least partially, professional judgment and knowledge of the content domain area. Using the general standards and guidelines for test use from the *Standards* document, we present criteria for evaluating the quality of norming, item scaling, and reliability and validity of scores yielded by intelligence tests.

EXPECTATIONS AND IDEALS FOR NORMING

Norm Samples

The foundation for the scientific study of intelligence is the natural phenomenon of individual differences in cognitive abilities; individuals of all ages differ in their level and speed of performance on cognitive tasks. In the practice of psychology, an understanding of these individual differences is derived from consideration of where an individual's test performance falls when compared to expectations established via a *norm sample*. A norm sample is ideally a large sample of persons whose characteristics are similar to those of the individual being tested (e.g., age); this sample produces results (i.e., *norms*) to which the individual's results can be compared. These norms allow for a better understanding of typical levels of performance (and variation around it) at different levels of development. Ideally, norm samples would include every individual in a population, but doing so is unfeasible. Instead, norm samples should be as large and representative of the targeted population as possible.

Sometimes the term *standardization sample* is used to refer to the norm sample. For the most part, these terms are used interchangeably, but *standardization* refers to the use of the same directions, sample items, practice trials, feedback, and scoring guidelines for everyone completing a test. Standardization is a necessity for accurate and comparable results to be obtained across administration of tests, and without it, accurate norms would be impossible. We suppose that criterion-referenced tests, which typically make no reference to the performance of comparable others, could stem from standardization samples and not norm samples; for most tests, however, standardization samples and norm samples are the same.

Evaluating Norm Samples

Norms affect the accuracy and meaningfulness of the most important data that you will derive from intelligence tests: their norm-referenced scores (see Chapter 6). Accordingly, it is important to scrutinize these tests' norm samples. Typically, norm samples are evaluated according to their recency, their representativeness, and their size. This information is typically provided in technical manuals accompanying tests, but you should also review the age ranges associated with specific norm groups—those forming the norms and presented in norm tables—to evaluate the appropriateness of norm samples.

Recency

The recency of norms can be evaluated based how near in time the data were collected. As described in the ethical standards discussed in Chapter 3, you should generally avoid using tests that are old and outdated. This recommendation is in place because outdated norms may no longer match the experiences and ability levels of those being tested. For one thing, older tests might include item content that is no longer valid for modern-day test takers, and this could produce biased scores. Furthermore, the evidence indicates rising ability levels across time in populations (called the *Flynn effect*; Flynn, 1984, 1987, 1999, 2007), with older norms producing inflated scores compared to more recent norms. Flynn has estimated that IQ scores increase an average of 3 points per decade, or 0.3 points per year. The increase in IQ implies that scores on older tests are likely to be inflated in comparison to those on newer tests with contemporary norms. Therefore, it is essential to use the most recently normed tests.

To evaluate the recency of norms, you should examine not only the date of a test's publication, but also, and more importantly, the period during which its norming data were collected. You should ideally select intelligence tests that have been normed within the past 10 years. Tests with norming data collected earlier should be used sparingly and should probably be avoided.

Representativeness

The representativeness of norms is equally important. It can be evaluated according to the extensiveness of sampling (1) across political regions (e.g., U.S. states) and across data collection sites; and (2) across demographic characteristics (i.e., gender, race, socioeconomic status, and community size). Of course, norming samples consisting only of participants from a single state or region would not meet the requirement of national norming and would fail to represent the targeted population. Some norms for intelligence tests stem from statistical weighting of contributions by specified subgroups to enhance the representativeness, but if such weighting is not used, a simple way to determine representativeness of the sample is to examine the match between the specific characteristics of the norm sample and those from the referenced census report used as a benchmark for norming. For example, comparisons could be made according to geographic characteristics (e.g., region of the country, population size, and urban vs. rural settings) and demographic characteristics (e.g., race, ethnicity, gender, and socioeconomic status). Discrepancies between specific characteristics of the norm sample and those from the respective census that are greater than 5 percentage points have been reported as indicating oversampling or undersampling (Floyd & Bose, 2003; Merrell, 2008). As discussed in Chapter 13, the absence of a particular individual's demographic group from the norming sample is *not* ipso facto evidence that a test is biased. The test may be biased, but it may not be. Evidence of bias can be determined only by empirical research.

It has been claimed that individuals with disabilities and those who receive extremely high and extremely low scores should be included in the norming samples—and some intelligence test samples make a point to ensure that such cases are included—but it is becoming increasingly common for *extrapolated norms* to be used. Extrapolated norms are derived from statistical manipulations of the distributions of test scores to ensure that they fully represent the population as a whole; they compensate for the fact that the norming data may not, in fact, represent the population well. For example, extrapolated norms can produce an IQ of 185 for children age 5 years old, although no one on the normative sample actually obtained an IQ that high. Fully representative norms based on expansive ability sampling are extremely difficult to obtain, because it is so hard to find sufficient numbers of people with extremely high IQs, and so hard to test those with extremely low IQs due to potentially confounding factors.

Developmental Sensitivity

The age range covered by each segment of the norms must be considered to ensure that they are sensitive to developmental differences, especially during the periods when cognitive growth is most rapid (i.e., up until about 16–20 years of age; see Chapter 2). That is, divisions of the norms should help to disentangle the effects of maturation and experience that are associated with age (as confounds) from individual differences in the display of the targeted abilities (as targeted by norm-referenced scores). Without an effort to eliminate these confounds, the norms would under-estimate the abilities of the youngest children at the targeted age level (producing lower scores) and overestimate the abilities of the oldest children in the targeted age level (producing higher scores; Flanagan, Ortiz, Alfonso, & Mascolo, 2006).

Although parents, teachers, and other professionals tend to ground their developmental expectations in a child or adolescent's whole age in years or whole grade levels in school, norm divisions representing narrower periods of time (e.g., a half year, a quarter, or a few months) are often necessary to produce the most accurate norm-referenced scores. Many tests (especially those targeting very young children) include norm level sample blocks representing rather narrow periods of time (e.g., 2 months and 3 months). In contrast, when developmental differences across age groups would not be anticipated (e.g., during the decade of the 30s), norm sample blocks are often much broader (e.g., 5 to 10 years; Flanagan et al., 2006). According to Bracken (2000), in addition to considering the breadth of these blocks, it is important to evaluate the actual norm tables to judge their adequacy—especially when a child is "on the very upper cusp of one age level and who is about to 'graduate' to the next age level" (p. 42). Bracken has shared that one way to evaluate this *sensitivity* of the norms is to review the norm tables and "examine the difference in standard scores associated with a given raw score as you progress from one table to the next. If the standard score increases by large amounts (e.g., +1$\frac{1}{3}$ standard deviations), the test may provide too gross an estimate of ability to instill much confidence in the resultant score" (p. 42). To address this issue, standard score values should be compared at levels near the mean, about one standard deviation above the mean, and about one standard deviation below the mean, beginning with the block associated with the age of the prospective examinee.

In recent decades, many test authors have addressed the developmental sensitivity of norms by using *continuous norming* procedures (see tables in Chapter 7). Rather than deriving norm-referenced scores from descriptive statistics based on individuals in large segments of the norms (e.g., children the same year in age), as previously indicated, sophisticated statistical methods (e.g., curve smoothing) are used to consider the performance across much smaller age segments and to integrate this information across ages, so that a picture of the developmental expectations within the larger grouping are well represented. Test norms developed by using these methods are note-worthy and superior to those developed via more traditional methods.

Norm Sample Size and Size of Norm Blocks

In general, larger norm samples indicate higher-quality norming and more trustworthy norm-referenced scores. It is important to consider the size of each age-based interval of the norms. According to common standards (e.g., Emmons & Alfonso, 2005; Flanagan & Alfonso, 1995; cf. Hammill, Brown, & Bryant, 1992), each 1-year age-based interval of the norms can be judged to be acceptable if it includes at least 100 individuals. This standard seems like a reasonable one to us. However, evaluating this characteristic is sometimes tricky, because some tests present norm sample sizes across wider age ranges (e.g., 1-year increments) in the body of the technical manuals, but rely on norm sample blocks representing narrower time segments (e.g., 3- to 6-month intervals), as previously discussed. In such cases, the mean number of participants per norm block can be estimated by dividing the number of participants reported across the wider age range by the number of norm-related segments by which it is divided. For instance, if 120 children age 4 were reported to compose a 1-year norm block, but norms were calculated in three 4-month blocks (4:0–4:3, 4:4–4:7, and 4:8–4:11), an average of 40 children per norm block would be assumed. This value would be unacceptable based on the goal of including at least 100 children in this group, and we believe that an acceptable absolute low-end standard should be 30 children per norm block.

> **In general, larger norm samples indicate higher-quality norming and more trustworthy norm-referenced scores.**

SCALING

Range of Norm-Referenced Scores

Because you may be called on to assess children or adolescents suspected of having intellectual disability (ID; see Chapter 10) or intellectual giftedness (see Chapter 11), it is important that you know the range of scores provided by the intelligence tests you are evaluating. In addition, in order to differentiate between ability levels at every point across this range, you should consider item gradients for intelligence test subtests.

Scale Floors

A *scale floor* refers to the lowest norm-referenced score that can be obtained. When these floors are too high, the full range of ability at its lowest levels cannot be assessed, because, at the subtest level, items are too difficult for individuals with low ability; there are too few "easy" items for them. As a result of such problems, even when a child performs poorly on a subtest, answering only one item (or no items) correctly, the child will earn a score that is relatively close to what is considered average. Subtest scores with insufficient floors will overestimate the abilities of those who are near the lowest end of the ability range, and this overestimation will be transferred to all of the composite scores to which that subtest contributes.

Floors for subtests can be evaluated by examining norm tables and using score software; if a raw score (i.e., the sum of item scores) of 1 does not yield a norm-referenced score equal to or exceeding two standard deviations below the normative mean (a deviation IQ score of 70 or lower, a T score of 30 or lower, or a scaled score of 4 or lower; see Chapter 6), a *floor violation* is evident (Bracken, 1987; Bracken, Keith, & Walker, 1998; Bradley-Johnson & Durmusoglu, 2005). For composite scores that stem from summing norm-referenced scores from subtests, floor violations are apparent if the lowest basic score (e.g., the sum of scaled scores) is associated with a norm-referenced score less than two standard deviations below the mean. Floor violations are most frequently apparent at the youngest age levels targeted by intelligence tests.

Scale Ceilings

A *scale ceiling* refers to the highest norm-referenced score that can be obtained. When ceilings are too low, the full range of ability at its highest levels cannot be assessed. This scenario is the opposite of the one occurring when children or adolescents with low ability are assessed. As a result of such problems with ceilings, those with high ability are likely to have their abilities underestimated. Even when a child performs extremely well on a subtest, answering every item correctly, the child will earn a score that is relatively close to what is considered average. There are too few "difficult" items on the subtest to sufficiently challenge such children at this level.

Ceilings for subtests can also be evaluated by examining norm tables and using score software; if the highest possible raw score does not yield a norm-referenced score equal to or exceeding two standard deviations above the normative mean (i.e., a deviation IQ score of 130 or higher, a *T* score of 70 or higher, or a scaled score of 16 or higher; see Chapter 6), a *ceiling violation* is evident (Bracken, 1987; Bracken et al., 1998; Bradley-Johnson & Durmusoglu, 2005). For composite scores, ceiling violations can be identified if the highest basic score (e.g., the sum of scaled scores) is associated with a norm-referenced score less than two standard deviations above the mean. Ceiling violations are most frequently identified at the oldest age levels targeted by intelligence tests.

Item Scaling

Test authors typically devote much time and effort to developing, selecting, and scaling items for their instruments. For most subtests on intelligence tests, items are selected and scaled from easiest to most difficult. Examinees begin with items that most individuals of the same age would successfully complete, progress through items that are neither too easy nor too difficult for them, and reach items that are on the threshold of their current knowledge and skills. In order to evaluate the quality of an intelligence test, you should consider the methods used to accomplish such scaling and should evaluate evidence suggesting effective scaling.

Scaling Techniques

Traditional techniques used for item scaling include *item difficulty analysis*, in which items are evaluated according to the percentage of examinees passing those items. After administering the preliminary set of items to large groups of individuals, test authors using these techniques can identify patterns of scores across items and then place the items in order from those passed by the most individuals to those passed by the least individuals. During the past 30 or 40 years, *item response theory* (often referred to as only IRT, although we continue to use the full term) techniques have replaced more traditional techniques like item difficulty analysis. Item response theory analysis considers not only item difficulty, but also the relation between passing the item and the sum of all the items considered in the analysis (often called *item discrimination*) and random error (often called *guessing*). One common type of item response theory analysis is referred to as *Rasch modeling* (Rasch, 1960). This analysis, focused on accurately measuring the latent trait (or ability) underlying performance on an item, produces a purer method of evaluating item difficulty than any other single traditional technique, and for most subtests, it is the optimal method for scaling items. When you review technical information about an intelligence test, you should expect authors to have used item response theory to scale items.

Item Gradients

Appropriately scaled items should not only proceed from easy to difficult, but should also do so without rapidly progressing from easy to difficult items. An example of inappropriate item scaling for an achievement test would be a math subtest that includes easy single-digit multiplication items, advanced trigonometry items, and no items of intermediate difficulty. Such inappropriate scaling, as revealed through *item gradient violations*, can also be identified by a careful review of norm tables.

Ideally, there should be a consistent relation between item scores and norm-referenced scores as they both increase; this relation is referred to as the *item gradient*. According to Krasa (2007), "When the item gradient . . . is too steep, it does not sufficiently absorb 'noise'—that is, errors irrelevant to the construct being tested (such as carelessness or distractibility) can lead to an abrupt change in standard score that does not reflect a true difference in the ability being tested" (p. 4). When this standard is not met, huge jumps in ability estimates (as evidenced by the norm-referenced scores) could be the product of guessing correctly on a single item. For example, with woefully inadequate item gradients, an individual could go from having a slightly-above-average norm-referenced score of 105 to a well-above-average norm-referenced score of 115 because he or she guessed correctly on one item. Conversely, failing one additional item would cause the score to drop precipitously.

Item gradient violations for subtests, which are most closely linked to item-level performance, can be identified if there is not at least one raw score point associated with each one-third of a standard deviation unit in the norms (Bracken, 1987). For example, deviation IQ scores should not change more than 5 points per 1 raw score point change; *T* scores should not change more than 3 points per 1 raw score point change; and scaled scores should not change more than 1 point per 1 raw score point change (see Chapter 6). Even though we do not recommend routine interpretation of norm-referenced scores derived from subtests (see Chapter 6), they should not be ignored, because subtest scores contribute to the more reliable and valid composite scores. However, composite scores, due to their pooling of variability across subtests, should absorb most of the "noise" associated with item gradient violations and other sources of error in measurement.

RELIABILITY

Definition

It is important that the results of your assessment be as precise and consistent as possible. Certainly, none of us would want scoring errors to affect test scores, and we would look askance if we learned that someone obtained an IQ in the Superior range one day and an IQ in the Low Average range the following day after taking the same test. The term *reliability* is used to represent this valued score characteristic—consistency across replications. Quantitative values targeting reliability represent the extent to which unexplained and apparently random inconsistency across replications, called *measurement error* or *random error*, affects test scores. These unpredictable fluctuations are unavoidable effects of assessment; no test produces a perfect, 100% replicable measurement of any phenomenon. Even in the natural sciences, tools targeting physical measurements are affected by error. For example, rulers and tape measures expand and contract as the temperature fluctuates; even quantum clocks, which are probably the most accurate measures of time, vary slightly (e.g., by 1 second in a billion years) under some conditions.

> The term *reliability* is used to represent this valued score characteristic—consistency across replications.

In testing, we most frequently attribute measurement error to the person taking the test, and particularly to the person's variation in determination, anxiety, and alertness from item to item or from day to day. Furthermore, guessing correctly (producing spuriously high scores) comes into play, as do memory retrieval problems (leading to incorrect responses and producing spuriously low scores). In the same vein, those taking the test may respond in different ways to items because of prior experiences. For instance, they may fail items that are typically easier for others (e.g., early presidents of the United States) because they are uninterested in the item content, but may answer items that are typically more difficult for others (e.g., earth science) because they have a special interest in that area. In addition to fluctuation due to the person, external factors may also produce these fluctuations. Examples include the time of day in which the test is taken, distractions in the testing environment, and examiners' deviations in administration and scoring.

Reliability is an important precondition for the validity of tests results and their interpretations. According to the *Standards* (AERA et al., 1999), "To the extent that scores reflect random errors of measurement, their potential for accurate prediction of criteria, for beneficial examinee diagnosis, and for wise decision making is limited" (p. 31). This relationship between reliability and validity is an important one. In fact, it is this relation that leads us and many other scholars to discourage interpretation of less reliable intelligence test subtest scores and encourage interpretation of more reliable composite scores, such as IQs (see Chapter 6).

Evaluating Reliability and Determining Effects of Error

Although we expect variability stemming from the characteristics of examinees and the circumstances external to them, we assume in our measurement that there is consistency in scores across replications. This consistency in intelligence test scores is typically evaluated by using three methods producing reliability coefficients: *internal consistency, test–retest reliability*, and *scorer consistency*. Coefficients close to 1.00 indicate high levels of reliability and acceptable levels of measurement error, whereas coefficients below .70 indicate low reliability and unacceptably high levels of measurement error (Hunsley & Mash, 2008). For scores from intelligence tests and high-stakes diagnosis and eligibility decisions, minimal standards for reliability should be far higher.

Internal Consistency

The type of reliability coefficient most often reported in test technical manuals focuses on item-level consistency evident in a single testing session. These internal consistency coefficients tend to be the highest of all reliability coefficients, and they are most frequently used to calculate confidence interval values (see Chapter 6). They are often reported as *Cronbach's coefficient alpha*, which represents the average item-to-item relations across the entire scale in question. Alternately, split-half reliability analysis, which examines the relations between odd and even items or between items from the first half and second half of a scale, may be employed. If we assume that all intelligence test subtest items are positively correlated, the greater number of items a subtest includes, the higher its internal consistency reliability coefficient will be. This phenomenon is predicted by the *Spearman–Brown prophecy formula* (Brown, 1910; Spearman, 1910). Although these reliability analyses are commonly used to determine the internal consistency of intelligence test subtests, the internal consistency of resulting composites, such as IQs, are often determined by using subtest internal consistency coefficients and subtest intercorrelation values (Nunnally & Bernstein, 1994).

In general, the closer the analysis of reliability is to the item level, the lower the reliability will be. Items are most strongly affected by measurement error, but these effects are diminished as more and more items are considered in concert—from subtest scores, to composite scores formed from only a few subtests, and to composite scores stemming from numerous subtests. Thus, the most global composites are always the most reliable. When high-stakes decisions are to be made, we suggest using a lower-end standard of .90 for internal consistency reliability coefficients (Bracken, 1987; McGrew & Flanagan, 1998); scores with values below .90 should not be interpreted. We recommend that scores with internal consistency reliability coefficients of .95 or higher should be targeted.

Test–Retest Reliability

Evaluation of consistency across replications is most apparent when the same instrument is administered twice across a brief period (typically a month or less). When the relations between scores stemming from these two administrations are quantified by using a statistical technique called the *Pearson product–moment correlation*, an understanding about reliability across time is yielded. To the surprise of some, this technique is an appropriate one, because it is insensitive to differences in the magnitude of scores from the initial testing to the follow-up testing. As a consequence, the resultant correlation value, the *Pearson coefficient*, will reflect only the extent of relative consistency.

Test–retest reliability coefficients are commonly reported for intelligence test subtests and composites, and they may be the only type of reliability coefficient reported for speeded subtests, because traditional internal consistency reliability coefficients cannot be calculated for speeded subtests (unless advanced item response theory techniques are used). Test–retest reliability coefficients are degraded by multiple influences; both the length of the interval between test and retest and the nature of the ability being targeted should be considered in evaluating them. Typically, the longer the interval between initial and follow-up testing (e.g., 1 month vs. 6 months), the lower the reliability coefficient will be. Furthermore, if the ability being targeted tends to vary because of influences associated with the examinee and the effects of testing environment (e.g., Processing Speed), test–retest reliability coefficients will tend to be lower than those for abilities that tend to be more resistant to these influences (e.g., Crystallized Intelligence). Test–retest reliability coefficients tend to be lower than internal consistency reliability coefficients, and when high-stakes decisions are to be made, we suggest using a lower-end standard of .90 (Bracken, 1987; McGrew & Flanagan, 1998).

Scorer Consistency

Those persons scoring intelligence tests also produce measurement error in scores—especially when scores are based on subjective judgments about the quality of responses. This type of measurement error is most frequently quantified by *interrater agreement* indexes and *interrater reliability* coefficients. Interrater agreement indexes stem from analysis of individual items across a subtest, and they are typically reported as a percentage (representing *percentage agreement*) and not as a coefficient. For example, if two raters agree that 5 of 10 responses should earn a point and that 3 of the remaining 5 responses should not earn a point, then their percentage agreement in scoring is 80%. In contrast, interrater reliability coefficients typically stem from analysis of summed item scores across items obtained from independent scoring of responses across two examiners; they are typically the result of Pearson product–moment correlations. To compare and contrast these two indexes of scorer consistency, review Table 5.1. Across the 15 items scored on a 3-point scale by two raters, the scores were almost identical: 17 for Rater 1 and 18 for Rater 2. Furthermore, the average item score for Rater 1 was 1.13, whereas it was 1.20 for Rater 2. When the item-by-item agreement in scoring was considered (see "Agreement" column in Table 5.1), the interrater agreement index (reported as percentage agreement) was 67%, because only 10 of the 15 items were scored exactly the same way. When the correspondence of the rank ordering of item-level scores above and below their respective rater-specific means was considered and reported as a Pearson coefficient, the interrater reliability coefficient of .76 was somewhat modest, but higher in magnitude than the interrater agreement index.

Based on standards for interrater reliability and interrater agreement for assessment instruments targeting child and adolescent behavioral and emotional problems (e.g., Achenbach, McConaughy, & Howell, 1987; Floyd & Bose, 2003; Hunsley & Mash, 2008), interrater reliability levels of .60 or higher and interrater agreement levels of 60% or higher are desirable. Because the range of responses is much narrower, and scoring tends to be clearer with intelligence tests subtests than many other assessment instruments, reasonable lower-end standards for scorer consistency should be .80 for interrater reliability and 80% for interrater agreement.

VALIDITY

Definition

Whereas *reliability* refers to consistency across replications (e.g., across items, across multiple administration of the same tests, or across scorers), *validity* refers to representing the concept or characteristic being targeted by the assessment instrument in a complete and meaningful way. According to the *Standards* (AERA et al., 1999),

> Validity refers to the degree to which evidence and theory support the interpretations of test scores by proposed uses of tests. Validity is, therefore, the most fundamental consideration in developing and evaluating tests. The process of validation involves accumulating evidence to provide a sound scientific basis for the proposed score interpretations. . . . When test scores are used or interpreted in more than one way, each intended interpretation must be validated. (p. 1)

As apparent in this definition, tests do not possess validity; it is a misnomer to refer to a "valid test." Instead, you should refer to "validity of score-based interpretations" and know that that this con-

TABLE 5.1. An Item-Scoring Example Yielding Interrater Agreement and Interrater Reliability Coefficients

Item number	Rater 1 score	Rater 2 score	Agreement analysis		Pearson product–moment correlation analysis				
			Agreement	Agreement score	Rater 1 deviation from M	Rater 2 deviation from M	Product of deviations from M	Squared Rater 1 deviation from M	Squared Rater 2 deviation from M
1	2	2	Yes	1	0.87	0.80	0.69	0.75	0.64
2	2	2	Yes	1	0.87	0.80	0.69	0.75	0.64
3	2	2	Yes	1	0.87	0.80	0.69	0.75	0.64
4	2	2	Yes	1	0.87	0.80	0.69	0.75	0.64
5	1	2	No	0	-0.13	0.80	-0.11	0.02	0.64
6	2	1	No	0	0.87	-0.20	-0.17	0.75	0.04
7	2	2	Yes	1	0.87	0.80	0.69	0.75	0.64
8	1	1	Yes	1	-0.13	-0.20	0.03	0.02	0.04
9	1	2	No	0	-0.13	0.80	-0.11	0.02	0.64
10	1	1	Yes	1	-0.13	-0.20	0.03	0.02	0.04
11	0	0	Yes	1	-1.13	-1.20	1.36	1.28	1.44
12	1	0	No	0	-0.13	-1.20	0.16	0.02	1.44
13	0	1	No	0	-1.13	-0.20	0.23	1.28	0.04
14	0	0	Yes	1	-1.13	-1.20	1.36	1.28	1.44
15	0	0	Yes	1	-1.13	-1.20	1.36	1.28	1.44
Sum	17	18		10			7.60	9.73	10.40
Average	1.13	1.20							

Percentage agreement

$$\frac{\text{Agreements}}{\text{Total items}} = \frac{10}{15} = .67, \text{ or } 67\%$$

Pearson correlation

$$r = \frac{\text{Sum of products of deviations for raters}}{\text{Square root of (squared Rater 1 Deviation from } M \text{ times squared Rater 2 deviation from } M)} = \frac{7.60}{\text{Square root of } (9.73 \times 10.40)} = .76$$

cept of validity is conditional, based on the intended uses of those scores. For example, an IQ from a test targeting high-ability preschool students might be valid for identifying intellectual giftedness (see Chapter 11), but if several of its subtests contributing to the IQ demonstrated floor violations, it would not be valid for identifying ID (see Chapter 10). Thus, details and conditions should be specified when you are discussing validity. Asking yourself, "Do I have solid evidence supporting my use of these scores to reach my goals?" addresses this issue well.

> **Validity** refers to representing the concept or characteristic being targeted by the assessment instrument in a complete and meaningful way.

As you consider validity evidence supporting uses and interpretations of intelligence tests scores, you should consider *construct validity* as an overarching conceptual framework. The term *construct* refers to the concept or characteristic that the assessment instrument is intended to measure, and in the case of intelligence tests, the construct is typically a cognitive ability. For example, measures of psychometric *g* represent abstract reasoning and thinking, the capacity to acquire knowledge, and problem-solving ability (Neisser et al., 1996). From this perspective, both test authors and test users should consider and articulate what construct is being targeted by all scores. In doing so, they must consider both (1) how fine-grained or global the intended interpretation is, and (2) what evidence has supported their favored interpretation. For example, does an intelligence test subtest requiring children to provide definitions to English words measure psychometric *g*, Crystallized Intelligence, word knowledge, the ability to articulate word definitions, listening ability, an enriched language environment, expressive language skills, long-term memory, concept formation, or executive system functioning? Of course, it is extremely rare that interpretations of scores are limited to only one meaning, but the wide array of constructs presented in this sample seems to represent what Kelley (1927) called the *jingle–jangle fallacy*. The *jingle fallacy* refers to using the same label to describe different constructs, and the *jangle fallacy*, which is more relevant to this example, refers to using different labels to describe similar constructs. Because of such problems in selecting the targeted construct, you must rely on theory and prior research (as described in Chapters 1 and 2) to develop an explicit statement of the proposed interpretation of your scores or score patterns. This validity argument can then be evaluated on the basis of existing evidence.

Evaluating Validity Evidence

Although the classic tripartite model of validity (focusing on apparently distinct types of validity—*content, criterion-related*, and *construct*) is still employed in some test technical manuals and in some of the psychology literature, this model is outdated. Modern conceptions of validity represent validity as a unitary concept; evidence of all types informs the construct validity of the inferences drawn from assessment results and subsequent decisions. Consistent with the *Standards* (AERA et al., 1999), this validity evidence can be compartmentalized into five validity strands: (1) evidence based on test content, (2) evidence based on response processes, (3) evidence based on internal structure, (4) evidence based on relations with other variables, and (5) evidence based on the consequences of testing.

A body of validity evidence should be evaluated by considering potential confounds in measurement that may undermine valid interpretations. The *Standards* document refers to these potential confounds as rival hypotheses and encourages consideration of both *construct under-representation* and *construct-irrelevant variance*. According to the *Standards* (AERA et al., 1999),

> Construct underrepresentation refers to the degree to which a test fails to capture important aspects of the construct. It implies a narrowed meaning of test scores because the test does not adequately sample some types of content, engage some psychological processes, or elicit some ways of responding that are encompassed by the intended construct. Take, for example, a test of reading comprehension intended to measure children's ability to read and interpret stories with understanding. A particular test might underrepresent the intended construct because it does not contain a sufficient variety of reading passages or ignored a common type of reading material. As another example, a test of anxiety might measure only physiological reactions and not emotional, cognitive, or situational components. (p. 10)

Construct irrelevance refers to the degree to which test scores are affected by processes that are extraneous to the test's intended construct. The test scores may be systematically influenced to some extent by components that are not part of the construct. On a reading comprehension test, construct-irrelevant components might include an emotional reaction to the test content, familiarity with the subject matter of the reading passages on the test, or the writing skill needed to compose a response. On an anxiety self-report instrument, a response bias leading to underreporting of anxiety might be a source of construct-irrelevant variance.

Using the concept of construct validity espoused in the *Standards*, and considering both construct underrepresentation and construct irrelevance as contributors to rival hypotheses, you should evaluate evidence for its contribution to interpretations and to revealing potential sources of invalidity. We discuss each type of validity evidence and address its contribution to identifying construct underrepresentation and construct irrelevance in the sections that follow.

Content

Evidence based on *test content* refers to substantiation that an instrument's items accurately represent the targeted construct or constructs in a complete, accurate, and unbiased manner. According to the *Standards* (AERA et al., 1999), "test content refers to the themes, wording, and format of the items, tasks, or questions on a test, as well as the guidelines for procedures regarding administration and scoring" (p. 11). As evident in Table 5.2, item development based on theory, prior literature, and existing diagnostic systems can support the validity of test items. After these items are developed, their evaluation by content experts and after use in item tryouts in the field contribute to such evidence. Although validity evidence based on content is often based on only human judgment, statistical methods may also be used to test validity arguments.

Response Processes

Evidence based on *response processes* refers to substantiation of the real or hypothesized behaviors that test takers follow when completing items. Typically, inferences made about psychological processes or cognitive operations must be drawn from responses to test stimuli. As evident in Table 5.2, these responses can be inferred from review of test stimuli. For example, cognitive tasks can be dissected into their component operations (see Carroll, 1993); reviewers can evaluate test items to determine their match with the targeted response processes; and text can be analyzed by using readability and cohesion metrics (Flesch, 1949; Graesser, McNamara, Louwerse, & Cai, 2004). Individuals taking the test can inform us about the accuracy of our validity arguments. For example, test takers may be asked to "think aloud" during test completion or to respond to questions about strategies they used (see Ericsson & Simon, 1993), and their responses can be evaluated to identify themes consistent with the targeted constructs. More sophisticated methods, such as eye-tracking technology and recording of response times (see Carpenter, Just, & Shell, 1990), also provide validity evidence based on response processes. Despite the promise of these methods, they are rarely applied to intelligence tests and almost never addressed in test technical manuals.

TABLE 5.2. Definitions of and Methods to Demonstrate the Five Strands of Validity Evidence

Evidence based on test content—substantiation that an instrument's items accurately represent the targeted constructs in a complete, accurate, and unbiased manner.
- Development of items based on strong theory, literature review, established educational or psychiatric diagnostic classifications, and review of case histories
- Expert analysis of gender, racial, cultural, or age bias in items
- Review and item tryouts by test users in applied settings
- Statistical analyses of items (e.g., differential item functioning, point–biserial correlations, and item characteristic curve analyses)

Evidence based on response processes—substantiation of the real or presumed behaviors that test takers exhibit when completing subtest items.
- Evaluation of instrument instructions and response formats
- Observations of test takers' behaviors (e.g., eye movements) during completion of items
- Interviews with test takers about thought processes during completion of subtest items
- "Think-aloud" protocols with test takers during completion of subtest items
- Task decomposition analyses of subtest items

Evidence based on internal structure—substantiation that an instrument's item-level or summative scores are related to other measures from the instrument in the manner expected.
- Correlations between items within a subtest
- Correlations between subtest scores
- Exploratory factor analysis (EFA)
- Confirmatory factor analysis (CFA)

Evidence based on relations with other variables—substantiation that item-level or summative scores from an instrument relate in a systematic way with other measures, such as scores from other instruments, demographic variables (e.g., age and gender), and educational or diagnostic classifications.
- Correlations with measures of the same or similar constructs
- Correlations with measures of distinct or dissimilar constructs
- Correlations with scores from well-validated instruments
- Prediction of current or future phenomena
- Group difference analyses (a.k.a. clinical group comparisons)

Evidence based on the consequences of testing—substantiation that scores and decisions based on them produce intended and not unintended consequences for those completing the test.
- Evaluation of treatment utility
- Evaluation of classification rates of racial/ethnic groups as disabled versus not disabled

Note. Content is based in part on Table 2 from Floyd and Bose (2003).

Internal Structure

Evidence based on internal structure refers to substantiation that a test's items or resultant scores are related to other variables from the test in the expected manner. (If the relations are with some other variables external to the test, another type of validity evidence is considered, as we discuss in the next section.) As evident in Table 5.2, correlations between item scores and subtest or composite scores, between subtest scores, and between composite scores provide such evidence. These correlations are typically Pearson correlations or variants of them. In some instances, correlations between item scores, as also evaluated in internal consistency analysis (described previously), contribute such validity evidence. Perhaps the most sophisticated methods for examining internal structure of tests are exploratory factor analysis (EFA) and confirmatory factor analysis (CFA), as described in Chapter 1. These analyses may use item scores to study the latent variables underlying patterns of correlations, but most of the research with intelligence tests (especially that presented in test technical manuals) focuses on relations between subtest scores. As made evident in Chapter 1, factor analysis has provided strong evidence for the structure of human cognitive abilities. It helped to form the foundation for psychometric theories of intelligence, and it continues to offer insights today (Keith & Reynolds, 2010, 2012).

External Relations

To establish the meaning of test scores, they must be related to external criteria. The main goal when investigating the *external relations* of a test is to examine the pattern of relations between measures of the constructs targeted by the test and other measures and variables, such as scores from other instruments, demographic variables (e.g., age and gender), and educational or diagnostic classifications. Construct validity is supported when the pattern of relations between test scores and the external criteria is both rational and consistent with hypotheses based on theory. Conversely, construct validity is not supported when the pattern of relations cannot be explained by hypotheses based on theory (Benson, 1998). This type of validity evidence seems to be most prevalent in test technical manuals and in the research literature; it often composes more than half of the validity evidence presented in test technical manuals.

Evidence of external relations includes correlations between measures of the same or similar constructs, often called *convergent relations*, as well as correlations between measures of dissimilar constructs, often called *discriminant relations*. Analysis of convergent and discriminant relations tends to be theoretically focused, whereas analysis of *criterion-related validity* tends to be more practical. For example, it makes sense that scores from a new intelligence test would correlate highly with those from an older "classic" intelligence test if both were administered to the same children over a brief period. Such evidence would yield *concurrent validity* evidence for the new test when compared to the "gold standard" criteria yielded by the older, classic intelligence test. Furthermore, when examining criterion-related validity, important social and educational outcomes may serve as criteria for comparison. For example, as described in Chapter 1, IQs demonstrate strong *predictive validity* evidence by yielding sizeable, positive correlations with long-term academic outcomes. Again, correlations reflecting convergent and discriminant relations and concurrent and predictive validity evidence are typically Pearson correlations. Finally, validity evidence from external relations can also surface from comparisons of known groups (often clinical groups, such as children with learning disabilities or attention-deficit/hyperactivity disorder [ADHD]) known to differ on the construct being measured. Such results produce what some researchers (e.g., Floyd, Shaver, & McGrew, 2003; Haynes, Smith, & Hunsley, 2012) call *discriminative validity* (not discriminant validity) evidence.

Consequences

Evidence based on the *consequences* of testing refers to substantiation that scores and decisions based on them produce intended and not unintended consequences for those taking the tests, depending on the purpose of the assessment. In terms of intended consequences, some assert that *treatment utility* (Hayes, Nelson, & Jarrett, 1987; Nelson-Gray, 2003)—evidence that measurable benefits stem from test interpretation—provides positive evidence supporting intended consequences. Others have argued that overrepresentation and underrepresentation of certain racial/ethnic minority groups in special education constitute evidence of invalidity in assessment. This type of validity evidence, however, is understudied and poorly understood (see Braden & Kratochwill, 1997; Cizek, Bowen, & Church, 2010). Many researchers are uncertain about the inclusion of this type of validity evidence along with the other four, because it does not appear to be a relevant criterion for evaluating the validity of certain instruments. For example, do yardsticks provide invalid measures of height because basketball players are taller on average than the general population? Obviously, they are not. On the one hand, we appreciate that the inclusion of this type of validity evidence challenges us to enhance the body of support for the positive outcomes of test results; on the other hand, we fear that excessive emphasis on negative consequences— without carefully designed scientific research studies and clear thinking—will lead to unfounded animosity directed toward testing in schools and related settings, due to presumed invalidity and bias. (See Chapter 13 for further discussion of test bias.)

Making Sense of Validity Evidence

As we have stated previously, when validity evidence is being considered, details and conditions should be specified. Asking, "Do I have solid evidence supporting my use of these scores to reach my goal?" ensures consideration of these details and conditions. According to the *Standards* (AERA et al., 1999), "A sound validity argument integrates various strands of evidence into a coherent account of the degree to which existing evidence and theory support the intended interpretation of test scores for specific uses" (p. 17). Many argue that the validation of any instrument and its scores is an ongoing process, but there is probably a point at which there is a "good enough" body of validity evidence for the provisional application of test score interpretation.

> **When validity evidence is being considered, details and conditions should be specified.**

SELECTING THE BEST TEST FOR YOUR NEEDS

Following the *Standards*, you should be able to (1) consider both the context of the assessment and the personal characteristics and background of each child or adolescent you are slated to assess and (2) select tests that most accurately measure the child or adolescent's cognitive abilities. However, doing so is no easy feat. You must first consider the stakes involved in the assessment. Most decisions involving intelligence tests are high-stakes decisions, such as diagnosis or eligibility determination. These decisions require higher standards of evidence, and this requirement should lead you to employ a more conservative approach to score interpretation. Then, you must consider the quality of the norms, the reliability of resultant scores, and validity evidence for the intelligence tests available to you. These steps can easily be completed in general, but you must also consider carefully the individual's characteristics, including age, presenting problems, sensory acuity, motor development, language proficiency, background characteristics, and so on, when selecting intelligence tests to administer to him or her.

In order to address these goals, you should seek out published test reviews of intelligence tests. Perhaps the best source for such reviews is the Buros Center for Testing *(www.buros.org)*, formerly the Institute for Mental Measurements, which publishes a series of *Mental Measurement Yearbooks*. Furthermore, several peer-reviewed journals—including *Assessment for Effective Intervention*, the *Canadian Journal of School Psychology*, and the *Journal of Psychoeducational Assessment*—publish test reviews. Although such narrative reviews do not provide systematic, objective evaluations of the tests they target, they can pave the way for your careful review of tests.

The benefit of reading a test's technical manual from cover to cover, however, cannot be understated. As you do, you should pay particular attention to the norming process, review the norm table for scaling problems, evaluate the reliability estimates for the scores you are likely to interpret, and consider the sources of validity evidence. Furthermore, you should consider these test properties and score properties for the specific child or adolescent you will be testing. You should, for example, compare your child's characteristics to those of the norm sample and consider scaling issues subtest by subtest, reliability estimates score by score, and validity evidence appropriate for the child's age and for the referral concern. To assist you in this process, we have reviewed, evaluated, and described characteristics of the most prominent full-length intelligence tests, nonverbal intelligence tests and related composites, and brief and abbreviated intelligence tests in Chapter 7. We have also provided, in Form 5.1, a form for evaluating and selecting the best intelligence test for your needs. This checklist addresses basic demographic characteristics, the referral concern, results from your screening (see Chapter 4), test norming, and measurement properties associated with varying score types.

SUMMARY

This chapter has highlighted standards guiding the selection and use of tests, and it has reviewed their most critical characteristics. We encourage you to promote measurement integrity through careful test reviews and test selection before you begin testing, rather than calling on this information after you have noticed an oddball score or two that does not fit with the remainder of the information from your assessment. The intelligence tests available to you are stronger than ever before. Your efforts to choose the best tests for your needs should yield dividends in your producing more accurate and meaningful results for those children or adolescents you test, as well as for their families and their educators.

Intelligence Test Measurement Properties Review Form

Name of child or adolescent: _____

Age in years and months: _____

Referral concern: _____

_____

Screening Results

☐ Visual acuity problems   ☐ Fine motor problems
☐ Color blindness   ☐ Noncompliance
☐ Auditory acuity problems   ☐ Limited English proficiency
☐ Articulation problems   ☐ Acculturation problems

Targeted intelligence test: _____

Norming Information

Last year of norming data collection (see tables in Chapter 7) _____

☐ 10 years ago or less   ☐ 15 years ago or less   ☐ More than 15 years ago

Age range of norm table block applicable to examinee (e.g., 3.0- to 3.3-year-olds or 7-year-olds):

_____

Number or estimated number of participants in norm table block (see Age unit/block in tables in Chapter 7)

☐ 100 or more   ☐ 50 to 99   ☐ 49 to 30   ☐ Under 30

Score Type

Stratum III composites (i.e., IQs)

Maximum norm-referenced score: _____   ☐ Ceiling violation

Minimum norm-referenced score: _____   ☐ Floor violation

Internal consistency reliability: _____   ☐ Under .95

Test–retest reliability: _____   ☐ Under .90

Validity evidence: ☐ Content   ☐ Response processes   ☐ Internal structure
                       ☐ External relations   ☐ Consequences

Stratum III composites (i.e., IQs)

Maximum norm-referenced score: _____   ☐ Ceiling violation

Minimum norm-referenced score: _____   ☐ Floor violation

Internal consistency reliability: _____   ☐ Under .95

Test–retest reliability: _____   ☐ Under .90

Validity evidence: ☐ Content   ☐ Response processes   ☐ Internal structure
                       ☐ External relations   ☐ Consequences

(continued)

Stratum II composites (e.g., broad ability composites)

        Score type: ☐ Deviation IQ score   ☐ *T* score   ☐ Scaled score

Composite 1: _____

Maximum norm-referenced score: _____   ☐ Ceiling violation

Minimum norm-referenced score: _____   ☐ Floor violation

Internal consistency reliability: _____   ☐ Under .95

Test–retest reliability: _____   ☐ Under .90

Validity evidence: ☐ Content   ☐ Response processes   ☐ Internal structure
                  ☐ External relations   ☐ Consequences

Composite 2: _____

Maximum norm-referenced score: _____   ☐ Ceiling violation

Minimum norm-referenced score: _____   ☐ Floor violation

Internal consistency reliability: _____   ☐ Under .95

Test–retest reliability: _____   ☐ Under .90

Validity evidence: ☐ Content   ☐ Response processes   ☐ Internal structure
                  ☐ External relations   ☐ Consequences

Composite 3: _____

Maximum norm-referenced score: _____   ☐ Ceiling violation

Minimum norm-referenced score: _____   ☐ Floor violation

Internal consistency reliability: _____   ☐ Under .95

Test–retest reliability: _____   ☐ Under .90

Validity evidence: ☐ Content   ☐ Response processes   ☐ Internal structure
                  ☐ External relations   ☐ Consequences

Composite 4: _____

Maximum norm-referenced score: _____   ☐ Ceiling violation

Minimum norm-referenced score: _____   ☐ Floor violation

Internal consistency reliability: _____   ☐ Under .95

Test–retest reliability: _____   ☐ Under .90

Validity evidence: ☐ Content   ☐ Response processes   ☐ Internal structure
                  ☐ External relations   ☐ Consequences

(continued)

Composite 5: _____

Maximum norm-referenced score: _____   ☐ Ceiling violation

Minimum norm-referenced score: _____   ☐ Floor violation

Internal consistency reliability: _____   ☐ Under .95

Test–retest reliability: _____   ☐ Under .90

Validity evidence: ☐ Content   ☐ Response processes   ☐ Internal structure
                            ☐ External relations   ☐ Consequences

Composite 6: _____

Maximum norm-referenced score: _____   ☐ Ceiling violation

Minimum norm-referenced score: _____   ☐ Floor violation

Internal consistency reliability: _____   ☐ Under .95

Test–retest reliability: _____   ☐ Under .90

Validity evidence: ☐ Content   ☐ Response processes   ☐ Internal structure
                            ☐ External relations   ☐ Consequences

Subtest scores

Ceiling violations (list subtests; see tables in Chapter 7 for indications): _____

_____

_____

_____

_____

Floor violations (list subtests; see tables in Chapter 7 for indications): _____

_____

_____

_____

_____

Item gradient violations (list subtests' and the raw scores associated with violations): _____

_____

_____

_____

_____

Notes:

CHAPTER 6

Interpreting Intelligence Test Scores

According to the *Merriam–Webster Dictionary*, the verb *interpret* means "to explain or tell the meaning of" and "to present in understandable terms," and the noun *interpretation* means "the act or the result of explanation." This chapter focuses on interpretation of an examinee's responses and resulting scores. It targets interpreting data from qualitative and quantitative perspectives, using interpretive strategies that are based on an understanding of the nature of and relations between cognitive abilities, and relying on the scientific research base. This chapter begins with discussion of general frameworks applied during interpretation, and it continues with discussion of scores commonly yielded by intelligence tests. It ends with a description of strategies for score interpretation that are consistent with standards for evidence-based practice.

FOUNDATIONS FOR INTERPRETATION

Interpretive frameworks for understanding performance on intelligence tests generally fall along two dimensions (see Floyd & Kranzler, 2012). One dimension reflects the contrast between interpretation of *qualitative* and *quantitative* data. Qualitative approaches draw meaning from differences in the kinds of behaviors exhibited by those being tested. Narrative descriptions of odd test behaviors, recordings of vocalizations, and patterns of errors across items are examples of qualitative data. In contrast, quantitative approaches draw meaning from the numbers derived from assessment. IQs and frequency counts are examples of quantitative data.

The second dimension reflects the contrast between *nomothetic* and *idiographic* interpretations (Allport, 1937). Nomothetic interpretations are based on comparison of attributes of an individual to a larger group (e.g., a *norm group*). These interpretations are interindividual in nature and reflect the relative standing of the individual on some measurement; they are norm-based. Idiographic interpretations are based on understanding the attributes of an individual—all other things being equal. For example, reviewing a child's developmental history and considering the types of errors made during completion of an intelligence test subtest are consistent with the idiographic approach. Furthermore, idiographic interpretations may also reflect the comparison of some of an individual's attributes to his or her other attributes. These interpretations are intra-individual in nature (a.k.a. person-relative). In this section of the chapter, we consider these two dimensions in concert as we organize discussion of interpretive methods and specific score types.

Qualitative Idiographic Approaches

There is a tradition of applying qualitative and idiographic approaches to interpretation of intelligence tests and related assessment instruments, and this tradition is particularly strong in clinical neuropsychology (Semrud-Clikeman, Wilkinson, & Wellington, 2005). These approaches make use of the extremely rich data that stem from testing sessions. In essence, every purposeful behavior and involuntary response by the person being tested produces qualitative and idiographic data that can be interpreted as meaningful and relevant to the presenting problem. An examinee's trembling voice, shaking hands, and sweat on the brow may indicate excessive anxiety and perhaps fear. Refusal to remain seated during testing, excessive fidgeting, and impulsive responding to test items may indicate attention-deficit/hyperactivity disorder (ADHD). Vocalized self-derision (e.g., "I am so stupid; I just can't do math") and statements indicating hopelessness (e.g., "I'll never be good at reading") may indicate a depressive disorder. Asking for orally presented items to be repeated may indicate a hearing problem, just as an examinee's moving his or her face closer to or farther away from words printed on a page may indicate a vision problem. Rare behaviors by examinees, such as frequent rotations on block construction tasks, cursing, and bizarre statements, may also reflect brain injuries or serious mental disorders. On the other hand, an examinee's behaviors may indicate adaptive strategies. For example, examinees may benefit from counting on their fingers or "writing" a math problem with a finger on the table. Others may benefit from closing their eyes to screen out distractions or using rehearsal strategies when asked to repeat orally presented information.

It is important to consider qualitative idiographic data during completion of a comprehensive assessment. Such data aid in understanding the whole child and in generating ideas for intervention strategies that might otherwise be overlooked if only quantitative data are considered. The one-on-one interactions between examiner and examinee during testing sessions provide opportunities—perhaps unique ones—for carefully studying behaviors that may be meaningful and relevant to the presenting problem. For example, an adolescent's facial tics or petit mal seizures may have previously been overlooked by teachers, parents, and other adults in his or her life, and keen observations of the adolescent during testing may lead to identification of associated disorders. The potential of these data for generating hypotheses to be evaluated via more objective and ecologically valid methods cannot be ignored.

> **Interactions between examiner and examinee during testing sessions provide opportunities to carefully study behaviors that may be meaningful and relevant to the presenting problem.**

In fact, there is little to no evidence supporting the validity or utility of such qualitative idiographic approaches for assessing high-incidence disabilities. In addition, there is a real threat of invalid inferences and other decision-making errors based on the nature of the assessment methods underlying them. These data are typically most useful in a highly limited manner for informing statements about the validity of the quantitative scores yielded by intelligence tests (see Chapter 4).

Quantitative Idiographic Approaches

Quantitative and idiographic methods to interpretation are relatively uncommon in the intelligence-testing literature. *Raw scores* from individual subtests also fall into this category; the adjective *raw* refers to the fact that the score is not changed in any way. The raw scores most typically mentioned in test manuals and research represent the number of correct responses, the number of points earned, or the number of errors made during a subtest; they are sums calculated from item-level scores. Everyone understands when these raw scores are used to calculate *percentage correct* (another quantitative idiographic variable). For example, a child who correctly completes 16 of 20 items receives a percentage correct score of 80%. Most intelligence test subtests include items that increase in difficulty, so it is extremely uncommon to calculate and report percentage correct scores based on item scores. Percentage correct scores should not be confused with percentile rank values, which are discussed later in this chapter.

There are substantial limitations in interpreting raw scores. Because item-based scores tend to be highly unreliable, notable variation in the total number of raw score points due to error should also be expected, and there is no easy way to adjust these raw scores to control for this error. By nature, raw scores also lack meaningfulness in determining whether the performance yielding them can be considered "normal" or "abnormal." For instance, a raw score of 10 on a subtest targeting vocabulary knowledge may be well above average for a 5-year-old in comparison to same-age peers, but well below average for an 18-year-old. The process of norm referencing addresses this limitation; raw scores are the foundation for the vast majority of the other scores in the quantitative nomothetic category.

In recent decades, advances in psychometrics, particularly item response theory (see Embretson & Reise, 2000), have permitted for the transformation of raw scores into more refined scores that have equal units along their scales. Examples include *ability scores* from the Differential Ability Scales—Second Edition (DAS-II; Elliott, 2007); *change-sensitive scores* from the Stanford–Binet Intelligence Scales, Fifth Edition (SB5; Roid, 2003); and *W scores* from the Woodcock–Johnson III Tests of Cognitive Abilities (WJ III COG; Woodcock, McGrew, & Mather, 2001; see Chapter 7 for more details about these tests). These scores are absolute in measuring the targeted ability (unlike norm-referenced scores) and may be useful in examining change in the abilities underlying test performance across time. However, most test users do not attend to and interpret these scores. Although such scores offer promise in evaluating change over time (e.g., in progress monitoring; see Chapter 9), intelligence tests were not developed for this purpose.

As described briefly in Chapter 4 and consistent with Feuerstein's test–teach–test method mentioned in Chapter 13, *testing of limits*, a technique conducted after completion of the standardized administration, can facilitate another type of quantitative idiographic interpretation. For example, if a child seems to misunderstand a lengthy question during standardized administration of a test of knowledge, you could reword that question—clarifying the points of confusion—and determine whether your rewording elicits the response that was targeted. Typically, performance after this testing-of-limits "intervention" is compared informally to that of the original performance—in a qualitative manner. Such methods have been standardized in some tests, such as the Wechsler Intelligence Scale for Children—Fourth Edition Integrated (WISC-IV Integrated; Kaplan et al., 2004), as described in Chapter 4; however, differences between the original and follow-up testing conditions are tainted by confounds, such as carryover effects and guessing.

Finally, this category includes *ipsative analysis*, an intraindividual or person-relative comparison of scores that is sometimes called *profile analysis*. Although the scores included in an ipsative analysis are typically based on reference to a norm group, it is the comparison of these scores for an individual that makes them idiographic. These scores may be subtest scores or composite scores, but the subtest-level ipsative analysis has historically been most common. Ipsative analysis has typically involved calculation of the average across subtest scores and subsequent comparison of each subtest score to that average. When the difference between a subtest score and the average of other scores is substantial and the subtest score in question is higher than the average, the subtest score is interpreted as indicating a *relative strength*. In contrast, when the difference between a subtest score and the average of other scores is substantial and the subtest score in question is lower than average, the subtest score is interpreted as indicating a *relative weakness*. In some schemes, these labels can be applied only if the difference between the average across scores and the score in question is not likely to have happened by chance (i.e., is statistically significant), and if such a difference can be considered rare.

Despite the intuitive appeal of conducting an ipsative analysis of subtest scores, a sizeable body of evidence has indicated that this practice is fraught with error and that it does not contribute to diagnostic or treatment utility (for a review, see Watkins, Glutting, & Youngstrom, 2005). Unlike the overall score on intelligence tests, patterns of relative strengths and relative weaknesses for individuals tend to have rather poor stability. In addition, as mentioned in Chapter 1, they add little to prediction of important criteria beyond psychometric *g*. Moreover, at the current time, the results of ipsative analysis do not improve diagnostic accuracy and do not help with treatment planning. Not only are patterns of subtests ineffective for group differentiation (e.g., those with and without

> **Conducting an ipsative analysis of subtest scores is fraught with error and does not contribute to diagnostic or treatment utility.**

specific learning disability [SLD]), but the average profile within any diagnostic category does not characterize the profiles of every member of that group. Specific profiles of a particular diagnostic group also may be characteristic of members in other groups. Although conducting ipsative analysis at the composite score level has been increasingly recommended over the past decade (e.g., see Flanagan & Kaufman, 2009; Lichtenberger & Kaufman, 2009)—in part due to the higher reliability estimates supporting composite scores than subtest scores, as well as closer ties to prominent models of cognitive abilities—the most salient criticisms of subtest-level profile analysis also apply to composite score profiles. Composite-level ipsative analysis methods have been evaluated far less than those at the subtest level, but at present there is very little evidence to suggest that the subtest or composite score differences on intelligence tests can be used to improve decisions about individuals.

Qualitative Nomothetic Approaches

Interpretive methods that focus on the kinds of behaviors—not numerical counts of them—exhibited during testing, and that compare these behaviors to some group-based standard, are extremely uncommon. In fact, by definition, all nomothetic approaches are necessarily quantitative; however, a few interpretive approaches come closest to representing this category. For example, examiners using the WISC-IV Integrated (Kaplan et al., 2004) can (1) observe and record qualitative behaviors, such as requests for item repetition, pointing responses, and use of extra blocks and breaks in the final configurations; and (2) determine how rare such behaviors are when compared to those observed in the normative group. In general, such interpretive approaches enhance the meaningfulness of more basic qualitative observations and are intriguing—but in the absence of a clear pattern of external correlates, test users should probably avoid them.

Quantitative Nomothetic Approaches

Intelligence test interpretation has strong quantitative and nomothetic foundations. As described in detail in Chapter 2, the foundation for understanding and measuring intelligence in the practice of psychology is the normal curve (see Figure 2.1). The normal curve represents very well the patterns of individual differences across cognitive abilities of varying levels of generality (Carroll, 1993). Individual differences in cognitive abilities are inferred from the deviation of the individual's performance from the average performance determined from testing large groups of individuals with similar characteristics (e.g., age). For intelligence tests, the expectation is that this group—the *norm group*—is large and representative of the population as a whole (see Chapter 5). Below, we address scores derived from such groups.

Age-Level and Grade-Level Referenced Scores

Some, but very few, modern intelligence tests yield both age and grade equivalent scores. Interpretation of these scores is reflective of a quantitative and nomothetic approach, but they differ in many ways from both (1) a focus on individual differences (as described earlier in the chapter) and (2) the most commonly used norm-referenced scores, standardized scores and percentile ranks (described later).

AGE EQUIVALENTS

Age equivalents typically represent the age level at which the typical score (i.e., the mean or median score) on a subtest is the same as an examinee's raw score. More specifically, they reflect the level of development at which the typical raw score earned by a particular age group equals the raw score earned by an individual. Age equivalents are typically expressed in years and months with a hyphen or dash between them, such as 7-1, 8-11, and 10-10. Traditionally (but erroneously), such scores have been interpreted as reflecting "mental age," and inferences indicating that a child has the "mind of a 2-year-old" have been drawn from them.

Age equivalents are gross representations of an individual's level of development inferred from cross-sectional patterns of scores from a norming sample. The comparisons across age levels are statistical and not necessarily related to particular developmental milestones; age equivalents do not reference criteria that should be met at a certain age (e.g., being able to speak in three-word sentences by age 2 or being able to identify all the continents by age 9). Because the reference point at every age level is the mean or median score for that small group, age equivalents also do not reference the range of individual differences in abilities at every age level. In the same vein, they do not indicate that about half of children at every age level (e.g., at 7 years, 1 month) would obtain a higher raw score and that about half of children at that age level would obtain a lower raw score. Nor do they indicate how deviant a child is from expectations based on comparisons to same-age peers. Finally, like the raw scores on which they are based, age equivalents have unequal units along their scale, and are prone to increases or decreases due to error in measurement. For example, a 1-point increase in a raw score may mean a 2-year increase in age equivalents at some age levels and $\frac{1}{3}$-year increase at other age levels. Although well-scaled items (due to improved scaling technology) have lessened problems with unequal units along age equivalent scales, these scores are particularly prone to overinterpretation because of the sensitivity of age equivalents to error in measurement.

GRADE EQUIVALENTS

Like age equivalents, grade equivalents typically represent the grade level at which the typical score on a subtest is the same as an examinee's raw score. More specifically, they reflect the particular point in the school year at which the typical raw score earned by a grade-based group equals the raw score earned by an individual. Grade equivalents are typically expressed in grade levels and months of the school year (10 months at most are considered; 0 is September), with a decimal point in between them, such as 7.1, 8.9, and 10.5. (If the value on the right side of the point exceeds 9, the score is probably an age equivalent.) Grade equivalents are more frequently interpreted when yielded by achievement tests than when yielded by intelligence tests. For example, one might conclude (albeit erroneously) that "My first grader is reading on a fifth-grade level."

Like age equivalents, the comparisons across grade levels and months of the school year are statistical and not content-related; grade equivalents do not reference criteria that should be met in a certain grade or school curriculum. They also do not indicate that about half of children at the grade level associated with the score in question would obtain a higher raw score and that about half of children at that grade level would obtain a lower raw score. Nor do they indicate how deviant a child is from expectations based on comparison to same-grade peers. They also have unequal units along their scale. Furthermore, their use assumes that growth in abilities is consistent across the academic year and across school years, and this is clearly not the case in the achievement areas (Nese et al., 2012; Skibbe, Grimm, Bowles, & Morrison, 2012). Grade equivalents are not produced by most intelligence tests; of all the intelligence tests described in Chapter 7, only the WJ III COG (Woodcock et al., 2001) produces grade equivalents.

Scores Derived from Age- and Grade-Based Norms

The most commonly used and useful scores from intelligence tests represent individual differences in abilities inferred from the deviation of the individual's performance from the average performance of a group to which they belong. They are *standardized scores* and *percentile ranks*, and they overcome many of the limitations of age equivalents and grade equivalents.

NORM GROUPS

As described in Chapter 5, norm groups are the products of field testing, standardization, and norming, and they allow for a better understanding of typical levels of performance and variation around it at different levels of development. Age-based norms are the most common type of norms used with intelligence tests. Some intelligence tests cover an extremely broad age range (from toddlerhood to late adulthood), whereas others cover a more narrow age range. In traditional norming procedures, as discussed in Chapter 5, a sizeable sample of volunteers at every age level completes the intelligence tests under standardized conditions. From their performance, descriptive statistics (e.g., means and standard deviations) are obtained; each raw score is transformed into a standardized score (sometimes through an intermediate score based on item response theory); and norm tables are constructed to link those raw scores to the norm-referenced scores for test users. First, we discuss the general class of norm-referenced scores called *standardized scores*, and then we discuss the associated *percentile ranks*.

STANDARDIZED SCORES

Standardized scores stem from the comparison of raw scores (or sums of any type of scores) to a mean score from a group with reference to the standard deviation of that group. Most graduate students and professionals with undergraduate training in statistics are familiar with the formula for calculating z scores as part of their training in use of statistical tests. For any distribution, z scores have a mean of 0 and a standard deviation of 1, and they typically range from −3.0 to 3.0. Positive z scores indicate that the raw score in question is higher in magnitude than the mean for the sample, and negative z scores indicate that the raw score in question is lower in magnitude than the mean for the sample.

> **Standardized scores stem from the comparison of raw scores (or sums of any type of scores) to a mean score from a group with reference to the standard deviation of that group.**

A z score for an individual can be calculated as a difference between an obtained score (X) and a sample mean (M) divided by the standard deviation (SD) from the sample.

$$z = \frac{X - M}{SD}$$

For example, if the average raw score across 100 third graders who completed a vocabulary subtest was 20 and the standard deviation for this group was 4, the following z scores would be produced.

- A child who receives a score of 20 receives a z score of 0.

$$z = \frac{X - M}{SD} = \frac{20 - 20}{4} = \frac{0}{4} = 0$$

- A child with a raw score of 28 receives a z score of 2.0.

$$z = \frac{X - M}{SD} = \frac{28 - 20}{4} = \frac{8}{4} = 2$$

- A child with a raw score of 14 receives a z score of −1.5.

$$z = \frac{X - M}{SD} = \frac{14 - 20}{4} = \frac{-6}{4} = -1.5$$

All standardized scores are calculated in essentially the same manner, but the means and standard deviations of these scores (not of the original raw score distributions) are somewhat arbitrarily set. As a result of such standardization of raw scores, each standardized score represents its proximity of the mean of the referenced norm group. As a result, individual differences in the targeted ability are represented in these standardized scores. The process of standardizing the score (making the raw scores higher and lower relative to their own mean) allows for comparisons to be made between scores from the same intelligence test or across scores from different tests. In contrast to age equivalents and grade equivalents, standardized scores have more equal units along the scale.

The most common type of standardized scores yielded by intelligence tests are *deviation IQ scores*; they are often called *standard scores*. They have a mean of 100 and a standard deviation of 15. Most IQs and closely associated composite scores across intelligence tests are scaled by using these deviation IQ scores (see Chapter 7). Intelligence tests are typically limited to a range of deviation IQ scores from four standard deviations below the mean to four standard deviations above the mean (i.e., 40–160). Score range labels often indicate that deviation IQ scores from approximately 10 points above and below 100 are in the *Average* range, and additional score range labels are applied to scores approximately 10 points above and below the Average range (e.g., 81–90 = *Low Average* and 110–119 = *High Average*). More information on these score labels is provided in Chapter 8.

In order to differentiate subtest scores from IQ and other composite scores, intelligence test authors have often had them yield other types of standardized scores. Some intelligence test subtests yield *T scores*, which have a mean of 50 and a standard deviation of 10; others employ *scaled scores*, which have a mean of 10 and a standard deviation of 3. As is evident in Figure 2.1 (in Chapter 2), these standardized scores are generally interchangeable with the deviation IQ scores. We believe that students should be able to quickly recall the means for deviation IQ scores, *T* scores, and scaled scores, as well as scores associated with one standard deviation below the mean (i.e., 85, 40, and 7, respectively), two standard deviations below the mean (i.e., 70, 30, and 4, respectively), one standard deviation above the mean (i.e., 115, 60, and 13, respectively), and two standard deviations above the mean (i.e., 130, 70, and 16, respectively).

Although these three types of standardized scores are typically interchangeable, the ranges of these scores and their scaling do make a difference. For example, as evident in Figure 2.1, scaled scores are limited to a lower end range of $3\frac{1}{3}$ standard deviations (i.e., a scaled score of 1), whereas deviation IQ scores and *T* scores can go many standard deviations lower before reaching a score of 0, the end point on the scale. In addition, scores with smaller standard deviations (e.g., scaled scores) rather than larger standard deviations (e.g., deviation IQ scores) lead to more abrupt score "jumps" between one area of the normal curve and another area with one score point difference. Because standardized scores tend to be limited to whole numbers, each scaled score spans $\frac{1}{3}$ of a standard deviation, each *T* score $\frac{1}{10}$ of a standard deviation, and each deviation IQ score $\frac{1}{15}$ of a standard deviation. That is, there are far wider gaps in the normal curve between scores for scaled scores than for deviation IQ scores. For example, as evident in Figure 2.1, the amount of area under the curve between a scaled score of 10 and a scaled score of 13 is almost 35%; in contrast, the difference between a deviation IQ score of 100 and a deviation IQ score of 103 is only about 3%. We consider these limitations in subtest scaling (vs. IQ and composite scores that tend to use deviation IQ scores) when recommending that subtest scores not typically be interpreted.

PERCENTILE RANKS

Percentile ranks also represent the degree of deviation of a score from the mean of the referenced group. Percentile ranks provide a representation of an examinee's relative position (following rank order) within the norm group. In particular, they indicate the percentage of the norm group that scored the same as or lower than the examinee. Percentile ranks are expressed as percentages (with a range from 0.1 to 99.9) that reflect the area under the normal curve (see Figure 2.1). Like standardized scores, they allow comparisons to be made between scores within and across intelligence tests. We believe that students should be able to quickly recall the percentile ranks at the upper and lower end of the Average range (i.e., percentile ranks of roughly 25 and 75) and at two standard deviations above and below the mean (i.e., percentile ranks of roughly 2 and 98). In addition, they should know the standardized scores roughly associated with certain percentile ranks, such as the

> **Percentile ranks provide a representation of an examinee's relative position (following rank order) within a group.**

10th percentile (81, 37, and 6 for deviation IQ scores, T scores, and scaled scores, respectively) and the 90th percentile (119, 63, and 14 for deviation IQ scores, T scores, and scaled scores, respectively).

Percentile ranks share some limitations with standardized scores, and they have some limitations of their own. Like some standardized scores, their range is somewhat limited. At least when percentile ranks as whole numbers are considered, they reach a ceiling at the 99th percentile and a floor at the 1st percentile. Scores higher or lower than these points will yield percentile rank differences of a fraction of a point (e.g., 99.53, 99.62, 99.69, 99.74, etc.) and at another point (approximately $3^{2}/_{3}$ standard deviations above or below the mean), the percentile ranks must be differentiated by thousandths of a point. These decimal fractions are challenging to explain clearly, but we discuss them further in Chapter 8. In contrast to standardized scores, percentile ranks have unequal units along their scale. As evident in Figure 2.1, a 10-point difference between percentile ranks near the mean (e.g., between percentile ranks of 40 and 50) would indicate small differences in standardized scores (i.e., deviation IQ scores of about 96 and 100) and would thus be of little importance, whereas in the tails of the normal curve, a 10-point difference between percentile ranks would indicate substantial and perhaps important differences.

CONFIDENCE INTERVALS FOR STANDARDIZED SCORES
AND PERCENTILE RANKS

As discussed in Chapter 5, reliability in measurement is an essential feature to consider in selecting tests and determining which test scores are likely to yield the best information during assessment. At the score level, reliability is akin to accuracy in measurement, and the flip side of reliability is *measurement error*. Measurement error is represented as the difference between a reliability estimate (especially an internal consistency reliability coefficient) and unity (i.e., 1.00). Such error can be incorporated into interpretation by considering *confidence intervals* surrounding scores.

Just as we commonly hear the results of polls followed by mention of the margin for error (e.g., "plus or minus 5 percentage points"), many norm-referenced scores can be surrounded by bands of error. The width of the bands of error tell us how much to expect a child's obtained score (the single norm-referenced score yielded by the test) to vary from his or her "true score" if the child was administered the same test repeatedly (assuming no practice effects, fatigue effects, or the like). Following a prominent analogy, picture two archers of varying skill levels shooting at a target on a calm day. Both archers aim at the target's center, the bull's-eye, and both shoot 10 arrows. Because neither archer is perfect and because environmental influences affect the trajectory of arrows, we would expect the arrows to be scattered about the target in a predictable pattern—with a higher density in the middle of the target and a lower density toward the borders of the target. However, these patterns will be likely to differ for the two archers. The more skilled archer will hit the bull's-eye occasionally and will have a greater number of arrows near it and relatively few arrows near the border. In contrast, the less skilled archer will hit near the bull's-eye with a couple of arrows but will scatter others around the target, with a greater number of arrows near the border and perhaps some arrows missing the target altogether.

The archers' skill level is equivalent to reliability. Less skilled archers scatter their arrows across a wider range of segments of the target than more skilled archers, and less reliable tests produce scores that are more likely to vary across the range of hypothetical administrations of the test than the scores of more reliable tests are. In addition, to continue with this metaphor, it is possible (although highly improbable) that the more skilled archer will miss the target altogether with one arrow, while hitting the bull's-eye with another and coming very close to it with the vast majority of their other arrows. In such a case, we could hypothesize that the one errant shot is due to "bad luck" or some extraneous, distracting influence, but we would understand that although it is not likely to happen again, such a bad shot is not outside the hypothetical range of possible shots. However, the shot does not appear to be representative of the archer's true skill level. Similarly, the less skilled archer may hit the bull's-eye while missing the target altogether across all other shots; this perfect shot could be considered a random, improbable occurrence (i.e., really good luck) within the hypothetical range of possible shots and not representative of the archer's true skill level. The most accurate estimates of an archer's skill level would stem from shooting multiple arrows across multiple trials. In the same vein, the most reliable scores stem from multiple items from multiple subtests considered together in a composite score.

In order to better understand confidence intervals, you must also understand the standard error of measurement (SE_m). The SE_m is based in part on the reliability coefficient (most commonly, the internal consistency reliability coefficient) described in Chapter 5, and the other key variable is the standard deviation of the score in question. Confidence intervals are most commonly reported for standardized scores (and specifically for deviation IQ scores), so we focus on them here. The formula for the SE_m requires that an estimate of error be obtained by subtracting the reliability coefficient from 1.0. The square root of this value is obtained, and it is multiplied by the standard deviation of the score (in the case of a deviation IQ score, 15).

If the reliability of a score is .97, and its standard deviation is 15, the formula can be applied in this manner:

$$SE_m = 15 \ (\text{SQRT}(1 - .97))$$
$$SE_m = 15 \ (\text{SQRT}(.03))$$
$$SE_m = 15 \ (.1732)$$
$$SE_m = 2.60$$

This SE_m is the standard deviation of the distribution of hypothetical *true scores* around, most frequently, the obtained score. True scores, according to classic test theory, are hypothetical entities that represent—with perfect accuracy—the targeted construct. If we consider the same normal curve discussed earlier in this chapter and presented in Figure 2.1, the same "rules" for area under the normal curve apply to the distribution of error around the obtained score. For example, because the SE_m is the standard deviation of the distribution of hypothetical true scores, we know that about 68% of the true scores would fall between 1 SE_m above the obtained score and 1 SE_m below the obtained score. For instance, considering a child's obtained IQ of 100 and a SE_m of 2.6, we can anticipate that the child's true IQ would fall within the range of 97.4 and 102.6 about two out of three times (i.e., 68% of the time) if he or she were able to take the test repeatedly (assuming no carryover effects, etc.).

Knowing the area under the curve, we can use the SE_m values to calculate *confidence intervals*, which represent the range of true scores around the obtained score beyond 1 SE_m. A confidence interval is calculated by multiplying the SE_m by standard deviation units expressed as z scores (see our discussion of z scores earlier in the chapter). For example, we would multiply the SE_m by 1.65 to obtain the 90% confidence interval, by 1.96 to obtain the 95% confidence interval, and by 2.58 to obtain the 99% confidence interval. For reference, the SE_m of 2.6 produces these confidence intervals:

90% confidence interval: ±4.29
95% confidence interval: ±5.10
99% confidence interval: ±6.71

Our review of intelligence tests in Chapter 7 indicates that most test authors center confidence intervals around an *estimated true score* versus the actual score earned by the examinee (a.k.a. the obtained score). This practice is apparent when the confidence interval values above and below the obtained score are not symmetrical. Estimated true scores (also called *regressed true scores*) are practically always closer to the mean of the population distribution than obtained scores. Obtained scores are more deviant from the mean in part because of error (i.e., chance) deviations due to guessing, "bad luck," or the like. Estimated true scores are derived by (1) multiplying the difference between the obtained score and the mean by the same reliability coefficient used to calculate the SE_m, and (2) adding this product to the mean. Because no measurement has perfect reliability, the difference from the population score mean (e.g., 100) for the estimated true score is always smaller in magnitude than the difference from the population score mean of the obtained score; it is a product of multiplying this difference by a value less than 1 (e.g., .95). In addition, as evident in Chapter 7, almost every prominent intelligence test produces confidence intervals based on adjustments to the SE_m by multiplying it by the same reliability coefficient to produce the *standard error of the estimated true score* (SE_E). The SE_E values are always smaller than the SE_m values, for the same reason explicated for the estimated true score: We are multiplying it by a number that is less than 1.0.

In many ways, confidence intervals seem to produce a paradoxical effect. In using them, we seem to sacrifice precision (as represented by a single obtained score) for confidence in estimating the true score. The more confident we are that the true score falls within the SE_m or SE_E interval (e.g., 95% confidence), the less precise we are; conversely, the less confident we are (e.g., 68% confidence), the

> **Confidence intervals seem to produce a paradoxical effect. In using them, we seem to sacrifice precision for confidence in estimating the true score.**

more precise we are. Confidence intervals show us that we may, in fact, better represent the abilities we have targeted by expressing performance as a range of scores. We encourage you to employ confidence intervals when reporting results (see Chapter 8).

ADVANCED QUANTITATIVE INTERPRETIVE METHODS

So far in this chapter, we have addressed general interpretive frameworks and the most basic score-based interpretations. This section is devoted to the most prominent methods for understanding patterns of quantitative nomothetic data yielded by tests. With the increasing sophistication of intelligence tests—which now yield a greater number of subtest and composite scores, and which target abilities at various levels of the three-stratum theory (Carroll, 1993)—test users may be overwhelmed with the wealth of information yielded by a single test. In order to make sense of all this information, we offer some general rules of thumb to follow and our KISS model of interpretation.

The First Four Waves of Interpretation

One of our reasons for writing this book is our belief that measurement and understanding of cognitive abilities in applied psychology have never been stronger. This greater understanding is reflected in the progression of prominent models of test score interpretation, detailed in Kamphaus, Winsor, Rowe, and Kim's (2012) description of the four waves of test interpretation. The first wave reflected the quantification of the general level of intelligence. During this wave of interpretation, a focus on psychometric g as measured by IQs was predominant, and individuals were placed in rank order primarily on a single scale measuring this ability. With advancing technology in the form of intelligence test subtests that each yielded norm-referenced scores, the second wave of interpretation emerged. It was characterized by clinical analysis of patterns of subtest scores in addition to the IQ, and idiographic and qualitative interpretations were highlighted. More specifically, subjective and idiosyncratic analysis of subtest profiles guided by psychoanalytic theory and clinical lore typified this approach. The third wave highlighted advances in psychometrics that guided (1) the application of factor analysis to test interpretation, and (2) ipsative analysis of subtest scores within the profiles of individuals using statistical tests to determine significant differences. In particular, this wave was reflected in greater consideration of the shared measurement properties of subtests (used to form specific-ability composites) and their unique components, as well as the evidence supporting the interpretation of profiles of IQ, composite, and subtest scores.

> We believe that measurement and understanding of cognitive abilities in applied psychology have never been stronger.

Finally, the fourth wave reflects the application of research-based models of cognitive abilities to the development of tests and score interpretation. The most prominent models guiding the fourth wave have stemmed from the theoretical models of Carroll (1993) and Horn (1991). Despite their differences, these two models have been integrated in the Cattell–Horn–Carroll (CHC) theory (as described in Chapter 1), and it has been promoted as the most well-supported and sophisticated psychometric model of intelligence (Newton & McGrew, 2010; Schneider &

McGrew, 2012). Furthermore, authors of prominent intelligence tests (e.g., Kaufman & Kaufman, 2004a; Woodcock et al., 2001) have developed tests and produced scores representing a number of the broad abilities described in the CHC theory.

We agree with Kamphaus et al. (2012) and others that this fourth wave, and the convergence of research and professional opinion on models like the CHC theory, afford the test user at least three benefits. First, scores from all intelligence tests can be interpreted by using these models; test users need not rely primarily on test-specific models, which may vary substantially from one test to another. Second, test users can select an intelligence test that best meets their needs. That is, their test selection need not be based only on their theoretical leanings or the differences in the quality of the tests per se. Instead, they can choose tests according to the age level and limitations of their typical clients, the clients' referral concerns, the breadth of specific-ability coverage, the time of administration, and other individual preferences. Third, they can benefit from training in understanding a general theoretical model and from books that promote its application to test score interpretation.

Making Meaning in the Fourth Wave and Considerations for a Fifth Wave

The most common approach to interpreting scores yielded by an intelligence test has been the *successive-levels approach*. In one classic model, Sattler (2008) has suggested that six levels of interpretation be addressed. First, the IQ is interpreted. Second, scores from lower-order composites are interpreted. Third, scores from subtests contributing to each lower-order composite are interpreted in isolation and in comparison to the average across subtests contributing to their respective lower-order composite. Fourth, scores from subtests are compared across the entirety of the test (including in meaningful pairs). Fifth, patterns of item-level scores are evaluated for each subtest. Finally, a qualitative idiographic analysis of item-level responses and other behaviors during the test sessions is conducted. In order to maximally apply the fourth wave of interpretation and to make the transition to more evidence-based practices, we encourage test users to attend to two psychometric considerations—reliability and *generality*—and we offer some additional points that may be considered in a fifth wave of interpretation.

Reliability

Following the principles discussed in Chapter 5, we know that scores closest to the item level (item-level scores and subtest scores) should not attract our attention to the extent that scores stemming from aggregation across numerous items and several subtests should. Composite scores that exceed minimal standards for internal consistency and test–retest reliability should be the focus of our attention. As apparent for every intelligence test evaluated in Chapter 7, stratum III composites (i.e., IQs) yield the highest reliability coefficients, followed by stratum II composites (e.g., factor indexes). Because reliability constrains validity, the most reliable scores from intelligence tests will yield the most dividends for predicting educational, occupational, and other life outcomes and addressing the most pressing referral concerns. Be choosy about which scores you interpret, and feel comfortable ignoring scores if they do not meet the highest standards of reliability and validity. Just because the test or its scoring software produces a score, you need not interpret it.

Generality

In a manner similar to reliability, we know that when scores from numerous items and multiple subtests are aggregated, the influences of specific item content and specific mental processes largely cancel out one another. As a result, more general abilities are measured. In contrast, based on our perceptions and common sense, intelligence test subtests measure abilities in very specific ways. For example, a subtest requiring examinees to respond to orally presented words by orally providing definitions of these words seems to measure vocabulary knowledge versus a more general ability associated with thinking abstractly and problem solving. Other subtests may also appear to measure the vocabulary knowledge via different methods, such as having the examinee (1) hear an orally presented word and point to a picture that represents the word, or (2) view pictures and name what they depict. These related subtests may share a common element—regardless of the assessment method used—that produces higher or lower scores across individuals. For example, that common element may, in fact, be vocabulary knowledge, which is a stratum I (or narrow) ability (Lexical Knowledge). These subtest scores also tend to be highly correlated with subtests measuring knowledge of cultural phenomena and the ability to reason using words. The vocabulary knowledge subtests and other related subtests measuring breadth of knowledge seem to tap into a more general ability that could be called Crystallized Intelligence at stratum II. In this case, the individual subtest characteristics—and even vocabulary knowledge more generally—reflect only pieces of the larger puzzle, because they are more specific than this stratum II (or broad) ability that produces higher and lower scores across similar subtests.

As described in Chapter 1, it is a known fact that almost every measure of cognitive abilities tends to be positively related to most every other measure of cognitive abilities, which suggests that they are measuring the same thing. How can this be? We can see how vocabulary knowledge subtests measure the same thing and how, on a broader level, Crystallized Intelligence subtests measure the same thing, but how is it possible that vocabulary knowledge subtests measure the same thing as subtests requiring the construction of designs with blocks or the identification of abstract patterns across images on a page? It's *uncommon sense*: Believing the evidence produced through more than 100 years of scientific research (without necessarily experiencing it; see Lilienfeld, Ammirati, & David, 2012) allows us to conclude that there is an extremely general superfactor, the *g* factor, that accounts for score variation across all such subtests. Subtests that look vastly different are apparently measuring the same things to a surprising degree.

As discussed in Chapter 1, we can conclude that the ability at the highest level of generality is the most powerful influence in producing higher or lower scores on intelligence tests, and that the measures best representing this ability tend to produce the strongest relations with important societal outcomes. As we focus on more and more specific abilities rather than this general ability, the explanatory and predictive power afforded by these specific abilities tends to decrease dramatically. Considerations of both reliability and generality lead us to conclude that the most accurate and most general scores from intelligence tests, the stratum III composites (the IQs), should be the focus of interpretation. Scores with lower levels of reliability and less generality are likely to produce the results that seem to have deep meaning, but research examining errors in clinical decision making

> **The most accurate and most general scores from intelligence tests, the stratum III composites (the IQs), should be the focus of interpretation.**

(in general) and in subtest score interpretation (more specifically) indicates that results from such scores most likely reflect only illusions of meaning (Lilienfeld et al., 2012; Watkins, 2009).

But can't the specific abilities represented in Carroll's three-stratum theory and CHC theory be measured? The answer is yes, but their effects cannot be isolated with accuracy when interpreting intelligence test scores (Gustafsson, 2002; Oh, Glutting, Watkins, Youngstrom, & McDermott, 2004). When we refer to *specific abilities*, we are considering influences on test scores that are independent of the g factor (see Chapter 1). In fact, when we are targeting specific abilities per se, variability due to the general factor can be considered construct-irrelevant. (The same may be true for measures of the g factor; we certainly do not want lots of specific-ability variance entering into the IQs.) In general, specific-ability variance estimates tend to be relatively low when compared to total variance and general factor variance; those measures that tend to be strongly influenced by the g factor tend to have weaker specific-ability estimates. Basically, very few subtests and only some composite scores measure a sufficient amount of specific-ability variance to warrant their interpretation as indicators of those more specific abilities.

We see only three options for interpreting scores as representing specific abilities, and all of these options have serious limitations:

1. *Interpret sufficiently reliable composite scores stemming from two or more subtest scores as representing specific abilities.* This practice is the most common, but it fails to consider that general factor variance in these composite scores is construct-irrelevant when the composite targets specific abilities. Moreover, many highly reliable composites tend to have more variance associated with the general factor than with specific abilities. This method is a very crude way to examine individual differences in specific cognitive abilities; it works primarily if the general factor is ignored during interpretation of these composites.

2. *Interpret scores from sufficiently reliable composites (stemming from two or more subtest scores) in a profile of related scores using an ipsative analysis. When composite scores differ significantly from the profile mean, it indicates that strengths or weaknesses in specific cognitive abilities are at play. If they are, place more emphasis on them during interpretation.* This practice is far less common than the first and it has some potential for carefully formulated profile analysis. However, it is limited in several ways. Because such composites tend to vary in the influence of the general factor on them and in their reliability, the amount of variance associated with specific abilities in each composite also varies substantially. One composite score may appear to be significantly different from the others, indicating a specific-ability strength or weakness, but this may be due in large part to its weaker reliability than the others. Furthermore, (1) these composite strengths and weaknesses are likely to be unstable across time (as that seen with subtests), and (2) we have no scientific evidence of benefits garnered by using this interpretive practice.

3. *Create specific ability factor scores (removing the construct-irrelevant influences of the* g *factor on them), and interpret them after they are norm-referenced.* We support the creation of such composite scores that represent separate abilities from varying strata of cognitive abilities (e.g., stratum III, stratum II, etc.) and are excited about recent advances in actualizing this promise (Schneider, 2012). At present, however, no intelligence tests produce composites representing specific abilities in this manner. We also suspect that the reliability of these scores will tend to be inadequate because they stem from such small slices of test score variance, but confidence interval

values could be applied to them (Schneider, 2013). At present, we have no good evidence supporting interpretation of such factor scores representing specific abilities and no evidence at all of the benefits stemming from their interpretation. We remain open-minded about the potential of this method and await the development of a strong body of validity evidence before recommending that it be applied during high-stakes testing, however.

A Fifth Wave

We believe that a fifth wave of interpretation will build on the strengths of the fourth wave and that it will rely on evidence-based and empirically supported interpretations that go beyond primarily factor-analytic research. Interpretation in this wave will promote more selective and focused intelligence testing. Consistent with the standards for validity evidence cited in Chapter 5, this wave may require test users to apply only those interpretations that are based on highly focused scientific evidence. This wave will probably lead to a vastly restrictive successive-levels approach that includes, at most, two levels of interpretation: stratum III scores (a.k.a. IQs) and selective lower-order (e.g., stratum II) composite scores that have been shown to have high-quality scientific research supporting their validity (e.g., incremental validity in prediction or treatment utility). Lower levels of interpretation will be cast aside in favor of (1) instruments designed to measures some of the constructs targeted in high-inference interpretation of subtest profiles and item-level responses, and (2) interpretation of only scores supported by a large body of reliability and validity evidence. Item-level scores and scores from intelligence test subtests will not be interpreted. Consistent with the sea change that has led to disregard of idiographic and qualitative interpretations of projective tests, the fifth wave may bring about the end of the wide-ranging qualitative idiographic "clinical interpretations" of intelligence test scores that have lingered on since their heyday in the second wave.

> A fifth wave of interpretation will rely on evidence-based and empirically supported interpretations that go beyond primarily factor-analytic research to promote more selective and focused intelligence testing.

The KISS Model in a Fifth Wave

> We offer a KISS—"Keep it simple and scientific" or "Keep it simple, scholar"—model to guide interpretation in a fifth wave of interpretation.

We offer a KISS model to guide interpretation in a fifth wave of interpretation. The acronym KISS may stand for "Keep it simple and scientific" or "Keep it simple, scholar." (Take your pick!) We think that it well represents empirically supported best practice in the field at the current time. We address each component of the model in turn.

Interpretation of the Stratum III Composite

Interpretation should begin with consideration of the most reliable, general, and empirically supported score yielded by the intelligence test: the IQ. The preponderance of evidence suggests that the fifth wave of interpretation should include the same focus as the first wave—consideration of the psychometric *g*—during interpretation. You are typically standing on solid ground when considering an individual's normative level of performance on IQs.

Ipsative analysis of composite and subtests scores has also been conducted to determine the "validity" or "interpretability" of more global scores (e.g., IQs and composites) when there is "scatter" in their constituent parts. When significant scatter is found, the practice has long been to discount the IQ and focus instead on interpreting the individual's profile of subtest or composite scores (Pfeiffer, Reddy, Kletzel, Schmelzer, & Boyer, 2000). In fact, Hale and Fiorello (2001) argued that one should "never interpret the global IQ score if there is significant scatter or score variability" (p. 132); the rationale is that you are figuratively mixing apples and oranges when combining scores that measure different abilities. Recent research, however, has failed to support this contention that the IQ is invalidated when there is significant variability among composite or subtest scores (Daniel, 2007; Freberg, Vandiver, Watkins, & Canivez, 2008; Kotz, Watkins, & McDermott, 2008; Watkins, Glutting, & Lei, 2007). Thus, research supports the interpretation of the IQ even when the scores contributing to it are not consistent.

Interpretation of Stratum II Composites as Measures of Specific Abilities

Interpretation of composite scores as measures of broad cognitive abilities has become increasingly popular in recent years (e.g., Flanagan & Kaufman, 2009; Prifitera, Saklofske, & Weiss, 2005), due in part to the lack of evidence supporting the interpretation of subtests and other problems with subtest-level interpretation (e.g., McDermott & Glutting, 1997; Watkins & Canivez, 2004). We know, though, that we are on more shaky ground now, due to the lessened reliability and lessened generality of these composites. Nevertheless, applying nomothetic quantitative interpretive strategies to these scores seems to paint a more descriptive picture of test performance than focusing on only the IQ. We believe that we should probably engage in selective and cautious interpretation of these composites after considering (1) their reliability (expecting internal consistency values of .90 or higher), (2) the influence of the psychometric *g* and specific abilities on them, and (3) evidence supporting the validity of their interpretation in addition to the IQ. However, without a more sophisticated framework to guide interpretation of these composite scores, we struggle to act on this belief.

Interpretation of Subtests

Most intelligence test subtests have reliability and validity far inferior to those of IQs and stratum II composites; this pattern has been well documented. Furthermore, subtests have two additional weaknesses. First, as mentioned previously, most subtests are scaled (with scaled scores or *T* scores), so that the measurement of ability is less precise than deviation IQ scores. Second, despite their inferior reliability, confidence interval values are extremely rarely applied to subtests; such values would allow for some control over the influences of error on their scores. For all of these reasons, subtest scores and profiles of these scores should not be the focus of interpretation. Norm-referenced subtest scores should be interpreted as indicators of broader and more general abilities—as contributors to IQs and stratum II composites—and not as representations of specific skills or narrow abilities per se.

Interpretation of Item-Level Responses

As we have conveyed elsewhere (Floyd & Kranzler, 2012), qualitative idiographic approaches to interpretation of item-level responses are not supported by enough evidence to recommend their routine use for high-stakes decisions. Moreover, item-level interpretation is fraught by substantial error in measurement. We are prone to critical thinking errors when evaluating item-level responses in isolation and in forming patterns across them. From a practical perspective, there is presently little convincing evidence that the devotion of additional time and effort to consider patterns of errors on intelligence test subtests yields dividends for clinicians or their clients.

SUMMARY

We understand the motives of those trying to obtain the most information possible from intelligence tests; these tests yield a wealth of information. We recognize that qualitative information from intelligence tests can seem to accurately reflect the patterns of strengths and weaknesses displayed by children and adolescents in their everyday lives and that such information can be used as part of a comprehensive assessment to inform effective interventions. Furthermore, we know that specific cognitive abilities have been evidenced by a very large body of research and that they are appropriately included in prominent theories of cognitive abilities. We understand the rationale for reviewing subtest task requirements and inferring what cognitive processes and abilities they measure; we see value in labeling subtests according to these inferences; and we feel that composite scores (and on rare occasions subtest scores) may be useful to interpret. All of this information, however, cannot be treated equally during interpretation, and we must evaluate it with a discerning eye. Our KISS model is a guide to doing so.

Results of recent research do not support the successive-levels-of-analysis approach for the interpretation of intelligence tests. Rather, the interpretation of intelligence tests should focus primarily on stratum III composites (i.e., IQs). Not only are these scores the best estimates of psychometric g, but they also are the most reliable and predictive scores yielded by intelligence tests. We encourage test users to focus their efforts on interpreting the norm-referenced scores for IQs and to reference broad confidence intervals surrounding them. We also encourage test users to consider the purpose of their assessment and to tailor their testing toward that purpose, as well as to refer to the evidence base that illuminates empirically supported practices. Interpretation may focus on select stratum II composites if there is strong empirical support for their interpretation as measures of specific abilities, but we do not advocate interpretation of all specific-ability composites yielded by intelligence tests or of specific-ability composite profiles, due to lack of evidence supporting these methods.

CHAPTER 7

A Review of Intelligence Tests

with Ryan L. Farmer

In this chapter, we provide an overview of the array of intelligence tests available to you. First, we target full-length multidimensional intelligence tests, which are the most well-known and commonly used in research and practice. (They are *multidimensional* in that they sample from more than a single stratum II ability domain and numerous stratum I ability domains across their component subtests.) Then we target full-length multidimensional nonverbal intelligence tests, which were designed to reduce the effects of English-language skills on test performance. In the same vein, we review language-reduced composite scores included in full-length multidimensional intelligence tests designed for the same purpose. Finally, we target brief multidimensional intelligence tests, as well as abbreviated multidimensional intelligence tests that are formed from a subset of subtests from their full-length counterparts. For each test, we provide a narrative description of its central features and offer, in a table, a summary of norming, score, and other measurement features (based in part on criteria presented in Chapter 5). We do not review interscorer consistency evidence or item gradient violations, because they are specific to subtests (and, for item gradient violations, to specific age groups) and not composites. We also do not review (1) test–retest reliability evidence, because variability in the time intervals between initial and follow-up testing makes reporting of results potentially misleading; or (2) bodies of validity evidence, because such evidence should be considered in light of specific validity questions. You should carefully evaluate this information, guided in part by Form 5.1, before you begin testing.

Consistent with the fourth wave of interpretation and our projections for the fifth wave (as described in Chapter 6), we highlight in this chapter the evidence supporting the use and interpretation of stratum III composites (i.e., IQs). We also address some stratum II composites that may be useful to consider in cases where sufficient validity evidence supports their interpretation.

Technical information presented in this chapter has been obtained from the technical manuals accompanying the tests unless otherwise noted.

FULL-LENGTH MULTIDIMENSIONAL INTELLIGENCE TESTS

Cognitive Assessment System

The Cognitive Assessment System (CAS; Naglieri & Das, 1997) is a full-length intelligence test designed for children ages 5 through 18. It includes 12 subtests (see Table 7.1). The CAS was developed to operationalize the central components of Planning, Attention, Simultaneous, and Successive (PASS) theory, which is based on Luria's neuropsychological model. Its scores, however, can be interpreted from the perspective of the three-stratum theory and the Cattell–Horn–Carroll (CHC) theory (see Keith, Kranzler, & Flanagan, 2001).

Norming data supporting the CAS were collected from 1993 to 1996 across 27 of the United States; the test developers followed a norming plan based on the 1990 U.S. Census. Use of continuous norming procedures was not noted. These dates of data collection make it appear likely that CAS scores are inflated somewhat (on an absolute scale and relative to other, more recently normed intelligence tests) due to the Flynn (1984, 1987, 1999, 2007) effect; the norm sample is too dated to use for high-stakes decision making. There are at least approximately 30 children per norm table block across all age levels, and these numbers are notably higher for younger children in the norm sample.

The CAS produces a stratum III composite called the Full Scale; this score is formed from 12 subtests in its Standard Battery and 8 subtests in its Basic Battery. The average internal consistency reliability value for the Full Scale was .96 across ages for the Standard Battery, and notably lower (.87) across ages for the Basic Battery. There are no ceiling violations for subtests contributing to the Full Scale, yet some subtest floor violations are evident at ages 6:11 and younger. The Planning and Attention composites and their subtests appear to measure Processing Speed; the Simultaneous composite and its subtests seem to measure Visual Processing; and the Successive composite and its subtests seem to measure Short-Term Memory (Keith et al., 2001; Kranzler & Keith, 1999). The average internal consistency reliability values for the composites fell below .90 for both the Planning and Attention composites.

Although the CAS was designed to measure abilities associated with PASS processes, we believe that there is ample evidence for interpreting its scores from the perspective of the three-stratum theory and CHC theory. The Full Scale score from the CAS Standard Battery is an IQ, with strong reliability and validity evidence supporting its use. In contrast, the Full Scale score from the CAS Basic Battery fails to meet the .90 standard for internal consistency reliability and should probably not be used routinely. The CAS seems to measure the abilities Visual Processing, Short-Term Memory, and (to a large extent) Processing Speed across its composites. The two composite scores measuring Processing Speed (i.e., Attention and Planning) do not meet the standard for internal consistency reliability across Standard and Extended batteries.

We are impressed with the CAS authors' use of theory to guide test construction, and we appreciate the ingenuity in the design of an intervention program linked to the CAS (i.e., the PASS Reading Enhancement Program and the Cognition Enhancement Training; Das, 1999, 2004). The CAS is also supported by a software program for scoring, but no report-writing software is available. Nevertheless, the CAS has some notable limitations when compared to other intelligence tests. Most notably, its dated norm sample prevents it from yielding the most accurate scores, but

TABLE 7.1. Cognitive Assessment System (CAS)

Publisher: Riverside Publishing

Publication date: 1997

Age range: 5:0–17:11

Completion time: 40–60 minutes

Norming Information

Norm sample *N*: 2,200

Dates collected: 1993–1996

Census data: 1990

Number U.S. states sampled: 27

Characteristics considered: Age, sex, race, ethnicity, geographic region, community setting, classroom placement, educational classification, and parental education level

Continuous norming: Not specified

Age unit/block: Ages 5:0–7:11, $n = {\sim}100$/block; ages 8:0–10:11, $n = {\sim}67$/block; and ages 11:0–17:11, $n = {\sim}34$/block

Scores Provided

Stratum III Composites

Full Scale (Standard Battery)
- 12 subtests with floor violations at ages 6:3 and younger, and no ceiling violations
- Yields standard score, PR, and CIs
- Standard score range: 40–160
- Mean internal consistency reliability = .96

Full Scale (Basic Battery)
- 8 subtests with floor violations at ages 6:11 and younger, and no ceiling violations
- Yields standard score, PR, and CIs
- Standard score range: 40–160
- Mean internal consistency reliability = .87

Stratum II Composites

Planning
- 3 (Standard Battery) or 2 subtests (Basic Battery)
- Yields standard score, PR, and CIs
- Standard score range: 45–155 (Standard Battery), 47–152 (Basic Battery)
- Mean internal consistency reliability = .88 (Standard Battery), .85 (Basic Battery)

Attention
- 3 (Standard Battery) or 2 subtests (Basic Battery)
- Yields standard score, PR, and CIs
- Standard score range: 45–155 (Standard Battery), 48–153 (Basic Battery)
- Mean internal consistency reliability = .88 (Standard Battery), .84 (Basic Battery)

Simultaneous
- 3 (Standard Battery) or 2 subtests (Basic Battery)
- Yields standard score, PR, and CIs
- Standard score range: 45–155 (Standard Battery), 46–152 (Basic Battery)
- Mean internal consistency reliability = .93 (Standard Battery), .90 (Basic Battery)

Successive
- 3 (Standard Battery) or 2 subtests (Basic Battery)
- Yields standard score, PR, and CIs
- Standard score range: 45–153 (Standard Battery), 49–152 (Basic Battery)
- Mean internal consistency reliability = .93 (Standard Battery), .90 (Basic Battery)

Subtests

- 12 subtests yielding scaled scores and age equivalents

Other Information

Item scaling: Traditional

Bias evaluation: Statistical analysis of item bias

Confidence intervals: Standard error of the estimated true score (SE_E) centered around the estimated true score

Scoring software: Yes

Report-writing software: No

Note. In all tables in this chapter: PR = percentile rank; CIs = confidence intervals.

an updated and renormed CAS is due for release in early 2014. More information about the CAS can be found in this training resource and this test review:

Naglieri, J. A. (1999). *Essentials of CAS assessment.* New York: Wiley.

Plake, B. S., & Impara, J. C. (Eds.). (2001). *The fourteenth mental measurements yearbook.* Lincoln, NE: Buros Institute of Mental Measurements.

Differential Ability Scales, Second Edition

The Differential Ability Scales, Second Edition (DAS-II; Elliott, 2007) is a full-length intelligence test comprising three age-specific batteries: one for those ages 2 and 3, another for those ages 3 through 6, and a final one for those ages 7 through 17. Across batteries, it includes 21 subtests. (See Table 7.2.) Norming data were collected from 2002 to 2005 across 49 of the United States; the test developer followed a norming plan based on the 2002 U.S. Census and used continuous norming procedures. There are at least approximately 50 children per norm table block across age levels, and there are at least approximately 100 children per block beginning at age 9:0.

The DAS-II produces a stratum III composite called General Conceptual Ability; for all batteries but that for the youngest children, this score is formed from six subtests. There are no floor or ceiling violations for any subtest contributing to the General Conceptual Ability at any age level. Average internal consistency reliability values for the General Conceptual Ability were .93 or higher across batteries. The DAS-II also produces stratum II composite scores labeled Verbal and Nonverbal for all age groups, and for the Upper-Level Early Years Battery and the School-Age Battery, it also produces stratum II composites labeled Spatial, Processing Speed, and Working Memory. Average internal consistency reliability values for only the Nonverbal (in both Early Years batteries), Processing Speed (in the Upper-Level Early Years battery), and Verbal composites (in the Upper-Level Early Years and School-Age Batteries) fell below .90. In the batteries for older children, the DAS-II stratum III composites seem to represent Crystallized Intelligence, Fluid Reasoning, Visual Processing, Processing Speed, and Short-Term Memory well (Keith, Low, Reynolds, Patel, & Ridley, 2010), and the DAS-II Verbal, Nonverbal, Spatial, and Working Memory composites possess both strong *g* loadings and sizeable specific-ability effects at most age levels. Only Processing Speed seems to measure proportionally more specific variance than general-factor variance (Maynard, Floyd, Acklie, & Houston, 2011).

The DAS-II has some noteworthy features, including scores formed from different subtests at varying ages, allowing for more developmentally sensitive assessment; provision of ability scores based on item response theory; and inclusion of child-friendly manipulatives. It is supported by a software program designed to facilitate scoring and report writing, and it produces a language-reduced composite called the Special Nonverbal Composite (see Table 7.14, below). More information about the DAS-II can be found in this training resource and these test reviews:

Dumont, R., Willis, J. O., & Elliott, C. D. (2008). *Essentials of DAS-II assessment.* Hoboken, NJ: Wiley.

Beran, T. N. (2007). Review of the Differential Ability Scales (2nd ed.). *Canadian Journal of School Psychology, 22,* 128–132.

Marshal, S. M., McGoey, K. E., & Moschos, S. (2011). Review of the Differential Ability Scales—Second Edition. *Journal of Psychoeducational Assessment, 29,* 89–93.

Spies, R. A., Carlson, J. F., & Geisinger, K. F. (Eds.). (2010). *The eighteenth mental measurements yearbook.* Lincoln, NE: Buros Institute of Mental Measurements.

TABLE 7.2. Differential Ability Scales, Second Edition (DAS-II)

Publisher: Harcourt Assessments (on release) and Pearson (current)

Publication date: 2007

Age range: 2:6–17:11

Completion time: 45–60 minutes

Norming Information

Norm sample *N*: 3,480

Date collected: 2002–2005

Census data: October 2002

Number U.S. states sampled: 49, excluding Hawaii

Characteristics considered: Age, sex, race, parental education level, and geographic region

Continuous norming: Yes

Age unit/block: Ages 2:6–4:11, $n = {\sim}88$/block; ages 5:0–8:11, $n = {\sim}50$/block; and ages 9:0–17:11 = ${\sim}100$/block

Scores Provided
Lower-Level Early Years Battery (Ages 2:6–3:5)

Stratum III Composite

General Conceptual Ability
- 4 subtests with no floor or ceiling violations
- Yields standard score, PR, and CIs
- Standard score range: 45–165
- Mean internal consistency reliability = .93

Stratum II Composites

Verbal
- 2 subtests
- Yields standard score, PR, and CIs
- Standard score range: 30–170
- Mean internal consistency reliability = .92

Nonverbal
- 2 subtests
- Yields standard score, PR, and CIs
- Standard score range: 32–170
- Mean internal consistency reliability = .87

Subtests

- 8 subtests yielding *T* scores, PRs, and Ability scores

Upper-Level Early Years Battery (Ages 3:6–6:11)

Stratum III Composite

General Conceptual Ability
- 6 subtests with no floor or ceiling violations
- Yields standard score, PR, and CIs
- Standard score range: 45–165
- Mean internal consistency reliability = .95

Stratum II Composites

Verbal
- 2 subtests
- Yields standard score, PR, and CIs
- Standard score range: 30–170
- Mean internal consistency reliability = .89

Nonverbal
- 2 subtests
- Yields standard score, PR, and CIs
- Standard score range: 32–170
- Mean internal consistency reliability = .86

Spatial
- 2 subtests
- Yields standard score, PR, and CIs
- Standard score range: 34–170
- Mean internal consistency reliability = .95

Processing Speed (not available until age 5:0)
- 2 subtests
- Yields standard score, PR, and CIs
- Standard score range: 30–170
- Mean internal consistency reliability = .89

Working Memory (not available until age 5:0)
- 2 subtests
- Yields standard score, PR, and CIs
- Standard score range: 33–169
- Mean internal consistency reliability = .93

Subtests

- 10 subtests yielding *T* scores, PRs, and Ability scores

(continued)

TABLE 7.2. *(continued)*

Differential Ability Scales, Second Edition
School-Age Battery (Ages 7:0–17:11)

Stratum III Composite

General Conceptual Ability
- 6 subtests with no floor or ceiling violations
- Yields standard score, PR, and CIs
- Standard score range: 45–165
- Mean internal consistency reliability = .96

Stratum II Composites

Verbal
- 2 subtests
- Yields standard score, PR, and CIs
- Standard score range: 31–169
- Mean internal consistency reliability = .89

Nonverbal
- 2 subtests
- Yields standard score, PR, and CIs
- Standard score range: 31–166
- Mean internal consistency reliability = .93

Spatial
- 2 subtests
- Yields standard score, PR, and CIs
- Standard score range: 32–170
- Mean internal consistency reliability = .95

Processing Speed
- 2 subtests
- Yields standard score, PR, and CIs
- Standard score range: 30–170
- Mean internal consistency reliability = .90

Working Memory
- 2 subtests
- Yields standard score, PR, and CIs
- Standard score range: 33–169
- Mean internal consistency reliability = .95

Subtests
- 14 subtests yielding T scores, PRs, and Ability scores

Other Information

Item scaling: Item response theory

Bias evaluation: Bias review panel, statistical analysis of item bias, and predictive bias evaluation of stratum III composite

Confidence interval method: Standard error of the estimated true score (SE_E) centered around the estimated true score

Scoring software: Yes

Report-writing software: No

Kaufman Assessment Battery for Children, Second Edition

The Kaufman Assessment Battery for Children, Second Edition (KABC-2; Kaufman & Kaufman, 2004a) is a full-length intelligence test for ages 3 through 18. It includes 18 subtests (see Table 7.3). The KABC-2 was developed by utilizing dual theoretical models: the Luria neuropsychological model, which parallels the PASS model used to develop the CAS, and the more mainstream CHC theory. Norming data were collected from September 2001 to January 2003 across 39 of the United States and the District of Columbia; the test developers followed a norming plan based on the 2001 U.S. Census and used continuous norming procedures. There are at least approximately 50 children per norm table block across age levels.

The KABC-2 produces a stratum III composite called the Fluid–Crystallized Index; for all ages above 3, this is formed from scores from 10 subtests. The average internal consistency reliability value for the Fluid–Crystallized Index ranged from .96 to .97 across ages. An alternative to the Fluid–Crystallized Index that omits the two subtests targeting the Crystallized Intelligence ability, called the Mental Processing Composite, has psychometric properties similar yet slightly inferior to those of the Fluid–Crystallized Index. For subtests contributing to these composites, floor violations are evident at ages 6:7 and younger, and ceiling violations are evident for approximately ages 15:6 and older. The KABC-2 also produces five stratum II composites, and they seem

TABLE 7.3. Kaufman Assessment Battery for Children, Second Edition (KABC-2)

AGS (on release) and Pearson (current)

Publication date: 2004

Age range: 3:0–18:0

Completion time: 35–70 minutes

Norming Information

Norm sample N: 3,025

Dates collected: September 2001–January 2003

Census data: March 2001

Number U.S. states sampled: 39, as well as D.C.

Characteristics considered: Age, sex, race, individual or parental education level, parental education within ethnic group, educational placement, educational status of 18-year-olds, and geographic region

Continuous norming: Yes

Age unit/block: Ages 3:0–3:11, $n = 50$/block; ages 4:0–4:11, $n = {\sim}63$/block; ages 5:0–14:11, $n = {\sim}67$/block; ages 15:0–17:11, $n = {\sim}75$/block; and age 18:0–18:11, $n = {\sim}63$/block

Scores Provided

Stratum III Composites

Fluid–Crystallized Index
- 7 (age 3), 9 (age 4–5), or 10 subtests (ages 6–18); floor violations at ages 6:7 and younger, and ceiling violations at ages 15:6 and older
- Yields standard score, PR, and CIs
- Standard score range: 40–160 (age 3:0–5:11, 10:0–12:11), 49–160 (age 6:0–6:11), 45–160 (ages 7:0–9:11), and 47–160 (ages 13:0–18:11)
- Mean internal consistency reliability = .96 (ages 3:0–6:11); .97 (ages 7:0–18:11)

Mental Processing Index
- 5 (age 3), 7 (ages 4–5), or 8 subtests (ages 4–18); floor violations at 6:7 and younger and ceiling violations at 15:6 and older
- Yields standard score, PR, and CIs
- Standard score range: 40–160 (ages 3:0–3:11, 5:0–5:11); 41–160 (ages 4:0–4:11); 48–160 (ages 6:0–6:11); 44–160 (ages 7:0–9:11); 43–160 (ages 10:00–12:11); and 48–160 (ages 13:00–18:11)
- Mean internal consistency reliability = .95 (ages 3:0–6:11); .95 (ages 7:0–18:11)

Stratum II Composites

Crystallized Intelligence
- 2 subtests
- Yields standard score, PR, and CIs

- Standard score range: 48–160 (ages 4:0–4:11, 10:0–18:11); 50–154 (ages 5:0–6:11); 44–160 (ages 7:0–9:11)
- Mean internal consistency reliability = .90 (ages 3:0–6:11); .92 (ages 7:0–18:11)

Fluid Intelligence
- 2 subtests
- Yields standard score, PR, and CIs
- Standard score range: 51–160 (ages 7:0–18:11)
- Mean internal consistency reliability = .88 (ages 7:0–18:11)

Long-Term Retrieval
- 2 subtests
- Yields standard score, PR, and CIs
- Standard score range: 48–160 (ages 4:0–18:11)
- Mean internal consistency reliability = .91 (ages 3:0–6:11); .93 (ages 7:0–18:11)

Short-Term Memory
- 2 subtests
- Yields standard score, PR, and CIs
- Standard score range: 49–158 (ages 4:0–18:11)
- Mean internal consistency reliability = .91 (ages 3:0–6:11); .89 (ages 7:0–18:11)

Visual–Spatial
- 2 subtests
- Yields standard score, PR, and CIs
- Standard score range: 40–160 (ages 4:0–4:11); 40–159 (ages 5:0–5:11); 52–158 (ages 6:0–6:11); 48–157 (ages 7:0–9:11); 43–160 (ages 10:0–12:11); 50–160 (ages 13:0–18:11)
- Mean internal consistency reliability = .92 (ages 3:0–6:11); .88 (ages 7:0–18:11)

Subtests
- 18 subtests yielding scaled scores

Other Information

Item scaling: Traditional

Bias evaluation: Statistical analysis of item bias

Confidence intervals: Standard error of the estimated true score (SE_E) centered around the estimated true score

Scoring software: Yes

Report-writing software: No

to represent similarly labeled CHC broad abilities well (Reynolds, Keith, Fine, Fisher, & Low, 2007). Average internal consistency reliability values below .90 are evident for only the Fluid Intelligence, Short-Term Memory, and Visual–Spatial composites.

The KABC-2 has some noteworthy features, including a dual theoretical interpretive framework; scores formed from different subtests at varying ages, allowing for more developmentally sensitive assessment; and inclusion of unique and engaging subtest activities. The KABC-2 is supported by a software program designed to facilitate scoring and report writing. It seems to assess a wider breadth of stratum II abilities than many other tests (with its inclusion of measures targeting Long-Term Retrieval), and it omits subtests measuring Processing Speed, which are usually affected by motor and visual acuity problems. It also produces a language-reduced composite called the Nonverbal Index (see Table 7.14, below). Test records also address qualitative indicators for each subtest (as addressed in Chapter 4), and it is linked to a co-normed and comprehensive achievement test. More information about the KABC-2 can be found in this training resource and these test reviews:

Kaufman, A. S., Lichtenberger, E. O., Fletcher-Janzen, E., & Kaufman, N. L. (2005). *Essentials of KABC-II assessment*. Hoboken, NJ: Wiley.

Bain, S. K., & Gray, R. (2008). Test reviews: Kaufman Assessment Battery for Children—Second Edition. *Journal of Psychoeducational Assessment, 26,* 92–101.

Spies, R. A., & Plake, B. S. (Eds.). (2005). *The sixteenth mental measurements yearbook*. Lincoln, NE: Buros Institute of Mental Measurements.

Reynolds Intellectual Assessment Scales

The Reynolds Intellectual Assessment Scales (RIAS; Reynolds & Kamphaus, 2003) is a full-length intelligence test for ages 3 through 94. It includes only six subtests (see Table 7.4). Norming data were collected from 1999 to 2002 across 41 of the United States; the test developers followed a norming plan based on the 2001 U.S. Census and used continuous norming procedures. The numbers of individuals per norm table block across age levels are smaller than those seen for most other intelligence tests we reviewed. For example, there is an average of 43 children per block across ages 3 through 18. For some age groups, these values fall below 30.

The RIAS produces a stratum III composite called the Composite Intelligence Index; for all ages, this score is formed from four subtests. The average internal consistency reliability value for the Composite Intelligence Index was .97 across ages. Floor violations for subtests contributing to the Composite Intelligence Index are evident at ages 5:7 and younger, but there are no ceiling violations for subtests. The RIAS also produces composite scores: the Verbal Intelligence Index, the Nonverbal Intelligence Index, and the Composite Memory Index. Average internal consistency reliability values for these composites were .95 across ages. These composites seem to be somewhat coarse from the perspective of three-stratum theory and CHC theory, and questions have surfaced regarding the extent to which the RIAS Verbal Intelligence Index and Nonverbal Intelligence Index measure specific abilities beyond psychometric *g* (Nelson & Canivez, 2012; Nelson, Canivez, Lindstrom, & Hatt, 2007).

The RIAS is somewhat unusual when compared to other full-length multidimensional intelligence tests. In particular, it includes far fewer subtests than most; in fact, it includes only as many as some brief intelligence tests (e.g., the Wechsler Abbreviated Scale of Intelligence—Second Edition; Wechsler, 2011). The RIAS has, however, some noteworthy features, including focused

TABLE 7.4. Reynolds Intellectual Assessment Scales (RIAS)

Publlisher: Psychological Assessment Resources

Publication date: 2003

Age range: 3–94

Completion time: 45–75 minutes

Norming Information

Norm sample *N*: 2,438

Dates collected: Summer 1999–January 2002

Census data: March 2001

Number U.S. states sampled: 41

Characteristics considered: Age, sex, race, parental or individual education level, and geographic region

Continuous norming: Yes

Age unit/block: Ages 3:0–3:11, 6:0–6:11, 8:0–8:11, and 10:0–10:11, $n = \sim34$/block; ages 4:0–4:11, $n = \sim57$/block; ages 5:0–5:11, $n = \sim42$/block; ages 7:0–7:11, $n = \sim36$/block; ages 9:0–9:11, $n = \sim38$/block; ages 11:0–12:11, $n = \sim26$/block; ages 13:0–14:11, $n = \sim22$/block; ages 15:0–16:11, $n = \sim61$/block; ages 17:0–19:11, $n = \sim84$/block; ages 20:0–54:11, $n = \sim163$/block; ages 55:0–74:11, $n = \sim41$/block; ages 75:0–94:11, $n = \sim45$/block

Scores Provided

Stratum III Composite

Composite Intelligence Index
- 4 subtests with floor violations at ages 5:7 and younger and no ceiling violations
- Yields standard score, PR, *T* score, *z* score, normal curve equivalent, stanine, and CIs
- Standard score range: 40–160
- Mean internal consistency reliability = .97

Stratum II Composites

Verbal Intelligence Index
- 2 subtests
- Yields standard score, PR, *T* score, *z* score, normal curve equivalent, stanine, and CIs
- Standard score range: 40–160
- Mean internal consistency reliability = .95

Nonverbal Intelligence Index
- 2 subtests
- Yields standard score, PR, *T* score, *z* score, normal curve equivalent, stanine, and CIs
- Standard score range: 40–160
- Mean internal consistency reliability = .95

Composite Memory Index
- 2 subtests
- Yields standard score, PR, *T* score, *z* score, normal curve equivalent, stanine, and CIs
- Standard score range: 40–160
- Mean internal consistency reliability = .95

Subtests

- 6 subtests yielding scaled scores

Other Information

Item scaling: Traditional

Bias evaluation: Bias review panel and statistical analysis of item bias

Confidence intervals: Standard error of the estimated true score (SE_E) centered around the estimated true score

Scoring software: Yes

Report-writing software: Yes

measurement of psychometric *g* across a broad age range. It omits manipulatives and paper-and-pencil tasks altogether, so its scores are not likely to be confounded by motor problems. The RIAS is supported by a software program designed to facilitate scoring and report writing, and it also includes an abbreviated intelligence test called the Reynolds Intellectual Screening Test (see Table 7.18, below). It is most problematic that the RIAS norming data are now somewhat dated. More information about the RIAS can be found in these test reviews:

Andrews, J. J. W. (2007). Review of RIAS: Reynolds Intellectual Assessment Scales. *Journal of Psychoeducational Assessment, 25,* 402–408.

Dombrowski, S. C., & Mrazik, M. (2008). Test review of RIAS: Reynolds Intellectual Assessment Scales. *Canadian Journal of School Psychology, 23,* 223–230.

Spies, R. A., & Plake, B. S. (Eds.). (2005). *The sixteenth mental measurements yearbook.* Lincoln, NE: Buros Institute of Mental Measurements.

Stanford–Binet Intelligence Scales, Fifth Edition

The Stanford–Binet Intelligence Scales, Fifth Edition (SB5; Roid, 2003) is a full-length intelligence test for ages 2 through 90. It includes 10 subtests (see Table 7.5). The SB5 was developed on the basis of CHC theory. Norming data were collected from 2001 to 2002 across 40 of the United States; the test developer followed a norming plan based on the 2001 U.S. Census and used continuous norming procedures. There are at least approximately 40 individuals per norm table block across age levels, and there are more than approximately 50 children per norm table block for ages 5 through 17.

The SB5 produces a stratum III composite called the Full Scale IQ; this score is formed from 10 subtests. The average internal consistency reliability value for the Full Scale IQ was .98 across ages. There are floor violations at ages 4:3 and younger, but there are no ceiling violations. From these same subtests, the SB5 produces Verbal IQ and Nonverbal IQ composite scores, each of which is formed from five subtests. Average internal consistency reliability values for these composites were .96 and .95, respectively. Like the RIAS stratum II composites, they are rather coarse indicators of CHC abilities, but their breadth of ability sampling indicates that they are probably stratum III composites. The SB5 also produces five stratum II composite scores; the average internal consistency reliability value for each was .90 or higher across ages. These composites seem to represent similarly labeled CHC broad abilities well; however, several studies have indicated that the SB5 measures little in terms of specific abilities beyond psychometric g (Canivez, 2008; DiStefano & Dombrowski, 2006).

The SB5 has some noteworthy features, including a broad age range; scores formed from different subtests items at varying ages, allowing for more developmentally sensitive assessment; provision of ability scores (i.e., change-sensitive scores) based on item response theory; and inclusion of child-friendly manipulatives. It includes routing subtests to estimate ability-based start points for later subtests, to promote expedited administration. The SB5 produces an abbreviated stratum III composite from the two routing subtests called the Abbreviated IQ (see Table 7.18, below) and a nonverbal composite from five subtests called the Nonverbal IQ composite (see Table 7.14, below). The SB5 is supported by a software program designed to facilitate scoring and report writing. Like the RIAS, the SB5 norming data are now somewhat dated. More information about the SB5 can be found in this training resource and these test reviews:

Roid, G. H., & Barram, A. (2004). *Essentials of Stanford–Binet Intelligence Scales (SB5) assessment*. Hoboken, NJ: Wiley.

Bain, S. K., & Allin, J. D. (2005). Review of the Stanford–Binet Intelligence Scales, Fifth Edition. *Journal of Psychoeducational Assessment, 23*, 87–95.

Janzen, H. L., Obrzut, J. E., & Marusiak, C. W. (2004). Review of the Stanford–Binet Intelligence Scales, Fifth Edition (SB:V). *Canadian Journal of School Psychology, 19*, 235–244.

Spies, R. A., & Plake, B. S. (Eds.). (2005). *The sixteenth mental measurements yearbook*. Lincoln, NE: Buros Institute of Mental Measurements.

Wechsler Adult Intelligence Scale—Fourth Edition

The Wechsler Adult Intelligence Scale—Fourth Edition (WAIS-IV; Wechsler, 2008) is a full-length intelligence test for ages 16 through 91. The WAIS-IV includes 15 subtests (see Table 7.6). Norming data were collected from March 2007 to April 2008 across 49 of the United States; the test

TABLE 7.5. Stanford–Binet Intelligence Scales, Fifth Edition (SB5)

Publisher: Riverside

Publication date: 2003

Age range: 2:0–89:11

Completion time: 45–75 minutes

Norming Information

Norm sample *N*: 4,800

Dates collected: 2001 and 2002

Census data: 2001

Number U.S. states sampled: 40

Characteristics considered: Age, sex, race, parental or individual education level, and geographic region

Continuous norming: Yes

Age unit/block: Ages 2:0–4:11, $n = \sim40$/block; ages 5–16, $n = \sim67$/block; ages 17:0–29:11, $n = \sim75$/block; ages 30:0–59:11, $n = \sim50$/block; ages 60:0–89:11, $n = \sim100$/block

Scores Provided

Stratum III Composites

Full Scale IQ
- 10 subtests with floor violations at age 4:3 and younger, and no ceiling violations
- Yields standard score, PR, age equivalency, change-sensitive scores, and CIs
- Standard score range: 40–160
- Mean internal consistency reliability = .98

Verbal IQ
- 5 subtests
- Yields standard score, PR, age equivalency, change sensitive scores, and CIs
- Standard score range: 43–156
- Mean internal consistency reliability = .96

Nonverbal IQ
- 5 subtests
- Yields standard score, PR, age equivalency, change-sensitive scores, and CIs
- Standard score range: 42–158
- Mean internal consistency reliability = .95

Stratum II Composites

Fluid Reasoning
- 2 subtests
- Yields standard score, PR, age equivalency, change-sensitive scores, and CIs

- Standard score range: 47–153
- Mean internal consistency reliability = .90

Knowledge
- 2 subtests
- Yields standard score, PR, age equivalency, change-sensitive scores, and CIs
- Standard score range: 49–151
- Mean internal consistency reliability = .92

Quantitative Reasoning
- 2 subtests
- Yields standard score, PR, age equivalency, change-sensitive scores, and CIs
- Standard score range: 50–149
- Mean internal consistency reliability = .92

Visual–Spatial Processing
- 2 subtests
- Yields standard score, PR, age equivalency, change-sensitive scores, and CIs
- Standard score range: 48–152
- Mean internal consistency reliability = .92

Working Memory
- 2 subtests
- Yields standard score, PR, age equivalency, change-sensitive scores, and CIs
- Standard score range: 48–152
- Mean internal consistency reliability = .91

Subtests

- 10 subtests yielding scaled scores

Other Information

Item scaling: Item response theory

Bias evaluation: Statistical analysis of item bias

Confidence intervals: Standard error of the estimated true score (SE_E) centered around the estimated true score

Scoring software: Yes

Report-writing software: Yes

TABLE 7.6. Wechsler Adult Intelligence Scale—Fourth Edition (WAIS-IV)

Publisher: Pearson

Publication date: 2008

Age range: 16:0–90:11

Completion time: 60–90 minutes

Norming Information

Norm sample N: 2,200

Dates collected: March 2007–April 2008

Census data: October 2005

Number U.S. states sampled: 49, excluding Alaska

Characteristics considered: Age, sex, race, individual or parental education level, and geographic region

Continuous norming: Yes

Age unit/block: Ages 16:0–69:11, $n = 200$/block; ages 70:0–90:11, $n = 100$/block

Scores Provided
Stratum III Composite

Full Scale IQ
- 10 subtests with no floor or ceiling violations
- Yields standard score, PR, and CIs
- Standard score range: 50–150
- Mean internal consistency reliability = .98

Stratum II Composites

Verbal Comprehension Index
- 3 subtests
- Yields standard score, PR, and CIs
- Standard score range: 50–150
- Mean internal consistency reliability = .96

Perceptual Reasoning Index
- 3 subtests
- Yields standard score, PR, and CIs
- Standard score range: 50–150
- Mean internal consistency reliability = .95

Working Memory Index
- 2 subtests
- Yields standard score, PR, and CIs
- Standard score range: 50–150
- Mean internal consistency reliability = .94

Processing Speed Index
- 2 subtests
- Yields standard score, PR, and CIs
- Standard score range: 50–150
- Mean internal consistency reliability = .90

Subtests
- 15 subtests yielding scaled scores

Other Information

Item scaling: Traditional

Bias evaluation: Bias review panel and statistical analysis of item bias

Confidence intervals: Standard error of the estimated true score (SE_E) centered around the estimated true score

Scoring software: Yes

Report-writing software: Yes

developers followed a norming plan based on the 2005 U.S. Census and used continuous norming procedures. There are 200 individuals per norm table block for ages 16 through 70, and 100 at ages 70 and older.

The WAIS-IV produces a stratum III composite called the Full Scale IQ; for all ages, this is formed from 10 subtests. There are no floor or ceiling violations for these subtests. The average internal consistency reliability value for the Full Scale IQ was .98 across ages. The WAIS-IV produces four stratum II composite scores that are generally supported by independent research (e.g., Canivez & Watkins, 2010a, 2010b). The Verbal Comprehension Index and Processing Speed Index seem to represent the abilities of Crystallized Intelligence and Processing Speed well, but there are questions about the ability composition of the Perceptual Reasoning Index and the Working Memory Index (e.g., Benson, Hulac, & Kranzler, 2010). Average internal consistency reliability values for these composites were .90 or higher across ages.

The WAIS-IV has some noteworthy features, including co-norming with the Wechsler Memory Scale—Fourth Edition. It is supported by software programs for scoring and report writing, and it produces an abbreviated stratum III composite called the General Ability Index (see Table 7.18, below). More information about the WAIS-IV can be found in these training resources and test reviews:

Holdnack, J. A., Dozdick, L. W., Weiss, L. G., & Iverson, G. (2013). *WAIS-IV/WMS-IV advanced clinical solutions*. San Diego, CA: Academic Press.

Lichtenberger, E. O., & Kaufman, A. S. (2012). *Essentials of WAIS-IV assessment* (2nd ed.). Hoboken, NJ: Wiley.

Weiss, L. G., Saklofske, D. H., Coalson, D., & Raiford, S. E. (2010). *WAIS-IV clinical use and interpretation: Scientist-practitioner perspectives*. London: Academic Press.

Climie, E. A., & Rostad, K. (2011). Test review: D. Wechsler, Wechsler Adult Intelligence Scale (4th ed.). San Antonio, TX—Psychological Corporation, 2008. *Journal of Psychoeducational Assessment, 29,* 581–586.

Hartman, D. E. (2009). Test review: Wechsler Adult Intelligence Scale IV (WAIS IV): Return of the gold standard. *Applied Neuropsychology, 16,* 85–87.

Spies, R. A., Carlson, J. F., & Geisinger, K. F. (Eds.). (2010). *The eighteenth mental measurements yearbook*. Lincoln, NE: Buros Institute of Mental Measurements.

Wechsler Intelligence Scale for Children—Fourth Edition

The Wechsler Intelligence Scale for Children—Fourth Edition (WISC-IV; Wechsler, 2003) is a full-length intelligence test for ages 6 through 17. The WISC-IV includes 15 subtests (see Table 7.7). Norming data were collected between March 2000 and March 2003 across 49 of the United States; the test developers followed a norming plan based on the 2000 U.S. Census and used continuous norming procedures. There are at least approximately 66 individuals per norm table block across age levels.

The WISC-IV produces a stratum III composite called the Full Scale IQ; for all ages, it is formed from 10 subtests. There are no floor or ceiling violations for these subtests. The average internal consistency reliability value for the Full Scale IQ was .97 across ages. The WISC-IV produces four stratum II composite scores that are largely supported by independent research (e.g., Keith, Fine, Taub, Reynolds, & Kranzler, 2006; Watkins, 2006). The Verbal Comprehension Index and the Working Memory Index seem to represent the abilities of Crystallized Intelligence and Short-Term Memory well, but there are questions about the ability composition of the Perceptual Reasoning Index and the Processing Speed Index (e.g., Keith et al., 2006). Average internal consistency reliability values below .90 were evident only for the Processing Speed Index.

The WISC-IV has some noteworthy features. It is supported by software programs for scoring and report writing. Alternate and extended versions of the WISC-IV include the WISC-IV Spanish and WISC-IV Integrated. The WISC-IV Spanish is administered in Spanish and promotes comparisons to the WISC-IV and U.S. English-speaking children, as well as to Spanish-speaking children with similar educational experiences in the United States. The WISC-IV is also supported by extended norms for use with individuals who reach the ceiling on two or more subtests (Zhu, Cayton, Weiss, & Gabel, 2008), and it produces an abbreviated stratum III composited called the General Ability Index (see Table 7.18, below). More information about the WISC-IV can be found in these training resources and test reviews:

Flanagan, D. P., & Kaufman, A. S. (2009). *Essentials of WISC-IV assessment* (2nd ed.). Hoboken, NJ: Wiley.

Prifitera, A., Saklofske, D. H., & Weiss, L. G. (2008). *WISC-IV clinical assessment and intervention* (2nd ed.). London: Academic Press.

Baron, I. S. (2005). Test review: Wechsler Intelligence Scale for Children—Fourth Edition (WISC-IV). *Child Neuropsychology, 11*(5), 471–475.

Kaufman, A. S., Flanagan, D. P., Alfonso, V. C., & Mascolo, J. T. (2006). Review of Wechsler Intelligence Scale for Children, Fourth Edition (WISC-IV). *Journal of Psychoeducational Assessment, 24,* 278–295.

Spies, R. A., & Plake, B. S. (Eds.). (2005). *The sixteenth mental measurements yearbook.* Lincoln, NE: Buros Institute of Mental Measurements.

Wechsler Preschool and Primary Scale of Intelligence—Third Edition

Because the Wechsler Preschool and Primary Scale of Intelligence—Fourth Edition (WPPSI-IV; Wechsler, 2012) was published while this book was being completed, we provide reviews of both

TABLE 7.7. Wechsler Intelligence Scale for Children—Fourth Edition (WISC-IV)

Publisher: Psychological Corporation (on release) and Pearson (current)

Publication date: 2003

Age range: 6:0–16:11

Completion time: 60–90 minutes

Norming Information

Norm sample *N*: 2,200

Dates collected: 2000–2003

Census data: March 2000

Number U.S. states sampled: 49, excluding Hawaii

Characteristics considered: Age, sex, race, parental education level, and geographic region

Continuous norming: Yes

Age unit/block: Ages 6:0–16:11, $n = $ ~66/block

Scores Provided

Stratum III Composite

Full Scale IQ
- 10 subtests with no floor or ceiling violations
- Yields standard score, PR, and CIs
- Standard score range: 40–160
- Mean internal consistency reliability = .97

Stratum II Composites

Verbal Comprehension Index
- 3 subtests
- Yields standard score, PR, and CIs
- Standard score range: 45–155
- Mean internal consistency reliability = .94

Perceptual Reasoning Index
- 3 subtests
- Yields standard score, PR, and CIs
- Standard score range: 45–155
- Mean internal consistency reliability = .92

Working Memory Index
- 2 subtests
- Yields standard score, PR, and CIs
- Standard score range: 50–150
- Mean internal consistency reliability = .92

Processing Speed Index
- 2 subtests
- Yields standard score, PR, and CIs
- Standard score range: 50–150
- Mean internal consistency reliability = .88

Subtests
- 15 subtests yielding scaled scores

Other Information

Item scaling: Traditional

Bias evaluation: Bias review panel and statistical analysis of item bias

Confidence intervals: Standard error of the estimated true score (SE_E) centered around the estimated true score

Scoring software: Yes

Report-writing software: Yes

the WPPSI-IV and the Wechsler Preschool and Primary Scale of Intelligence—Third Edition (WPPSI-III; Wechsler, 2002) in this chapter. We begin with the WPPSI-III.

The WPPSI-III is a full-length intelligence test for children ages 2:6 through 7:3. It includes 14 subtests (see Table 7.8). Norming data were collected in 2000 across approximately 47 of the United States; the test developers followed a norming plan based on the 2000 U.S. Census and used continuous norming procedures. There are at least approximately 100 children per norm table block for most age levels, and in the others, there are approximately 67 per block.

The WPPSI-III produces a stratum III composite called the Full Scale IQ; for ages 3:11 and younger, this score is formed from four subtests, and for ages 4 years and older, this score is formed from seven subtests. For the battery targeting younger children, subtest floor violations are evident for ages 2:11 and younger; for the battery targeting older children, floor violations are evident for ages 4:8 and younger. No subtest ceiling violations are evident. The average internal consistency reliability values for the Full Scale IQ were .95 and .97, respectively, for the two batteries. The WPPSI-III also produces stratum II composite scores labeled Verbal IQ, Performance IQ, and Processing Speed Quotient. Average internal consistency reliability values for the Verbal IQ and Performance IQ were above the .90 criterion, but the Processing Speed Quotient did not meet this criterion.

We suggest that users of the WPPSI-III begin using the WPPSI-IV as soon as they are able. Because the WPPSI-III was normed 10–12 years earlier than the WPPSI-IV, we expect it, due to the Flynn effect, to produce a Full Scale IQ that is on average 3 or 4 points higher than that derived from the WPPSI-IV. This expectation is supported by results presented in the WPPSI-IV materials. More information about the WPPSI-III can be found in this training resource and these test reviews:

Lichtenberger, E. O., & Kaufman, A. S. (2003). *Essentials of WPPSI-III assessment*. New York: Wiley.
Gordon, B. (2004). Review of the Wechsler Preschool and Primary Scale of Intelligence, Third Edition (WPPSI-III). *Canadian Journal of School Psychology, 19*, 205–220.
Hamilton, W. B., & Thomas, G. (2003). Review of WPPSI-III: Wechsler Preschool and Primary Scale of Intelligence (3rd ed.). *Applied Neuropsychology, 10*, 188–190.
Spies, R. A., & Plake, B. S. (Eds.). (2005). *The sixteenth mental measurements yearbook*. Lincoln, NE: Buros Institute of Mental Measurements.

Wechsler Preschool and Primary Scale of Intelligence—Fourth Edition

The Wechsler Preschool and Primary Scale of Intelligence—Fourth Edition (WPPSI-IV; Wechsler, 2012) is a full-length intelligence test for children ages 2:6 through 7:7 that includes 7 subtests at ages 2:6–3:11 and 15 primary subtests at ages 4:0–7:7 (see Table 7.9). Norming data were collected in 2010–2012 across approximately 48 of the United States; the test developers followed a norming plan based on the 2010 U.S. Census and used continuous norming procedures. There are at least approximately 100 children per norm table block for most age levels, and in the others, there are approximately 67 per block.

The WPPSI-IV produces a stratum III composite called the Full Scale IQ; for ages 3:11 and younger, this score is formed from five subtests, and for ages 4 years and older, this score is formed from six subtests. For the battery targeting younger children, subtest floor violations are evident for ages 2:11 and younger; for the battery targeting older children, no floor violations are evident (in contrast to the WPPSI-III). No subtest ceiling violations are evident. The average internal

TABLE 7.8. Wechsler Preschool and Primary Scale of Intelligence—Third Edition (WPPSI-III)

Publisher: Psychological Corporation (on release) and Pearson (current)

Publication date: 2002

Age range: 2:6–7:3

Completion time: 30–45 minutes (ages 2:6–3:11) and 45–60 minutes (ages 4:0–7:3)

Norming Information

Norm sample *N*: 1,700

Date collected: 2000

Census data: October 2000

Number U.S. states sampled: Not specified; ~47

Characteristics considered: Age, sex, race, parental education level, and geographic region

Continuous norming: Yes

Age unit/block: Ages 2:6–5:11 and ages 7:0–7:3, n = ~100/block; ages 6:0–6:11, n = ~67/block

Scores Provided

Ages 2:6–3:11

Stratum III Composite

Full Scale IQ
- 4 subtests with floor violations at ages 2:11 and younger, and no ceiling violations
- Yields standard score, PR, and CIs
- Standard score range: 41–155
- Mean internal consistency reliability = .95

Stratum II Composites

Verbal IQ
- 2 subtests
- Yields standard score, PR, and CIs
- Standard score range: 49–150
- Mean internal consistency reliability = .95

Performance IQ
- 2 subtests
- Yields standard score, PR, and CIs
- Standard score range: 48–150
- Mean internal consistency reliability = .90

Subtests
- 5 subtests yielding scaled scores

Ages 4:0–7:3

Stratum III Composite

Full Scale IQ
- 7 subtests with floor violations at ages 4:8 and younger, and no ceiling violations
- Yields standard score, PR, and CIs
- Standard score range: 40–160
- Mean internal consistency reliability = .97

Stratum II Composites

Verbal IQ
- 3 subtests
- Yields standard score, PR, and CIs
- Standard score range: 46–155
- Mean internal consistency reliability = .95

Performance IQ
- 3 subtests
- Yields standard score, PR, and CIs
- Standard score range: 45–155
- Mean internal consistency reliability = .95

Processing Speed Quotient
- 2 subtests
- Yields standard score, PR, and CIs
- Standard score range: 46–150
- Mean internal consistency reliability = .86

Subtests
- 14 subtests yielding scaled scores

Other Information

Item scaling: Traditional

Bias evaluation: Bias review panel and statistical analysis of item bias

Confidence intervals: Standard error of the estimated true score (SE_E) centered around the estimated true score

Scoring software: Yes

Report-writing software: Yes

TABLE 7.9 Wechsler Preschool and Primary Scale of Intelligence, Fourth Edition

Publisher: Psychological Corporation (on release) and Pearson (current)

Publication date: 2012

Age range: 2:6–7:7

Completion time: 30–45 minutes (ages 2:6–3:11) and 45–60 minutes (ages 4:0–7:7)

Norming Information

Norm sample N: 1,700

Dates collected: 2010–2012

Census data: October 2010

Number U.S. states sampled: Not specified; ~47

Characteristics considered: Age, sex, race, parental education level, and geographic region

Continuous norming: Yes

Age unit/block: Ages 2:6–5:11 and ages 7:0–7:7, $n =$ ~100/block; ages 6:0–6:11, $n =$ ~67/block

Scores Provided
Ages 2:6–3:11
Stratum III Composite

Full Scale IQ
- 5 subtests with floor violations at ages 2:11 and younger, and no ceiling violations
- Yields standard score, PR, and CIs
- Standard score range: 40–160
- Mean internal consistency reliability = .96

Stratum II Composites

Verbal Comprehension
- 2 subtests
- Yields standard score, PR, and CIs
- Standard score range: 45–155
- Mean internal consistency reliability = .94

Visual Spatial
- 2 subtests
- Yields standard score, PR, and CIs
- Standard score range: 45–155
- Mean internal consistency reliability = .89

Working Memory
- 2 subtests
- Yields standard score, PR, and CIs
- Standard score range: 45–155
- Mean internal consistency reliability = .93

Subtests
- 8 subtests yielding scaled scores

Ages 4:0–7:7
Stratum III Composite

Full Scale IQ
- 6 subtests with no floor or ceiling violations
- Yields standard score, PR, and CIs
- Standard score range: 40–160
- Mean internal consistency reliability = .96

Stratum II Composites

Verbal Comprehension
- 2 subtests
- Yields standard score, PR, and CIs
- Standard score range: 45–155
- Mean internal consistency reliability = .94

Visual Spatial
- 2 subtests
- Yields standard score, PR, and CIs
- Standard score range: 45–155
- Mean internal consistency reliability = .89

Fluid Reasoning
- 2 subtests
- Yields standard score, PR, and CIs
- Standard score range: 45–155
- Mean internal consistency reliability = .93

Working Memory
- 2 subtests
- Yields standard score, PR, and CIs
- Standard score range: 45–155
- Mean internal consistency reliability = .91

Processing Speed Quotient
- 2 subtests
- Yields standard score, PR, and CIs
- Standard score range: 45–150
- Mean internal consistency reliability = .86

Subtests

- 13 subtests yielding scaled scores

Other Information

Item scaling: Traditional

Bias evaluation: Bias review panel and statistical analysis of item bias

Confidence intervals: Standard error of the estimated true score (SE_E) centered around the estimated true score

Scoring software: Yes

Report-writing software: Yes

consistency reliability value for the Full Scale IQ was .96 for the two batteries. The WPPSI-IV battery targeting younger children produces three stratum II composite scores labeled the Verbal Comprehension Index, the Visual Spatial Index, and the Working Memory Index, and the battery targeting older children produces two additional composites labeled the Fluid Reasoning Index and the Processing Speed Index. Average internal consistency reliability values for the Verbal Comprehension Index, the Fluid Reasoning Index, and the Working Memory Index were above the .90 criterion, but the Visual Spatial Index did not meet this criterion in either battery, and the Processing Speed Index did not meet this criterion in the battery for older children.

The WPPSI-IV offers some noteworthy features. It produces, among other indexes, a Nonverbal Intelligence Index (see Table 7.14, below) and a General Ability Index (see Table 7.18, below). Notable improvements in the WPPSI-IV battery for younger children over the same battery from the WPPSI-III are evident: The total number of subtests has been increased from five to eight, and the WPPSI-IV Full Scale IQ stems from five rather than four subtest scores. In general, the WPPSI-IV offers five new subtests, a wider sampling of abilities across domains, and a greater number of stratum II composites. Some of the new subtests and composites focusing on working memory measure visual–spatial memory ability rather than auditory immediate memory abilities (a.k.a. Short-Term Memory), as most other working memory tasks do. They are likely to measure the same stratum II ability (Visual Processing) as subtests contributing to the Visual Spatial Index. The WPPSI-IV is supported by software programs for scoring and report writing. We look forward to reading additional research reports, training manuals, and test reviews focusing on the WPPSI-IV.

Woodcock–Johnson III Tests of Cognitive Abilities Normative Update

The Woodcock–Johnson III Tests of Cognitive Abilities, Normative Update (WJ III COG NU; Woodcock, McGrew, & Mather, 2001; Woodcock, McGrew, Schrank, & Mather, 2007) is a full-length intelligence test for ages 2 through 90 and older. It includes 20 subtests distributed across both a Standard Battery and an Extended Battery (see Table 7.10). The WJ III COG NU was the first intelligence test developed on the basis of CHC theory. Norm-referenced scores (viz., age and grade equivalent scores) can be obtained only by using scoring software.

The WJ COG III norming data were collected from September 1996 to August 1999 across approximately 27 of the United States and 100 U.S. communities; the test developers followed a norming plan based on the projected 2000 U.S. Census and used continuous norming procedures. In 2007, new scoring software was published referencing updated normative statistics (hence the phrase "Normative Update" in the new title). Through advanced statistical analyses, including weighting procedures, the original normative data were altered so that the Normative Update sample reflected the 2005 U.S. Census data. Because norm-referenced scores from the WJ III COG NU can be obtained only by entering the raw scores into scoring software, the norm tables were unavailable for review. As a result, the size of the age unit per block of the norms, floor violations, and ceiling violations are not reported. See Krasa (2007) for information about these issues as they affected WJ III COG scores before the Normative Update.

The WJ III COG NU produces two stratum III composites called General Intellectual Ability. The General Intellectual Ability—Extended is formed from 14 subtests, and the General Intellectual Ability—Standard is formed from 7 subtests. Both of these composites are derived from weighting of subtest scores according to their g loadings in an effort to increase the quality of measurement of psychometric g. All other intelligence tests included in this chapter's review use equal

TABLE 7.10. Woodcock–Johnson III Tests of Cognitive Abilities, Normative Update (WJ III COG NU)

Publisher: Riverside

Publication date: Original, 2001; Normative Update, 2007

Age range: 2:0–90+

Completion time: 35–45 minutes

Norming Information

Norm sample N: 8,782 (age) and 5,902 (grade)

Dates collected: September 1996–August 1999

Census data: 2005

Number U.S. states sampled: 27

Characteristics considered: Geographic region, community size, sex, race, type of school/college/university, parental or individual education level, occupational status of adults, occupation of adults in the labor force, and foreign-born status

Continuous norming: Yes

Age unit/block: Unknown

Scores Provided

Stratum III Composites

General Intellectual Ability—Extended
- 14 subtests
- Yields standard score, PR, CIs, W score, and age and grade equivalents scores
- Mean internal consistency reliability = .98

General Intellectual Ability—Standard
- 7 subtests
- Yields standard score, PR, CIs, W score, and age and grade equivalents scores
- Mean internal consistency reliability = .97

Stratum II Composites

Comprehension–Knowledge
- 2 subtests
- Yields standard score, PR, CIs, W score, and age and grade equivalents scores
- Mean internal consistency reliability = .95

Long-Term Retrieval
- 2 subtests
- Yields standard score, PR, CIs, W score, and age and grade equivalents scores
- Mean internal consistency reliability =.88

Visual-Spatial Thinking
- 2 subtests
- Yields standard score, PR, CIs, W score, and age and grade equivalents scores
- Mean internal consistency reliability = .81

Auditory Processing
- 2 subtests
- Yields standard score, PR, CIs, W score, and age and grade equivalents scores
- Mean internal consistency reliability = .91

Fluid Reasoning
- 2 subtests
- Yields standard score, PR, CIs, W score, and age and grade equivalents scores
- Mean internal consistency reliability = .95

Short-Term Memory
- 2 subtests
- Yields standard score, PR, CIs, W score, and age and grade equivalents scores
- Mean internal consistency reliability = .88

Subtests

- 20 subtests yielding standard scores, PRs, CIs, W scores, and age and grade equivalents scores

Other Information

Item scaling: Item response theory

Bias evaluation: Statistical item bias analysis

Confidence intervals: Standard error of measurement (SE_m) centered around estimated true score

Scoring software: Yes

Report-writing software: Yes

weighting procedures to yield stratum III composites; in this way, the WJ III COG NU General Intellectual Ability composites are unique. The average internal consistency reliability values for the General Intellectual Ability—Extended and the General Intellectual Ability—Standard were .98 and .97, respectively.

The WJ III COG NU also produces the widest range of stratum II composites. It includes seven composites, and they appear to measure the CHC broad abilities of the same or similar names. Average internal consistency reliability values for four of these composites were .90 or higher across ages, but Long-Term Retrieval, Visual–Spatial Thinking, and Short-Term Memory did not meet this standard. Several of these composites, including Visual–Spatial Thinking, Auditory Processing, and Processing Speed, seem to measure proportionally more specific-ability variance than general factor variance (Floyd, McGrew, Barry, Rafael, & Rogers, 2009); this supports their interpretation as measures of specific abilities.

The WJ COG III NU has several notable features. It omits manipulatives altogether; all items are presented orally, via test easel pages, or via response booklets. It includes subtests measuring Auditory Processing, which is unique to the intelligence tests reviewed here, but the subtests targeting this ability make it particularly susceptible to the effects of hearing problems. Like the SB5, it produces ability scores (i.e., *W* scores) based on item response theory. It also yields an abbreviated stratum III composite called Brief Intellectual Ability (see Table 7.18, below). It was co-normed with a popular achievement test, the WJ III Tests of Achievement NU, as well as additional subtests that constitute the WJ III Diagnostic Supplement. Across the more than 50 subtests included in these tests, a variety of composites can be formed and interpreted. Co-norming with the Tests of Achievement also permits sophisticated discrepancy analyses to be conducted between measures of general ability and achievement domains. The WJ III COG NU is supported by software programs designed to facilitate scoring and report writing. More information about the WJ III COG and the WJ III COG NU can be found in these training resources and test reviews:

Schrank, F. A., & Flanagan, D. P. (2003). *WJ III clinical use and interpretation: Scientist-practitioner perspectives.* San Diego, CA: Academic Press.

Schrank, F. A., Miller, D. C., Wendling, B. J., & Woodcock, R. W. (2010). *Essentials of WJ III cognitive abilities assessment* (2nd ed.). Hoboken, NJ: Wiley.

Blackwell, T. L. (2001). Test review: Review of the Woodcock–Johnson III test. *Rehabilitation Counseling Bulletin, 44*, 232–235.

Bradley-Johnson, S., Morgan, S. K., & Nutkins, C. (2004). A critical review of the Woodcock–Johnson III. *Journal of Educational Assessment, 22*, 261–274.

Plake, B. S., Impara, J. C., & Spies, R. A. (Eds.). (2003). *The fifteenth mental measurements yearbook.* Lincoln, NE: Buros Institute of Mental Measurements.

Full-Length Multidimensional Nonverbal Intelligence Tests

In this section, we review four full-length multidimensional nonverbal intelligence tests. By *nonverbal*, we refer to the process by which an examiner uses the test's items to collect data about an examinee's intelligence. According to McCallum, Bracken, and Wasserman (2001), *nonverbal* in this sense indicates "a test administration process in which no receptive language or expressive language demands are placed on *either* [emphasis in original] the examinee or the examiner. . . . There should be no spoken test directions and there should be no spoken responses required [from] the examinee" (p. 8). Although not all of the tests we review below meet this strict criterion, all four were developed to promote such nonverbal assessment of ability. We have omitted unidimensional nonverbal intelligence tests that use primarily one method (i.e., matrix reasoning tasks) to measure intelligence (see also McCallum et al., 2001).

Leiter International Performance Scale—Revised

Because the Leiter International Performance Scale—Third Edition (Leiter-3; Roid, Miller, Pomplun, & Koch, 2013) was published only a few months before this book was completed, we provide reviews of both the Leiter-3 and the Leiter International Performance Scale—Revised (Leiter-R; Roid & Miller, 1997) in this chapter. We begin with the Leiter-R. The Leiter International Performance Scale—Revised (Roid & Miller, 1997) is a full-length nonverbal intelligence test for ages 2 through 21 that includes 10 subtests (see Table 7.11). The Leiter-R is administered primarily in pantomime via gestures (although some orally administered instructions are included), and examinees respond by moving cards and foam shapes, making marks with a pencil, and pointing. Norming data were collected during the early to mid-1990s across an unspecified number of the United States; the test developers followed a norming plan based on the 1993 U.S. Census. This information suggests that scores from the Leiter-R are likely to be inflated (on an absolute scale and relative to other, more recently normed intelligence tests), due to the Flynn effect; the norm sample is too dated to use for high-stakes decision making. Use of continuous norming procedures was not noted. The number of children per norm table block is small for many age groups. In fact, for ages 6 through 10 and ages 12 through 15, these values are less than 30.

The Leiter-R produces a stratum III composite called the Full IQ; this composite is formed from six subtests. For the battery targeting ages 2:0–5:11, subtest floor violations are evident at ages 4:8 and younger, and no ceiling violations are evident. For the battery targeting ages 6:0–20:11, subtest floor violations are evident at ages 7:8 and younger, and ceiling violations are evident at ages 9:0 and older. Average internal consistency reliability values for the Full IQ were .92 both for the 2:0–5:11 battery and for the 6:0–20:11 battery. The Leiter-R also produces two stratum II composites for each battery. Average internal consistency reliability values for the Fluid Reasoning composite did not exceed .90 for either battery, whereas the Fundamental Visualization and Spatial Visualization composites met this standard.

The Leiter-R has some noteworthy features, including an accompanying battery designed to assess the constructs of attention and memory; a rating scale for examiners targeting test session behavior; and a self-report rating scale and rating scales for parents and teachers targeting social, cognitive, and emotional domains. In addition, it produces ability scores based on item response theory. Although there are many things to like about the Leiter-R, it also displays notable weaknesses. For example, floor or ceiling violations exist on many of its subtests. Its dated norm sample prevents it from yielding the most accurate scores. It should not be used routinely for making high-stakes decisions. We suggest users of the Leiter-R begin using the Leiter-3 as soon as they are able. More information about the Leiter-R can be found in this training resource and this test review:

McCallum, R. S., Bracken, B. A., & Wasserman, J. (2001). *Essentials of nonverbal assessment.* New York: Wiley.

Plake, B. S., & Impara, J. C. (Eds.). (2001). *The fourteenth mental measurements yearbook.* Lincoln, NE: Buros Institute of Mental Measurements.

TABLE 7.11. Leiter International Performance Scale—Revised (Leiter-R)

Publisher: Stoelting

Publication date: 1997

Age range: 2:0–20:11

Completion time: 25–40 minutes

Norming Information

Norm sample *N*: 1,719 (typical), 692 (atypical)

Date collected: Not specified

Census data: 1993

Number U.S. states sampled: Not specified

Characteristics considered: Sex, race, ethnicity, socioeconomic status, age, community size, geographic region, and special education status

Continuous norming: Not specified

Age unit/block: Ages 2:0–2:11, $n = \sim 30$/block; ages 3:0–3:11, $n = \sim 32$/block; ages 4:0–4:11, ~ 48/block; ages 5:0–5:11, $n = \sim 45$/block; ages 6:0–6:11, $n = \sim 26$/block; ages 7:0–7:11, $n = \sim 26$/block; ages 8:0–8:11, $n = \sim 25$/block; ages 9:0–9:11, $n = \sim 26$/block; ages 10:0–10:11, $n = \sim 24$/block; ages 11:0–11:11, $n = \sim 49$/block; ages 12:0–13:11, $n = \sim 26$/block; ages 14:0–15:11, $n = \sim 25$; ages 16:0–17:11, $n = \sim 50$/block; ages 18:0–20:11, $n = \sim 31$/block

Scores Provided
Ages 2:0–5:11
Stratum III Composite

Full IQ
- 6 subtests with floor violations at ages 4:8 and younger, and no ceiling violations
- Standard score, growth score, PR, CIs, and age equivalent
- Standard score range: 30–170
- Mean internal consistency reliability = .92

Stratum II Composites

Fluid Reasoning
- 2 subtests
- Standard score, PR, CIs, and age equivalent
- Standard score range: 48–153
- Mean internal consistency reliability = .88

Fundamental Visualization
- 2 subtests
- Standard score, PR, CIs, and age equivalent

- Standard score range: 48–155
- Mean internal consistency reliability = .92

Subtests

- 6 subtests yielding scaled scores

Ages 6:0–20:11
Stratum III Composite

Full IQ
- 6 subtests with floor violations at ages 7:8 and younger, and ceiling violations at ages 9:0 and older
- Standard score, PR, CIs, and age equivalent
- Standard score range: 30–170
- Mean internal consistency reliability = .92

Stratum II Composites

Fluid Reasoning
- 2 subtests
- Standard score, PR, CIs, and age equivalent
- Standard score range: 48–153
- Mean internal consistency reliability = .89

Spatial Visualization
- 3 subtests
- Standard score, PR, CIs, and age equivalent
- Standard score range: 45–155
- Mean internal consistency reliability = .91
- Available for only ages 11:0–20:11

Subtests

- 7 subtests yielding scaled scores

Other Information

Item scaling: Item response theory

Bias evaluation: Statistical analysis of item bias

Confidence intervals: Standard error of the estimated true score (SE_E) centered around the estimated true score

Scoring software: No

Report-writing software: No

Leiter International Performance Scale—Third Edition

The Leiter-3 (Roid, Miller, Pomplun, & Koch, 2013) is the recently published edition of the Leiter. This edition covers a much broader age range (ages 3 through 75) but includes half the subtests of the Leiter-R (see Table 7.12). Like the Leiter-R, the Leiter-3 is administered primarily in pantomime via gestures, and examinees respond by moving blocks and foam shapes, making marks with a purple marker, and pointing. The Leiter-3 addresses the problem of outdated norms evident in the Leiter-R; norming data for the Leiter-3 were collected in 2011 using continuous norming procedures. The number of children per norm table block is small for many age groups. In fact, for ages 6 through 20 and ages 13 through 15, these values were less than 30.

The Leiter-3 produces a stratum III composite called the Nonverbal IQ; it is formed from scores from four subtests. There were no floor or ceiling violations for any of these subtests. The average internal consistency reliability value for the Nonverbal IQ was .96 across ages. This reliability value is notably higher than any other stratum III composite yielded by the multidimen-

TABLE 7.12. Leiter International Performance Scale—Third Edition (Leiter-3)

Publisher: Stoelting

Publication date: 2013

Age range: 3:0–75:0+

Completion time: 20–45 minutes

Norming Information

Norm sample *N*: 1,603 (typical), 548 (atypical)

Date collected: 2011

Number of U.S. states sampled: 36

Characteristics considered: Age, sex, race, ethnicity, socioeconomic status, community size, geographic region, special education or gifted/ESL status

Continuous norming: Yes

Age unit/block: ages 3:0–4:11, n = ~19/block; ages 5:0–6:11, n = ~18/block; ages 7:0–8:11, n = ~20/block; ages 9:0–10:11, n = ~19/block; ages 11:0–12:11, n = ~35/block; ages 13:0–14:11, n = ~24/block; ages 15:0–16:11, n = ~40/block; ages 17:0–19:11, n = ~40/block; ages 29:0–29:11, n = ~55/block; ages 30:0–39:11, n = ~88/block; ages 40:0–49:11, n = ~101/block; ages 50:0–59:11, n = ~98/block; ages 60–70:0+, n = ~43/block

Scores Provided

Stratum III Composite

Nonverbal IQ
- 4 core subtests with no floor or ceiling violations
- Standard score, growth score, PR, normal curve equivalent, CIs, and age equivalent
- Standard score range: 30–170
- Median internal consistency reliability = .96

Stratum II Composites

Nonverbal Memory:
- 2 subtests
- Standard score, growth score, PR, normal curve equivalent, CIs, and age equivalent
- Standard score range: 48–153
- Median internal consistency reliability = .95

Processing Speed:
- 2 subtests
- Standard score, Growth Score, PR, normal curve equivalent, CIs, and age equivalent
- Standard score range: 48–156
- Median internal consistency reliability = .86

Subtests

- 5 subtests yielding scaled scores

Other Information

Item scaling: Item response theory

Bias evaluation: Statistical analysis of item bias

Standard error of measurement (SE_E) centered around the observed score

Scoring software: Yes

Report-writing software: No

sional nonverbal intelligence tests reviewed in this chapter. The Leiter-3 also produces two stratum II composites: Nonverbal Memory and Processing Speed. The average internal consistency reliability value for the Processing Speed composite did not exceed .90, whereas the Nonverbal Memory composites met this standard.

Like the Leiter-R, the Leiter-3 has some noteworthy features, including an accompanying battery designed to assess attention and memory and a rating scale for examiners targeting test session behaviors. The Leiter-3 does not include a self-report rating scale and rating scales for parents and teachers targeting social, cognitive, and emotional domains like its predecessor. The Leiter-3, like the Leiter-R, SB5, and WJ III COG, also produces ability scores based on item response theory. A scoring software program is available. The Leiter-3 appears to have overcome many of the limitations of the Leiter-R and offers, at the time of this book's publication, the most recently normed nonverbal intelligence test.

Universal Nonverbal Intelligence Test

The Universal Nonverbal Intelligence Test (UNIT; Bracken & McCallum, 1998) is a full-length nonverbal intelligence test for ages 5 through 18 that includes six subtests distributed across three batteries. (See Table 7.13.) The UNIT is administered entirely in pantomime via gestures, and examinees respond by moving chips and blocks, drawing lines with a pencil, and pointing. Norming data were collected during the mid-1990s across 38 of the United States; the test developers followed a norming plan based primarily on the 1995 U.S. Census. This information suggests that scores from the UNIT are likely to be inflated (on an absolute scale and relative to other, more recently normed intelligence tests), due to the Flynn effect; the norm sample is too dated to use for high-stakes decision making. Use of continuous norming procedures was not noted. For most age levels, there are approximately 60 children per norm table block; only at the oldest age block do they number approximately 30.

The UNIT produces a stratum III composite called the Full Scale; this score is formed from six subtests in its Extended Battery and four subtests in its Standard Battery. There are subtest floor violations at ages 6:7 and younger for both batteries, but no ceiling violations. The average internal consistency reliability value for the Full Scale was .93 for each battery. The UNIT also produces four stratum II composite scores, which are obtained by combining the six subtests into partially overlapping groups. Average internal consistency reliability values were less than .90 for most of these composites.

There are many things to like about the UNIT, but it also displays notable weaknesses. In particular, the UNIT's dated norm sample prevents it from yielding the most accurate scores, but an updated and renormed UNIT is due for release in 2014. In addition, many of its stratum II composites do not appear to display sufficient reliability for routine interpretation. It should not be used routinely for making high-stakes decisions. More information about the UNIT can be found in this training resource and these test reviews:

McCallum, R. S., Bracken, B. A., & Wasserman, J. (2001). *Essentials of nonverbal assessment*. New York: Wiley.

Fives, C. J., & Flanagan, R. (2002). A review of the Universal Nonverbal Intelligence Test (UNIT): An advance for evaluating youngsters with diverse needs. *School Psychology International, 23*, 425–448.

Plake, B. S., & Impara, J. C. (Eds.). (2001). *The fourteenth mental measurements yearbook*. Lincoln, NE: Buros Institute of Mental Measurements.

TABLE 7.13. Universal Nonverbal Intelligence Test (UNIT)

Publisher: Riverside

Publication date: 1998

Age range: 5:0–17:11

Completion time: 45 minutes (Extended) and 30 minutes (Standard)

Norming Information

Norm sample *N*: 2,100

Date collected: Not specified

Census data: March 1995 (additional educational and federal sources were considered)

Number U.S. states sampled: 38

Characteristics considered: Age, sex, race, parental education level, special education services, classroom placement, community size, and geographic region

Continuous norming: Not specified

Age unit/block: Ages 5:0–15:11, $n = $ ~59/block; ages 16:0–17:11, $n = $ ~30/block

Scores Provided

Stratum III Composite

Full Scale (Extended)
- 6 subtests with floor violations at ages 6:7 and younger, and no ceiling violations
- Yields standard score, PR, and CIs
- Standard score range: 40–159
- Mean internal consistency reliability = .93

Full Scale (Standard)
- 4 subtests with floor violations at ages 6:7 and younger, and no ceiling violations
- Yields standard score, PR, and CIs
- Standard score range: 41–159
- Mean internal consistency reliability = .93

Stratum II Composites

Memory Quotient
- 2 subtests
- Scaled score and age equivalents
- Standard score range: 44–156 (Extended) and 49–152 (Standard)
- Mean internal consistency reliability = .90 (Extended) and .88 (Standard)

Reasoning Quotient
- 2 subtests
- Scaled score and age equivalents
- Standard score range: 40–157 (Extended) and 50–152 (Standard)
- Mean internal consistency reliability = .86 (Extended) and .90 (Standard)

Symbolic Quotient
- 2 subtests
- Scaled score and age equivalents
- Standard score range: 44–156 (Extended) and 49–153 (Standard)
- Mean internal consistency reliability = .89 (Extended) and .87 (Standard)

Nonsymbolic Quotient
- 2 subtests
- Scaled score and age equivalents
- Standard score range: 42–157 (Extended) and 47–152 (Standard)
- Mean internal consistency reliability = .87 (Extended) and .91 (Standard)

Subtests
- 6 subtests yielding scaled score and age equivalents

Other Information

Item scaling: Traditional

Bias evaluation: Bias review panel and statistical analysis of item bias

Confidence intervals: Standard error of the estimated true score (SE_E) centered around the estimated true score

Scoring software: Yes

Report-writing software: No

Wechsler Nonverbal Scale of Ability

The Wechsler Nonverbal Scale of Ability (WNV; Wechsler & Naglieri, 2006) is a full-length non-verbal intelligence test for ages 4 through 21 that includes six subtests (see Table 7.14). The WNV is administered primarily by using gestures and pictorial directions (although some orally administered instructions are included). Examinees respond by moving cards and puzzle pieces, pointing to blocks, drawing symbols with a pencil, and pointing. The WNV has two age-specific batteries, one for ages 4:0–7:11 and another for ages 8:0–21:11. Norming data were collected during the early to mid-2000s across all 50 of the United States, plus Puerto Rico and Canada; the test developers followed a norming plan based on the 2003 U.S. Census and 2001 data collected by Statistics Canada. Use of continuous norming procedures was not noted. For most age levels, there are approximately 50 children per norm table block, and at the oldest age levels, they exceed 100. Only at age 16 does this number fall below 30.

The WNV produces a stratum III composite, the Full Scale Score-4; this score is formed from scores from four subtests. Only two subtests (i.e., Matrices and Coding) are shared across those subtests that form the FSIQ-4. No subtest floor or ceiling violations are evident. The average internal consistency reliability value across both batteries for the Full Scale Score-4 was .91. The WNV does not produce stratum II composite scores. No supporting software programs are available. More information about the WNV can be found in this training resource and these test reviews:

TABLE 7.14. Wechsler Nonverbal Scale of Ability (WNV)

Publisher: Psychological Corporation (on release) and Pearson (current)

Publication date: 2006

Age range: 4:0–21:11

Completion time: 45 minutes

Norming Information

Norm sample N: 1,323 (U.S.) and 875 (Canada)

Date collected: Not specified

Census data: 2003 (U.S.)/2001 (Canada)

Number U.S. states sampled: 50, as well as Puerto Rico; standardization occurred simultaneously in Canada

Characteristics considered: Age, sex, race, parental or individual education level, and geographic region

Continuous norming: Not specified

Age unit/block: Ages 4:0–4:11, $n = $ ~50/block; ages 5:0–5:11, $n = $ ~37/block; ages 6:0–10:11 and 12:0–12:11, $n = $ ~50; ages 11:0–11:11, $n = $ ~66/block; ages 13:0–15:11, $n = $ ~ 42/block; ages 16:0–16:11, $n = $ ~21/block; 17:0–19:11, $n = $ ~186; ages 20:0–21:11, $n = $ ~148/block

Scores Provided

Stratum III Composite

Full Scale Score-4
- 4 subtests (ages 4:0–7:11 and 8:0–21:11); floor violations at ages 4:11 and younger and no ceiling violations
- Yields standard score, PR, and CIs
- Standard score range: 30–160 (ages 4:0–7:11 and 8:0–21:11);
- Mean internal consistency reliability = .91 (ages 4:0–7:11); .91 (ages 8:0–21:11)

Subtests
- 6 subtests yielding T scores

Other Information

Item scaling: Traditional

Bias evaluation: Bias review panel

Confidence intervals: Standard error of the estimated true score (SE_E) centered around the estimated true score

Scoring software: No

Report-writing software: No

Brunnert, K. A., Naglieri, J. A., & Hardy-Braz, S. T. (2008). *Essentials of WNV assessment.* Hoboken, NJ: Wiley.

Massa, I., & Rivera, V. (2009). Test review of Wechsler Nonverbal Scale of Ability. *Journal of Psychoeducational Assessment, 27,* 426–432.

Spies, R. A., Carlson, J. F., & Geisinger, K. F. (Eds.). (2010). *The eighteenth mental measurements yearbook.* Lincoln, NE: Buros Institute of Mental Measurements.

LANGUAGE-REDUCED COMPOSITES FROM FULL-LENGTH MULTIDIMENSIONAL INTELLIGENCE TESTS

In addition to reviewing full-length multidimensional nonverbal intelligence tests, we have reviewed composites yielded by full-length multidimensional intelligence tests that target the assessment of general ability via methods that reduce the influence of language on subtest performance. In most cases, these tests include spoken directions offered by the examiner, but no spoken responses are required from the examinee. More detailed information about the full-length batteries has been described previously, so we refer you to new information in Table 7.15.

BRIEF AND ABBREVIATED MULTIDIMENSIONAL INTELLIGENCE TESTS

We have also reviewed brief and abbreviated multidimensional intelligence tests to feature these focused measures of stratum III ability, psychometric *g*. Whether an intelligence test is considered *brief* or *abbreviated* depends on the amount of time required to administer it, as well as the breadth of abilities targeted by it (Homack & Reynolds, 2007). A *brief* intelligence test is a stand-alone test composed of only a few subtests that are administered in standard order and scored in reference to the test's independent norm sample. An *abbreviated* intelligence test is composed of select subtests from a full-length intelligence test (sometimes administered out of standard order) and yields scores based on the norm sample from the full-length intelligence test. Thus, a brief intelligence test is normed as a whole, whereas the abbreviated intelligence test derives its norm-based scores from norming of a more comprehensive intelligence test.

We believe that abbreviated intelligence tests are particularly important to consider before testing with full-length intelligence tests—when subtests from these full-length tests are inappropriate for the examiner in question (e.g., due to motor impairment)—and after testing with full-length intelligence tests—when subtests from these full-length tests have been invalidated (e.g., due to examiner error or other problems in the testing session). For abbreviated tests, because detailed information about the full-length tests from which they were derived has been described earlier in the chapter, we have presented their information in Table 7.19 and highlighted two abbreviated IQs in the text.

Kaufman Brief Intelligence Test, Second Edition

The Kaufman Brief Intelligence Test, Second Edition (KBIT-2; Kaufman & Kaufman, 2004b) is a brief intelligence test for ages 4 through 90. It includes three subtests (see Table 7.16). Norm-

TABLE 7.15. Language-Reduced Composites Embedded in Full-Length Multidimensional Intelligence Tests

Differential Ability Scales, Second Edition (DAS-II)

See Table 7.2 for complete information.

Upper-Level Early Years Battery (3:6–6:11)

Special Nonverbal Composite
- 4 subtests with no floor or ceiling violations
- Yields standard score, PR, and CIs
- Standard score range: 30–170
- Mean internal consistency reliability = .94

School-Age Battery (7:0–17:11)

Special Nonverbal Composite
- 4 subtests with no floor or ceiling violations
- Yields standard score, PR, and CIs
- Standard score range: 30–170
- Mean internal consistency reliability = .96

Kaufman Assessment Battery for Children, Second Edition (KABC-2)

See Table 7.3 for complete information.

Nonverbal Index
- 4 (ages 3–4) subtests with floor violations at ages 4:11 and younger and no ceiling violations; 5 (age 5) subtests with floor violations at ages 5:8 and younger; 6 (age 5) subtests with floor violations at age 6:7 and younger; and 5 (ages 7–18) subtests with no floor violations and ceiling violations
- Yields standard score, PR, and CIs
- Standard score range: 40–160 (ages 3:0–5:11, 7:0–9:11); 46–159 (ages 6:0–6:11); 47–160 (ages 10:0–18:11)
- Mean internal consistency reliability = .90 (ages 3:0–6:11); .92 (ages 7:0–18:11)

Stanford–Binet Intelligence Scales, Fifth Edition (SB5)

See Table 7.5 for complete information.

Nonverbal IQ
- 5 subtests with floor violations at age 3:7 and younger, and no ceiling violations
- Yields standard score, PR, and CIs; additional scores such as age equivalency and change sensitive scores can be derived
- Standard score range: 42–158
- Mean internal consistency reliability = .95

Wechsler Preschool and Primary Scale of Intelligence, Fourth Edition

See Table 7.9 for complete information.

Nonverbal
- 4 subtests with floor violations at ages 3:2 and younger and no ceiling violations
- Yields standard score, PR, and CIs
- Standard score range: 40–160 (ages 2:6–3:11); 40–160 (ages 4:0–7:7)
- Mean internal consistency reliability = .95 (ages 2:6–3:11); 95 (ages 4:0–7:7)

ing data were collected in 2002 and 2003 across approximately 34 of the United States; the test developers followed a norming plan based on the 2001 U.S. Census. Use of continuous norming procedures was not noted. The numbers of individuals per norm table block across age levels are smaller than those seen for most other intelligence tests included in this review. For example, there is an average of only approximately 42 children per block across ages 5 through 10, and only approximately 34 across ages 12 to 15. For some age groups, such as 4-year-olds, these values fall below 30.

The KBIT-2 produces a stratum III composite called the IQ Composite; this score is formed from three subtests. There are no floor or ceiling violations for these subtests. The average internal consistency reliability value for the IQ Composite was .93. The KBIT-2 also produces stratum II composites labeled Verbal and Nonverbal, but it is notable that the Nonverbal composite stems from performance on only one subtest. As a consequence, only the Verbal composite demonstrated an average internal consistency reliability coefficient across age groups that was above .90. The KBIT-2 was normed alongside the Kaufman Brief Achievement Test. No supporting

TABLE 7.16. Kaufman Brief Intelligence Test, Second Edition (KBIT-2)

Publisher: AGS (on release) and Pearson (current)

Publication date: 2004

Age range: 4:0–90:11

Completion time: 15–30 minutes

Norming Information

Norm sample N: 2,120

Dates collected: May 2002–May 2003

Census data: March 2001

Number U.S. states sampled: 34

Characteristics considered: Age, sex, parental or individual education level, race/ethnicity, and geographic region

Continuous norming: Not specified

Age unit/block: Ages 4:0–4:11, $n = \sim17$/block; ages 5:0–10:11, $n = \sim42$/block; ages 11:0–11:11 and ages 19:0–25:11, $n = \sim34$/block; ages 12:0–15:11 and ages 76:0–80:11, $n = \sim50$/block; ages 16:0–16:11, $n = 75$/block; ages 17:0–18:11, $n = \sim38$/block; ages 26:0–45:11, $n = 200$/block; ages 56:0–75:11, $n = \sim40$/block; and ages 81:0–90:11, $n = \sim25$/block

Scores Provided

Stratum III Composite

IQ Composite
- 3 subtests with no floor or ceiling violations
- Yields standard score, PR, and CIs
- Standard score range: 40–160
- Mean internal consistency reliability = .93

Stratum II Composites

Verbal
- 2 subtests
- Yields standard score, PR, and CIs
- Standard score range: 40–160
- Mean internal consistency reliability = .91

Nonverbal
- 1 subtest
- Yields standard score, PR, and CIs
- Standard score range: 40–160
- Mean internal consistency reliability = .88

Subtests

- 3 subtests yielding *T* scores

Other Information

Item scaling: Not specified

Bias evaluation: Items were evaluated, but method not specified

Confidence intervals: Standard error of measurement (SE_m) centered around estimated true score

Scoring software: No

Report-writing software: No

software programs are available. More information about the KBIT-2 can be found in these test reviews:

Bain, S. K., & Jaspers, K. E. (2010). Review of Kaufman Brief Intelligence Test, Second Edition. *Journal of Psychoeducational Assessment, 28,* 167–174.
Geisinger, K. F., Spies, R. A., Carlson, J. F., & Plake, B. S. (Eds.). (2007). *The seventeenth mental measurements yearbook.* Lincoln, NE: Buros Institute of Mental Measurements.

Wechsler Abbreviated Scale of Intelligence—Second Edition

The Wechsler Abbreviated Scale of Intelligence–Second Edition (WASI-II; Wechsler, 2011) is a brief intelligence test for individuals ages 6 through 90. It includes four subtests that parallel those included in other Wechsler intelligence tests, such as the WAIS-IV and WISC-IV (see Table 7.17). Norming data were collected from 2010 to 2011 across approximately 45 of the United States;

TABLE 7.17. Wechsler Abbreviated Scale of Intelligence—Second Edition (WAIS-II)

Publisher: Pearson
Publication date: 2011
Age range: 6:0–90:0
Completion time: 15 minutes

Norming Information
Norm sample N: 2,300
Dates collected: January 2010–May 2011
Census data: March 2008
Number U.S. states sampled: ~45
Characteristics considered: Age, sex, race, parental or individual education level, and geographic region
Continuous norming: Yes
Age unit/block: Ages 6:0–19:11, $n = \sim34$/block; ages 20:0–90:11, $n = 100$/block

Scores Provided
Full Scale–4
- 4 subtests with no floor or ceiling violations
- Yields standard score, PR, and CIs
- Standard score range: 40–160
- Mean internal consistency reliability = .96

Full Scale–2
- 2 subtests with no floor or ceiling violations
- Yields standard score, PR, and CIs
- Standard score range: 45–160
- Mean internal consistency reliability = .93

Stratum II Composites
Verbal Comprehension
- 2 subtests
- Yields standard score, PR, and CIs
- Standard score range: 45–160
- Mean internal consistency reliability = .94

Perceptual Reasoning
- 2 subtests
- Yields standard score, PR, and CIs
- Standard score range: 45–160
- Mean internal consistency reliability = .93

Subtests
- 4 subtests yielding T scores

Other Information
Item scaling: Traditional
Bias evaluation: Statistical analysis of item bias
Confidence intervals: Standard error of the estimated true score (SE_E) centered around the estimated true score
Scoring software: No
Report-writing software: No

the test developers followed a norming plan based on the 2008 U.S. Census and used continuous norming procedures. There are at least 67 individuals per norm table block across age levels; beginning at age 16, there are at least 100 individuals per block.

The WASI-II produces a stratum III composite called the Full Scale–4; this composite is formed from all available subtests. There are no floor or ceiling violations for these subtests. The average internal consistency reliability value, as reported in Wechsler (2011), for the Full Scale–4 was .96. The WASI-II also produces a second stratum III composite called the Full Scale–2; this composite is formed by two of the four subtests contributing to the Full Scale-4. The average internal consistency reliability value for the Full Scale-2 (.93) was slightly lower than that for the Full Scale-4, but it was still above the .90 standard. The WASI-II produces two stratum II composites; average internal consistency reliabilities were .93 or higher across ages.

The WASI-II is the most recently updated brief intelligence test, and its stratum III composites demonstrate excellent psychometric properties. No supporting software programs for it are available. More information about the WASI-II can be found in these reviews:

Irby, S. M., & Floyd, R. G. (in press). Review of the test Wechsler Abbreviated Scales of Intelligence, Second Edition. *Canadian Journal of School Psychology.*
McCrimmon, A. W., & Smith, A. D. (2013). Review of the Wechsler Abbreviated Scale of Intelligence, Second Edition (WASI-II). *Journal of Psychoeducational Assessment, 31,* 337–341.

Wide Range Intelligence Test

The Wide Range Intelligence Test (WRIT; Glutting, Adams, & Sheslow, 2000) is a brief intelligence test for ages 4 through 86. It includes four subtests (see Table 7.18). Neither dates nor locations for norming data collection were disclosed. For the data collection, the test developers followed a norming plan based on the 1997 U.S. Census. This information suggests that scores from the WRIT are likely to be inflated (on an absolute scale and relative to other, more recently normed intelligence tests) due to the Flynn effect; the norm sample is too dated to use for high-stakes decision making. The numbers of individuals per norm table block across age levels are smaller than those seen for most other intelligence tests included in this review. For example, there is an average of only approximately 25 children per block across ages 6 through 16. The WRIT produces a stratum III composite called the General IQ; this score is formed from four subtests. Subtest floor violations are evident for ages 4:11 and younger, but no ceiling violations are evident. The average internal consistency reliability value was .95 across ages. The WRIT also produces two stratum II composites; average internal consistency reliability coefficients for these composites were .92 or higher across ages.

The WRIT has the most dated normative data of the three brief intelligence tests reviewed in this section, and this issue prevents it from yielding the most accurate scores. We are unaware of any renorming of the WRIT. No supporting software programs are available. More information about the WRIT can be found in this training resource and this test review:

Homack, S. R., & Reynolds, C. R. (2007). *Essentials of assessment with brief intelligence tests.* Hoboken, NJ: Wiley.
Plake, B. S., Impara, J. C., & Spies, R. A. (Eds.). (2003). *The fifteenth mental measurements yearbook.* Lincoln, NE: Buros Institute of Mental Measurements.

TABLE 7.18. Wide Range Intelligence Test

Publisher: Wide Range

Publication date: 2000

Age range: 4:0–85:11

Completion time: 20–30 minutes

Norming Information

Norm sample *N*: 2,285

Date collected: Not specified

Census data: 1997

Number U.S. states sampled: Not specified

Characteristics considered: Age, sex, race, parental or individual education level, and geographic region

Continuous norming: Not specified

Age unit/block: Ages 4:0–5:11, *n* = ~44/block; ages 6:0–16:11, *n* = ~25/block; ages 17:0–24:11, *n* = ~118/block; ages 25:0–84:11, *n* = ~50/block

Scores Provided

Stratum III Composite

General IQ
- 4 subtests with floor violations at ages 4:11 and younger, and no ceiling violations
- Yields standard score, PR, and CIs
- Standard score range: 35–155
- Mean internal consistency reliability = .95

Stratum II Composites

Verbal IQ
- 2 subtests
- Yields standard score, PR, and CIs
- Standard score range: 35–155
- Mean internal consistency reliability = .94

Visual IQ
- 2 subtests
- Yields standard score, PR, and CIs
- Standard score range: 35–155
- Mean internal consistency reliability = .92

Subtests

- 4 subtests yielding *T* scores

Other Information

Item scaling: Not specified

Bias evaluation: Bias review panel and statistical analysis of item bias

Confidence intervals: Standard error of the estimated true score (SE_E) centered around the estimated true score

Scoring software: No

Report-writing software: No

Abbreviated IQs

Information about abbreviated IQs from full-length multidimensional intelligence tests is presented in Table 7.19. We highlight two of these IQs here because much of the information about them is not included in the test manuals supporting the tests from which they are derived.

WAIS-IV General Ability Index

The WAIS-IV produces a stratum III composite called the General Ability Index. This score is formed from six subtests (appearing first, second, fourth, fifth, sixth, eighth, and ninth in the WAIS-IV) that demonstrate no floor or ceiling violations (see Table 7.6). These subtests form the Verbal Comprehension Index and the Perceptual Reasoning Index from the WAIS-IV. The average internal consistency reliability value of the WAIS-IV General Ability Index was .97 (Lichtenberger & Kaufman, 2009).

WISC-IV General Ability Index

The WISC-IV also produces a stratum III composite called the General Ability Index (Raiford, Weiss, Rolfhus, & Coalson, 2005; Saklofske, Prifitera, Weiss, Rolfhus, & Zhu, 2005). This score is

TABLE 7.19. Abbreviated Stratum III Composites from Full-Length Multidimensional Intelligence Tests

Leiter International Performance Scale—Revised (Leiter-R)

See Table 7.11 for complete information.

Brief IQ
- 4 subtests with floor violations at 4:5 and younger, and ceiling violations at 9:0 and older
- Yields standard score, PR, CIs, and age equivalent
- Standard score range: 36–169
- Mean internal consistency reliability = .89

Reynolds Intellectual Screening Test (RIST; based on Reynolds Intellectual Assessment Scales [RIAS])

See Table 7.4 for complete information.

RIST Index
- 2 subtests with floor violations at ages 5:3 and younger, and no ceiling violations
- Yields standard score, *T* score, *z* score, normal curve equivalent, stanine, PR, and CIs
- Standard score range: 40–160
- Mean internal consistency reliability = .95

Stanford–Binet Intelligence Scales, Fifth Edition (SB5)

See Table 7.5 for complete information.

Abbreviated IQ
- 2 subtests with no floor or ceiling violations
- Yields standard score, PR, and CIs
- Standard score range: 47–153
- Mean internal consistency reliability = .91

Universal Nonverbal Intelligence Test (UNIT)

See Table 7.12 for complete information.

Abbreviated Full Scale
- 2 subtests with floor violations at ages 6:7 and younger, and no ceiling violations
- Yields standard score, PR, and CIs
- Standard score range: 45–153
- Mean internal consistency reliability = .91

Wechsler Adult Intelligence Scale—Fourth Edition (WAIS-IV)

See Table 7.6 for complete information.

General Ability Index
- 6 subtests with no floor or ceiling violations
- Yields standard score, PR, and CIs

- Standard score range: 40–160
- Mean internal consistency reliability = .97

Wechsler Intelligence Scale for Children—Fourth Edition (WISC-IV)

See Table 7.7 for complete information.

General Ability Index
- 6 subtests with no floor or ceiling violations
- Yields standard score, PR, and CIs
- Standard score range: 40–160
- Mean internal consistency reliability = .96

Wechsler Nonverbal Scale of Ability

See Table 7.14 for complete information.

Full Scale Score–2
- 2 subtests with floor violations at 4:11 and younger, and no ceiling violations
- Yields standard score, PR, and CIs
- Standard score range: 30–160
- Mean internal consistency reliability = .89 (ages 4:0–7:11); .91 (ages 8:0–21:11)

Wechsler Preschool and Primary Scale of Intelligence—Fourth Edition (WPPSI-IV)

See Table 7.9 for complete information.

General Ability Index
- 4 subtests with floor violations at ages 2:11 and younger, and no ceiling violations (ages 2:6–3:11) and 4 subtests with no floor or ceiling violations (ages 4:0–7.7)
- Yields standard score, PR, and CIs
- Standard score range: 40–160 (ages 2:6–3:11), 40–160 (ages 4:0–7.7)
- Mean internal consistency reliability = .95 (ages 2:6–3:11), .95 (ages 4:0–7.7)

Woodcock–Johnson III Test of Cognitive Abilities, Normative Update (WJ III COG NU)

See Table 7.10 for complete information.

Brief Intellectual Ability
- 3 subtests
- Standard score, PR, CIs, *W* score, age and grade equivalent scores
- Standard score range: Not specified
- Mean internal consistency reliability = .96

formed from six subtests (appearing first, second, fourth, sixth, eighth, and ninth in the WISC-IV) that demonstrate no floor or ceiling violations (see Table 7.7). As in the WAIS-IV General Ability Index, these subtests form the Verbal Comprehension Index and the Perceptual Reasoning Index from the WISC-IV. The mean reliability of the WISC-IV General Ability Index is .96 for ages 6 to 16 (Saklofske et al., 2005). A free Microsoft Excel application is available for calculating the WISC-IV General Ability Index (Raiford, Weiss, Rolfhus, & Coalson, 2010).

SUMMARY

As we have stated in Chapter 6, one of our reasons for writing this book is our belief that the understanding and measurement of cognitive abilities in applied psychology have never been stronger. The information presented in this chapter supports our contention. For example, most of the tests we have reviewed demonstrate few measurement flaws. Most include up-to-date norms; have no (or very few) subtest floor and ceiling violations; and were developed via advanced norming and measurement procedures, such as continuous norming, item response theory, and sophisticated calculations of confidence intervals. This information also demonstrates that stratum III composites (i.e., IQs) are consistently more reliable than more narrowly focused composite scores from multidimensional intelligence tests, and it is notable that stratum III composites from brief and abbreviated tests also demonstrate strong measurement properties. Our general review of tests in this chapter should provide a solid foundation for you to evaluate the evidence supporting the uses and interpretations of tests and their scores, according to the specific guidelines for selecting tests described in Chapter 5.

CHAPTER 8

Sharing the Results of Intellectual Assessments

Sharing the results of your assessment is an important and challenging activity. This sharing of results is usually accomplished through (1) psychological assessment reports and (2) face-to-face contact with the parents or caregivers of the children or adolescents completing the assessment. We have focused this chapter on these two pathways by which assessment results are shared. In order to address the needs of those in training, we also describe the process of sharing assessment results with supervisors during supervision meetings.

PSYCHOLOGICAL ASSESSMENT REPORTS

Structure

Psychological assessment reports provide a permanent record of the results of your assessment. They address the referral questions and summarize the child or adolescent's history and current functioning. They also list options for intervention based on the results (with your knowing that others will probably be tasked with selecting, implementing, and monitoring these interventions). There is some variation in how these reports are structured. We occasionally see lengthy reports (about 10–12 pages in length) that contain paragraphs about every test and every subtest, a detailed summary, and list of recommendations. On the other hand, we occasionally see reports that are filled primarily with tables presenting test results that are preceded by a sentence introducing each test and followed by a brief (two- to three-sentence) presentation of the most meaningful aspects of the results. Across styles, typical reports follow a format like that presented in Box 8.1. We discuss each section of these reports in the paragraphs that follow.

BOX 8.1. Sample Psychological Assessment Report

Anywhere Psychological Center

Psychological Assessment

Confidential

Name: Meredith Rosenbaum

Date of Initial Assessment: 03/20/2013

Date of Birth: 02/14/2006

Chronological Age: 7 years, 1 months

Parents: Nancy and Thomas Rosenbaum

School: Armstrong Elementary

Grade: Second

Examiner: Sophia Livingston, MA

Reason for Referral

Meredith Rosenbaum was referred to the Anywhere Psychological Center by Meredith's teacher, Mrs. Susan Benton. Meredith's mother reported that Meredith is a very bright girl, but sometimes her grades do not reflect this fact. This year, she reported seeing a drop in Meredith's reading and mathematics scores on classroom assignments. Ms. Rosenbaum reported that Meredith is sometimes lost in thought and that she frequently brings home incomplete classwork. She has seen these problems worsen since Meredith enrolled in elementary school.

Background Information

Meredith is a 7-year-old girl who is currently in the second grade at Armstrong Elementary School. She resides in Any City, Anystate with her parents and sibling. Meredith's father is a tax lawyer, and her mother is a stay-at-home mom. Meredith has a younger sister, Emily, who is 4 and attends a local Montessori program 5 days a week.

According to Ms. Rosenbaum, her pregnancy with Meredith was full-term. Ms. Rosenbaum stated that Meredith was born naturally, was of average weight, and experienced no serious medical conditions. Ms. Rosenbaum reported that Meredith met all developmental milestones within normal limits and has had no illnesses or injuries beyond those typical in childhood.

According to Ms. Rosenbaum, Meredith began attending the MidSouth Academy Preschool at the age of 3 and continued at the school through her kindergarten year. Her teachers noted no problems. Meredith began attending Armstrong Elementary School in first grade. Review of Meredith's most recent report card shows that she achieved M's (Meets Standards) or E's (Exceeds Standards) in all areas. However, Meredith's teacher, Mrs. Benton, noted on her report card that Meredith needs to use her class time more productively. Ms. Rosenbaum reported that Meredith scored in the 99th percentile for reading on the Standardized Test for Assessment of Reading (STAR) diagnostic test in February of 2013. Ms. Rosenbaum stated that even though this STAR diagnostic test score is extremely high, she has noticed Meredith's weekly reading scores varying dramatically. Ms. Rosenbaum added that Meredith frequently loses points on her classwork because items are incomplete.

Ms. Rosenbaum reported that Meredith is, and has always been, a very bright child. She stated that Meredith is generally happy and that she loves to read books (especially the Harry Potter series). She shared that Meredith has recently complained that school is no fun, and added that she whines about and protests going to school about twice a week.

(continued)

Meredith had not been previously tested, and her hearing and vision screenings are up to date. The date for her most recent hearing and vision screening exams was September 2012. She passed both screening exams.

Assessment Techniques

Interview with Meredith's mother, Ms. Rosenbaum
Reynolds Intellectual Assessment Scale (RIAS)
Woodcock-Johnson III Tests of Achievement
Behavior Assessment System for Children, Second Edition (BASC-2)
    Parent Rating Scales (completed by Mr. Rosenbaum)
    Teacher Rating Scales (completed by Ms. Benton)
Behavioral observations in the classroom
Behavioral observations during testing
Review of records
Review of class assignments

Behavioral Observations during Testing and Validity of Assessment

Meredith completed three sessions during the course of the assessment following an interview with her mother, Ms. Rosenbaum. Meredith's conversational proficiency seemed advanced for her age level; she used several advanced vocabulary words when describing her hobbies and her pet dog. Although Meredith appeared confident and self-assured throughout the examination, she was sometimes distracted. She was very inquisitive and often asked the examiner questions about herself and the clinic setting. During testing, she would sometimes immediately say she did not know the answer to an item, but after being prompted (especially on the RIAS) she would often answer correctly. On the BASC-2 rating scales, all validity indexes were within the Acceptable range. Overall, it is believed that the results of this assessment are valid estimates of Meredith's overall intellectual, academic, and psychosocial functioning.

Assessment Results

Cognitive Abilities

General Intelligence. Meredith completed the Reynolds Intellectual Assessment Scales (RIAS). Meredith's RIAS Composite Intelligence Index score places her in the Extremely High range when compared to other children her age (standard score [SS] = 152). The chances are 9 out of 10 that Meredith's true score falls within the range from 145 to 155. This score indicates that fewer than 1 in 1,000 children her age would be expected to obtain a score higher than hers (percentile rank [PR] = 99.9).

Specific Intelligences. Meredith's score on the RIAS Verbal Intelligence Index places her in the high end of the Extremely High range when compared to other children her age (SS = 157). Meredith's score on the Nonverbal Intelligence Index was significantly lower, but her score is still in the high end of the High range when compared to other children her age (SS = 128).

[Additional sections of results are omitted due to space limitations.]

(continued)

Summary

Cognitive difficulties were ruled out as the cause of Meredith's struggles at school by the measure of general intelligence from the Reynolds Intellectual Assessment Scale (RIAS). In fact, Meredith's scores from the RIAS indicate that she has extremely high general intelligence when compared to others her age. [Additional assessment results are not summarized due to space limitations.]

Recommendations

1. The information in this report should be shared with an Individualized Education Program (IEP) team at Armstrong Elementary School, to determine whether Meredith's current level of services is consistent with her educational needs.
2. Meredith's eligibility for the Gifted and Talented program at Armstrong Elementary should be considered.
3. Ms. Rosenbaum and Meredith's current teacher, Ms. Benton, should work together to enhance Meredith's intellectual, emotional, and personality strengths.
4. Ms. Rosenbaum should consider finding Meredith a mentor in the area of her interest. This mentor might help conceptualize career fields and expertise. A great program that could provide mentors is Mensa International (*www.mensa.org*).
5. Ms. Rosenbaum should continue to encourage Meredith to read as a hobby.
6. Meredith's parents should continue to expose her to a variety of cultural stimuli, in order to enrich her life and to help her gain knowledge from new and different experiences.
7. Meredith's parents should incorporate specific rewards tailored to Meredith's personality when she brings home schoolwork that is the product of much effort and ingenuity.

Sophia Livingston, MA

Sophia Livingston, MA
Intern

James R. Wener, Ph.D.

James R. Wener, PhD
License # FL3825347
Health Services Provider

Score Tables

Reynolds Intellectual Assessment Scales (RIAS) Age-Based Scores

Composite Scores	Standard Score	Percentile Rank	Range Based on Age
Composite Intelligence Index	152	99.97	Extremely High
Verbal Intelligence Index	157	99.99	Extremely High
Nonverbal Intelligence Index	128	97	High
Subtest	*T* Score		
Guess What	73		Very High
Verbal Reasoning	91		Extremely High
Odd-Item Out	67		High
What's Missing	62		High Average

[Additional score tables are not included due to space limitations.]

Headings

Most reports begin with a heading labeling the report and a heading labeling the results as confidential. These headings are sometimes placed under the letterhead of the clinic, hospital, or school district through which the assessment was conducted. These introductory headings are followed by a table presenting demographic information about the child or adolescent, and it is typical that the examiner's name is listed as well.

Reason for Referral

The first narrative section of the report is the Reason for Referral. This section addresses the referral questions in a clear manner. These questions may include the following: Why is this child not doing well at school? Is it a learning disability? Is it lack of motivation? Is he bored? Although we have referred to referral *questions* here, it is rare that sentences in this section are written in interrogative form; the concerns that guide the assessment and the referral agents, however, are typically addressed. This section is typically relatively brief.

Background Information

The second section is often lengthy, because it addresses the child or adolescent's history. It typically includes four general categories of content. First, demographic information is presented in narrative form and extended. Often, the first sentence provides the child or adolescent's age, gender, grade, and school. It is followed by a description of the family unit, listing the names of parents or other caregivers and siblings. Second, the child or adolescent's developmental history and medical history are addressed. Issues such as developmental delays, injuries, surgeries, previous mental health diagnoses, and prescription medications are summarized. Third, the child or adolescent's educational history is described. Results such as previous test scores, grades, and benchmark assessment results, as well as prior interventions (e.g., tutoring), are described. Finally, current functioning is described. Recent problems are detailed; content should increase understanding of the reason for referral. In this final section, a description of the child or adolescent's areas of strength and interests is sometimes provided, to underscore the importance of protective factors.

Assessment Techniques

Most reports have a section that lists the tests and other assessment techniques (e.g., interviews, review of records, and classroom observations) used to yield results during the assessment. As evident in Box 8.1, these techniques are listed and not written in complete sentences. Published instruments are capitalized (but not italicized), whereas unpublished and informal techniques are not marked with special formatting.

Behaviors during Testing Session and Validity of Assessment

Many reports include a section called Observations or Behavior Observations preceding the test results. Typical content in this section includes descriptions of behaviors during the testing session, and frequently this sections ends with a validity statement. This validity statement is the "stamp of approval" for the testing results. Often it reads like this: "The results of the standardized testing appear to be valid estimates of John's cognitive abilities and achievement." The labels Observations and Behavior Observations are not descriptive or accurate enough to represent the content of this section, however. For one thing, these section labels are too general; systematic direct observations of behavior may have been completed in settings other than the testing room (e.g., the general education classroom). Second, the typical section label fails to address the key components of this section: (1) the description of the behaviors that may have influenced the meaningfulness of the scores produced by the tests and interactions between the examiner and the child or adolescent; and (2) the results of screening conducted before testing (see Chapter 4). We prefer the more descriptive title Behaviors during Testing Session and Validity of Assessment.

Assessment Results

The foundation of the report is typically the section presenting the results of the formal assessment (in contrast to more informal methods, such as loosely structured interviews). In this section, many report writers include descriptions of all tests administered, the scores they produced, and their meaning. Typically, this section begins with the results of intelligence testing; continues to focus on the results of achievement testing; and ends with a focus on behaviors and emotions, assessed via techniques such as caregiver rating scales, direct observations, and self-report inventories. Each subsection is marked by a heading describing either the construct targeted (e.g., Intelligence or Reading) or the test administered (e.g., Wechsler Intelligence Scale for Children—Fourth Edition). Occasionally, score tables will be inserted within each section.

Summary

Many reports will conclude with a Summary section. In this section, the most important results from the prior sections are grouped. Most often, this section will include one sentence representing each subsection of the Assessment Results section. It is rare that it will contain a synthesis of results, but it will sometimes conclude with sentences addressing diagnosis or eligibility for special education.

Recommendations

The last section containing connected text in most reports is usually devoted to recommendations for parents, other caregivers, and teachers. These recommendations may address special education eligibility processes, additional assessment, home-based and classroom interventions, therapeutic services in clinic settings, and medical interventions. Typically, these recommendations are bulleted or numbered.

Signatures and Score Tables

The final two sections of a standard psychological assessment report include the signature of the report's author (and perhaps that of his or her supervisor), as well as tables providing scores from the assessment. It is standard practice for these signatures to follow the body of the report, and they signal that its content has been approved by its author (and the author's supervisor). We have seen no evidence of a transition to electronic psychological reports (e.g., with scanned signatures and saved as a .pdf); reports are still primarily distributed as hard copies. Many reports conclude with score tables following the signatures. These score tables tend to contain the norm-referenced scores for all relevant subtests and for composites on which interpretations are based.

Considerations in Writing a Psychological Report

Writing for Multiple Audiences

Different audiences may require different reports (Kamphaus, 2001; Ownby, 1997), and you should tailor your report to the intended readers and the settings in which you are working. For example, parents and other caregivers typically require that the report be written in an accessible manner, and they are likely to desire information about what they can do to improve the child or adolescent's learning and functioning. In addition, they will probably appreciate your highlighting some of the child or adolescent's positive characteristics. Teachers and special educators are likely to desire information about relative levels of performance and approximation of grade-level skills, the match of the results to special education eligibility criteria, and recommendations for evidence-based interventions. Reports may also be written for

> **Tailor your report to the intended readers and the settings in which you are working.**

supervisors, therapists, physicians, or judges (see Tallent, 1993). For these audiences, more technical terms and abbreviations may be acceptable, and the report is likely to be more focused. For example, a report written for a residential facility might focus on an adolescent's suicidal ideation or probability of relapse, whereas a report written as part of a forensic evaluation might emphasize whether a child is prepared to stand trial. We advocate a flexible style of report writing that can be tailored to multiple audiences—a "happy-medium report."

Regardless of the intended audience, you should write your report so that it is clear and accessible to most readers (Ownby, 1997). For instance, you should avoid technical terms that many readers may not understand. In particular, you should avoid using only acronyms; spell the terms out with each use, or define each acronym and use the acronym afterward. Harvey (1997) has asserted that the best marker of an accessible report is a relatively low readability score. Readability of text is most often measured via the Flesch–Kincaid Grade Level formula. This formula produces a score ranging roughly from 1 to 16 and reflecting the U.S. grade level of reading skill necessary in order to comprehend the analyzed text. Lower scores indicate greater reading ease, and readability values should be kept as low as possible (almost certainly < 12 when the report targets parents). Key variables to understanding readability are the average number of syllables per word and the average number of words per sentence (Flesch, 1948, 1949); accessible reports will exclude multisyllabic words and include relatively brief sentences.

You should include the child or adolescent's name and the names of all involved in the assessment (e.g., parents and teachers) in the report, in order to make the sources of the information clear and to contextualize the results. In our reports, we refer to the child or adolescent by first name and refer to adults by their last names, preceded by *Ms.*, *Mr.*, *Mrs.*, *Dr.*, and the like. Finally, you should strive to focus on the meaning of the results, and not on the assessment instruments and the numbers they produce. Kamphaus (2001) has shared that "one way to think of the scores is a means to an end, the end being better understanding of the child" (p. 502). We concur with this wise statement.

General Rules of Writing

The *Publication Manual of the American Psychological Association*, sixth edition (American Psychological Association [APA], 2010b) is an excellent source for recommendations for and modeling of grammar and style. When most students and some professionals think about APA style, they think narrowly about correctly formatting citations and references. They fail to consider all of the other issues addressed in the publication manual: general writing style; using the correct terms for gender, age, and race/ethnicity; appropriate use of punctuation, numbers, and abbreviations; and grammar and word selection. Table 8.1 summarizes some of the most important recommendations from the publication manual (APA, 2010b) that are relevant to writing psychological reports (plus some recommendations of our own), but you should carefully review Chapters 2 and 3 of the manual for more detailed explanations and a greater number of examples. In particular, read these chapters to enhance your technical writing skills before you begin writing reports.

Avoiding Foolish Mistakes

Your report may be the only way that many consumers of the information you provide "see you." To ensure that consumers of your reports are not left with a negative impression of your work—or, worse, that the child or adolescent you assessed is incorrectly described or misdiagnosed in your report—you should engage in multiple proofing strategies to prevent costly errors. Based on our review of the literature (e.g., Pagel, 2011), we recommend that you enter the proofing and editing phase of report generation with the belief that your draft report contains at least one costly error, which you must identify.

> **To ensure that consumers of your reports are not left with a negative impression of your work, you should engage in multiple proofing strategies to avoid costly errors.**

First, you should check and double-check the scores and the labels applied to them in your report. You should review your scores in text and scores in the score tables against those from test protocols or scoring software output. You should also compare every score to the label you provide for it (e.g., a standard score of 125 is in the High range). Your heightened neuroticism during this stage will prevent a lot of embarrassment later on.

Second, take advantage of electronic text analysis functions in your word processing program. For example, first use the Spelling and Grammar functions in Microsoft Word or other word-processing programs. In particular, you should make sure that you select the box "Use contextual spelling" to identify potential errors associated with homophone use (e.g., using *there* vs. *their*) in Microsoft Word in Word Options. However, if you do not uncheck the boxes in Word Options to "Ignore words in UPPERCASE" and "Ignore words that contain numbers" when checking for spelling errors, you may overlook a spelling error involving an acronym or test abbreviation. You should definitely uncheck them. In addition, based on excellent research by Harvey (1997), you should obtain readability statistics for your report document. In Word Options in Microsoft Word, make sure that you check the box "Show readability statistics." If the value is too high (>12), reduce sentence length and reduce the frequency of lengthy words as much as possible.

TABLE 8.1. Recommendations for General Writing Style and Word Selection in Reports

General Writing Style
- Remember that clear communication is the goal of report writing.
- Do not set a goal to be "creative," "witty," or "lively" in your report writing.
- Choose words with care, and do not vary them when describing the same concept.
- Use simple language and a straightforward writing style. Write in short, simple sentences. Avoid lots of clauses, and use semicolons and dashes sparingly. When you struggle to make a long sentence clear, break it up into shorter sentences.
- Write concisely. Eliminate needless words.
- Avoid jargon and technical terms (including medical terms). Use the most accessible terms, or define the most technical ones (e.g., *trichotillomania* as hair pulling).
- Reduce the frequency of long words. Usually, the more letters a word includes, the more difficult it is for readers to "process" it.
- Either (1) define abbreviations and acronyms initially and then use the abbreviation or acronym, or (2) spell them out each time and avoid them altogether.
- In contrast to the APA (2010b) recommendations, avoid writing in the first person (i.e., using *I* and *we*). If you must refer to yourself, write in the third person, calling yourself *the examiner* or the like.
- Emphasize words rather than numbers when describing results.
- Headings are important in reports, and they should be parallel across sections. Although centered headings and left-justified headings seem appropriate for reports, the indented headings followed by periods as recommended by the APA (2010b) are cumbersome and can easily be avoided.

Using the Optimal Terms
- Describe individuals as specifically as possible.
- Typically refer to children as *boys* and *girls*, and adults as *men* and *women*. In the case of adolescents, consider *adolescent males* and *adolescent females*, or *young man* and *young woman*.
- When referring to sexual orientation, use *gay*, *lesbian*, and *bisexual* as adjectives.
- When referring to race or ethnicity, capitalize the designation: *Black* or *African American*; *White* or *European American*; *Asian American*; *Hispanic* or *Latino/Latina*; and *American Indian*, *Native American*, or *Native North American*. When it is possible to be more specific by referring to a family's country of origin, do so.
- Capitalize languages (e.g., English, Spanish, and Mandarin Chinese).
- Avoid referring to people solely in terms of their educational, psychiatric, or medical conditions (e.g., "a class for the learning-disabled"); use person-first language instead (e.g., "a class for students with learning disabilities").
- Spell out disorders in lowercase (e.g., attention-deficit/hyperactivity disorder) but, when necessary, abbreviate in uppercase (e.g., ADHD). However, special education eligibility categories can be capitalized (e.g., Intellectual Disability and Learning Disability).
- Avoid loaded terms or those that might be misunderstood (e.g., *borderline, suffering from*).

Note. Based on American Psychological Association (APA) (2010b), except as noted.

Third, you should carefully read through your report from beginning to end while it is on your computer screen (i.e., in the word-processing program). Proofread both for content errors and for mechanical errors (moving your cursor below each word and reading text aloud as you do so). After you make edits to the text, read the sentence before each edit, the sentence containing the edit, and the sentence that follows to ensure that you have not introduced errors.

Finally, you should print and proofread at least one hard copy; some research indicates that proofreading is more accurate when conducted in the print medium (e.g., Wharton-Michael, 2008). Furthermore, you should monitor your attention to detail (and, conversely, fatigue) when proofreading; accuracy in identifying errors wanes during the reading of lengthy documents (see

Wharton-Michael, 2008). Knowing this fact may lead you to proofread from beginning to end on the computer screen, and to proofread from the end (section by section) to the beginning in hard-copy form. While you are proofreading the hard copy, you should also review page breaks to ensure that headings are not dissociated from the text that follows, and that lists and tables are not split across pages.

Reporting Content in Specific Sections

We now address four sections of the report that typically contain the most information and that require the most time and effort to complete: the Background Information section, the Behaviors during Testing Session and Validity of Assessment section, the Assessment Results section, and the score tables. We provide guidelines and sample scripts to apply in your report writing. We end with an introduction to a method for summarizing assessment findings that one of us (RGF) has used for 15 years in practice and training. Before moving forward, we want to express that there are practically no prohibitions against using text from this book, or from other prominent texts focusing on report writing—including Kamphaus (2001), Lichtenberger, Mather, Kaufman, and Kaufman (2004), Mather and Jaffe (2002), and Sattler (2008)—in your psychological assessment reports. In fact, we encourage you to use the scripts and more specific text included in this book. To appropriately include the most descriptive and clear wording in your reports, you must overcome the feeling that you are plagiarizing.

Background Information

In addressing the child or adolescent's history, you should summarize and highlight information that may affect the child or adolescent's functioning in school, home, or community settings. Doing so means that you must select the most pertinent information from a variety of sources, but a careful report writer must follow certain rules. First, you should clearly indicate the source of the information you are reporting. Two methods address this goal: (1) including a general statement at the beginning of this section, and (2) referring to the sources when specificity is needed. In many reports, we begin the Background Information section with a statement like this one: "Background information was obtained about Miranda's family, developmental, medical, psychological, and educational history through an interview with Miranda's mother, Mrs. Perez, and review of school records."

After the inclusion of this content, we then identify the source of information by using phrases like "According to Mrs. Perez," and using a variety of verbs following the informant's name to indicate what was reported. You should (1) vary these verbs, such as by using *said, stated, reported, conveyed, indicated, communicated, described, gave details about, acknowledged, articulated,* or *recounted,* versus using only one (e.g., *reported*); and (2) use past-tense verbs versus "clinical-ese," which employs primarily present-tense verbs (e.g., "Ms. Perez reports that . . . "). In general, if you are writing about things that happened in the past and that are not happening currently, use the past tense (e.g., "Miranda completed 2 years of tutoring" or "Miranda's mother reported that her pregnancy with Miranda was filled with medical problems"). If the behaviors or conditions of interest still continue, use present tense (e.g., "Miranda is currently in the second grade" and "Ms. Perez reported that Miranda reads each night before going to sleep").

Second, you should include the information in this section only if it has any potential impact on the child in relation to the referral concern. For example, the existence of a family pet, the family's religious affiliation, and the child or adolescent's favorite television shows, books, or video games need not be addressed if they are not relevant to this concern. As you consider the relevance of the content in this section, weigh issues related to the child's and the family's privacy against this relevance. Do not "air out dirty laundry"; instead, consider whether the content is too personal or too peripheral to the presenting problem to include. For example, in many cases information about children's parents, such as their mental health history (e.g., prior hospitalizations and addiction treatments) and their relationship history (e.g., prior marriages), will be too personal and too peripheral to the referral concern to include. Although we encourage comprehensive descriptions of the background information, you should be mindful of your own value judgments in your writing of this section, and take care to avoid biased terms (see Table 8.1 and APA, 2010b).

Third, you should summarize prior assessment results in this section. Prior assessments may be formal ones like the one you are describing in your report—from school districts, community mental health agencies, and the like. You should report previous psychological assessment results in summary form (and refer to the dates of prior assessments, the report authors, and the agency through which assessments were completed). In addition, lots of other assessment information is often available. For example, report card grades, discipline reports, and academic screening results may be available from the child's teacher or through a review of records. You should pepper this section with reference to time markers. You may choose to report the age of the child, the grade level, or the year (or some combination of them) when events occurred to support your chronological sequencing of events across this section.

Behaviors during Testing Session and Validity of Assessment

In the section on test session behaviors and assessment validity, you should describe in some detail the examinee's reaction to the testing environment. To accomplish this goal, you will probably include several pieces of qualitative idiographic information about the examinee (see Chapter 6 and Box 8.2). First, you should consider the importance of describing the examinee's appearance and dress. Such data may be relevant to the referral concern or educational outcome (e.g., if the child is extremely overweight or wearing obviously dirty clothes), or they may not be relevant. We do not recommend typically including content related to appearance and dress in this section—at least in part due to fear of making inappropriate value judgments—but it is a matter of professional style and judgment. Second, you should consider the examinee's behaviors that may have affected performance (for better or worse) during testing (see Chapter 4 for a detailed discussion of these issues). Because testing sessions are typically poor representations of children's typical behaviors, you should attend to behaviors during testing, such as social skills, attention, and conversational proficiency, but do not place too much trust in them as representing the "real things" in home and school settings. Do consider and place more emphasis on behaviors affecting item-level responding (and ultimately test scores). In technical terms, describe the child's test session behavior in the past tense. When you appraise or make judgment about a behavior (e.g., "Gracie appeared nervous during testing"), you should ideally support this statement with quotes and descriptions of the child's behaviors (e.g., describing trembling hands, foot tapping, and inappropriate laughter).

Perhaps the most important component of this section is its ending. According to the APA's Ethical Principles of Psychologists and Code of Conduct (APA, 2002, 2010a):

> When interpreting assessment results . . . psychologists take into account the purpose of the assessment as well as the various test factors, test-taking abilities and other characteristics of the person being assessed, such as situational, personal, linguistic and cultural differences, that might affect psychologists' judgments or reduce the accuracy of their interpretations. They indicate any significant limitations of their interpretations. (Component 9.06)

You must make a judgment about the meaningfulness of the test results—concluding that construct-irrelevant influences did not affect the test scores. For example, for children and youth from diverse backgrounds, it is important to rule out cultural and linguistic factors (e.g., opportunity to learn test content English-language proficiency) before interpreting intelligence test standard scores that are well below average as representing low general intelligence (see Chapter 13). In this section of the report, you may summarize the results of your direct screening for vision, hearing, fine motor, and articulation problems and color blindness via the Screening Tool for Assessment (see Chapter 4). And you may describe accommodations made to the standard test administration to address these problems (see Box 8.2). When all has gone well, we typically include a brief validity statement as follows: "The results from the testing appear to be valid estimates of Miranda's current cognitive abilities and academic achievement." When construct-irrelevant influences did affect the test scores, do not report or interpret those that are invalid. There are a number of ways to address construct-irrelevant influences on test scores and invalid scores; several examples are included in Box 8.2.

BOX 8.2. Examples of Text from the Behaviors during Testing Session and Validity of Assessment Section

Example 1

Zahan completed two sessions during the course of the assessment. His conversational proficiency in English was typical for his age and grade level. Zahan appeared at ease and comfortable during each session. Zahan's vision, hearing, fine motor skills, and the intelligibility of his speech were all found to be adequate for testing based on the Screening Tool for Assessment. Zahan noticeably increased his level of effort for difficult tasks, but at times, he responded too quickly, which led to errors. During achievement subtests requiring him to write sentences, Zahan sometimes stopped to stretch his hand as if it was hurting him. However, this same behavior was not observed during timed subtests on intelligence tests requiring rapid responses. The results of testing appear to be valid estimates of Zahan's current cognitive abilities, reading skills, and math skills. There is, however, some question about whether the results of the extended writing subtests accurately reflect Zahan's ability to quickly generate short sentences and to write sentences to clearly convey meaning to potential readers.

(continued)

Example 2

Oliver completed one session with the examiner. He completed the Screening Tool for Assessment, and his vision, hearing, and articulation were all found to be adequate for testing. However, Oliver had difficulties accurately tracing a straight line, a circle, and a star. In addition, in order to print letters neatly, Oliver wrote very slowly. As a result of these screening tests, the Wechsler Intelligence Scale for Children—Fourth Edition (WISC-IV) Coding subtest was replaced by the WISC-IV Cancellation subtest. Because of this modification to the standard battery of the WISC-IV, the results presented in this report are valid estimates of Oliver's general intelligence.

Example 3

Pretti completed three sessions during the course of the assessment, following an interview with her parents. During the first testing session, Pretti was administered the Woodcock–Johnson III Tests of Cognitive Abilities (WJ III COG). She reported that she was very tired because she had stayed up late to finish a paper for one of her classes. Pretti appeared drowsy and was slow in responding, and her performance was far below what was expected from her background information. The results were thought to be invalid in representing her day-to-day display of cognitive abilities. As a result, Pretti was also administered the Wechsler Adult Intelligence Scale—Fourth Edition (WAIS-IV). Pretti's performance on the WAIS-IV produced scores that were closer to what was expected, and scores were more congruent with those on the Woodcock–Johnson III Tests of Achievement; therefore, Pretti's scores from the WJ III COG are not included in this report. During all other testing, Pretti's level of conversational proficiency and cooperation were typical for her age. She was slow and careful in responding, and she generally persisted with difficult tasks. Overall, results presented in this report are valid estimates of Pretti's overall intellectual, academic, and psychosocial functioning.

Example 4

Rachelle completed three test sessions during the course of assessment. During each session, she was cooperative and maintained attention to the tasks, and she required no breaks in testing. Her conversational proficiency was typical for her age. Rachelle appeared at ease and comfortable throughout the assessment, and she generally persisted with difficult tasks.

After all testing sessions had been completed, Rachelle's mother, Mrs. Freedman, notified the clinic that Rachelle had just been prescribed reading glasses. Her prescription revealed spherical refractive error of +3.50 for the right eye and +3.00 for the left eye, indicating moderate hyperopia or farsightedness. Although Rachelle displayed no notable behaviors during testing that indicated that she had trouble seeing the letters and numbers presented to her, it is possible that her test results may have been affected by her hyperopia. In the absence of additional testing, which was declined, it cannot be concluded that the results of the current assessment are valid estimates of Rachelle's intellectual and academic functioning.

Assessment Results

With knowledge of the measurement properties of your assessment instruments (see Chapters 5 and 7) and score interpretation strategies (see Chapter 6), you should craft text to convey the meaning of your results. Typically, this section highlights nomothetic and quantitative results. In doing so, you should follow reporting conventions for standardized scores, score ranges, confidence intervals, and percentile ranks.

STANDARDIZED SCORES AND SCORE LABELS

The norm-referenced standardized scores yielded from the testing—be they deviation IQ scores ($M = 100$, $SD = 15$), T scores ($M = 50$, $SD = 10$), or scaled scores ($M = 10$, $SD = 3$)—are the data from which meaning is most typically derived. You should pair these scores with score labels that indicate their true meaning. We agree with Kamphaus (2001) that score-labeling terminology should be consistent across tests; using varied terms proposed by test authors and publishers for the same scores can only lead to errors on your part and to confusion on the part of your report's consumers. Following Schneider's (2011b) *High–Low* range labels, Table 8.2 includes a summary of narrative classifications of scores for the most commonly produced standardized scores. In Form 8.1, this summary is expanded to address narrative classifications of scores for each score type and to provide narrative descriptions of percentile ranks. It is noteworthy that the narrative classifications offered by Schneider begin and end similarly for scores above the mean and below the mean. Although we have often included score labels in our reports that are not only descriptive of performance but also may be considered somewhat snobby, such as *Superior* and *Exceptional*, we suggest using score classifications that do not have such connotations. Furthermore, we do not condone the use of the classification *Borderline* to label standard scores ranging from 70 to 79. It may be confused with *borderline personality disorder* (American Psychiatric Association, 2000), and it also indicates that about 10% of the population has either intellectual disability (ID) or *borderline* ID (see Chapter 10). The term has surplus meaning, and to us it seems outdated.

TABLE 8.2. Summary of Narrative Classifications Associated with Varying Standardized Scores

Narrative classification	Standard scores	T scores	Scaled scores
Extremely High	140+	77+	18–19
Very High	130–139	70–76	16–17
High	120–129	64–69	14–15
High Average	110–119	57–63	12–13
Average	91–109	44–56	9–11
Low Average	81–90	37–43	7–8
Low	71–80	31–36	5–6
Very Low	61–70	24–30	3–4
Extremely Low	≤60	≤23	1–2

Note. Based on Schneider's (2011b) High–Low range labels.

We believe that (1) capitalizing score classifications and (2) making frequent and explicit reference to the norm group on which scores are based are wise practices. For example, you can report that "Phillip's Full Scale IQ is in the Low range when compared to others his age," and then follow such statements with brief references to standardized scores and percentile ranks in parentheses. Furthermore, you can make reference to the high end or low end of a score range and occasionally report dual score ranges (Average to High Average) if the standard score is within 3 points of another score range or the *T* score is within 2 points of another score range. Examples of text used to describe standard scores and their associated score ranges appear in Box 8.3.

CONFIDENCE INTERVALS

We encourage you to employ confidence intervals during interpretation and reporting of results. As described in Chapter 6, norm-referenced scores from intelligence tests are never perfectly accurate. To account for this less-than-perfect accuracy, report a band of uncertainty around scores by using confidence intervals.

BOX 8.3. Text for Standardized Scores, Confidence Intervals, and Percentile Ranks

Standardized Scores

- According to age-based norms, Jill's overall cognitive ability is in the Very Low range.
- Juan's knowledge of word meanings and general information is in the Average range when compared to that of others his age (WISC-IV Verbal Comprehension Index = 103).

Confidence Intervals

- The chances are 9 out of 10 that Antwan's true IQ falls within the range of 101 to 109 when compared to others his age.
- Cedric obtained a WISC-IV Full Scale IQ of 122, and we can be 90% confident that his true WISC-IV Full Scale IQ falls within the range of 117–125.
- Ivy's DAS-II General Conceptual Ability score was 91 (±7).
- When considering that general intelligence cannot be measured perfectly, Mallory's RIAS Composite Intelligence Index score falls between 95 and 105 with 95% confidence.

Percentile Ranks

- According to age norms, about 98% of Jill's age-mates would be expected to have earned a higher score (percentile rank = 2).
- Sarah scored as high as or higher than only approximately 10% of children her age.
- Kay's percentile rank of 99.5 indicates that only 5 in 1,000 children her age would have a score higher than hers.
- Sally scored at the 28th percentile; she scored as high as or higher than only about one-quarter of children her age.

Confidence intervals are reported in a number of ways, and there appears to be no convention for doing so. As evident in Box 8.3, they may be reported as a range of scores following the obtained score, or with a plus or minus indicating what number was added to and subtracted from an obtained score. We often include another sentence following the initial report of the standardized score (e.g., the IQ) that addresses the confidence interval in a more detailed manner. We believe that either the 90% confidence interval (as recommended by Kamphaus, 2001) or the 95% confidence interval should be applied. We have found that the 90% confidence interval seems to be easier to describe (referring to the probability as 9 out of 10 times) and understand than the 95% confidence interval (referring to the probability as 19 out of 20 times).

> **Norm-referenced scores from intelligence tests are never perfectly accurate. To account for this less-than-perfect accuracy, report a band of uncertainty around scores by using confidence intervals.**

PERCENTILE RANKS

Remember that percentile ranks represent some of the same information about normative variation as standard scores, and the same score labels can be applied to them (see Form 8.1 and Box 8.3). They seem to be more easily understood by parents and teachers than standardized scores, so their judicious use in reports is wise (Wiener & Constaris, 2011). Typically, these scores are reported to reflect the percentage of children the same age (if age-based norms were used) who would have performed the same or lower on a task. Reporting that "Samantha's performance on the Wechsler Intelligence Scale for Children—Fourth Edition Full Scale IQ exceeded that of approximately 25% of children her age" is appropriate. Alternatively, the *reflected* percentile rank value can be used when scores are very low or very high. For example, a percentile rank of 1 indicates that 99% (100% − 1% = 99%) of children would score higher. Conversely, a percentile rank of 99 indicates that only 1% of children would score higher. Narrative descriptions used to describe percentile ranks appear in Form 8.1.

TEST INFORMATION

We recommend that you consistently capitalize the names of tests and subtests, but not capitalize words like *subtest, composite, index,* or *cluster,* unless such a word is part of the proper noun (e.g., the Verbal Comprehension Index). (Note that we have used italics here to mark linguistic examples; there is no need to use italics for these terms in reports.) Unlike Kamphaus (2001) and others, we do not believe that there is much utility in describing the structure of and intended use of intelligence tests. For example, many authors will include a full paragraph describing the number of subtests included in an intelligence test, the age range for which it is appropriate, and the range of score types yielded. Just as you are probably not concerned about the calibration of the electronic thermometer used in your primary care physician's office or the method used to determine your cholesterol levels, we believe that most consumers are not interested in the specifics of the test you used.

We encourage you to develop text to describe the meaning stemming from interpretation of the most reliable and valid scores produced by the intelligence tests (see Chapter 6). One of the benefits of increased understanding of the relations among cognitive abilities is that you may offer interpretations that are more theoretical than concrete (i.e., subtest- or test-based) by making reference (1) to the cognitive abilities being targeted; and (2) to deviance from the mean, when you are interpreting norm-referenced scores (see Ownby, 1997). On the other hand, from a qualitative and idiographic perspective, we understand the desire to examine patterns of errors when norm-referenced scores are lower than expected. In accordance with our KISS model, however, patterns of errors from intelligence tests should typically not be interpreted (see Chapter 6). When describing item content in a report, you must also walk a fine line between maintaining test security (e.g., by not revealing item content in your report) while also describing the child's behavior in response to items. Ideally, rather than quoting or describing specific items from such tests, you should develop descriptions of close parallels or describe patterns in general terms. In general, we believe that describing item-level behaviors as reflecting skills that have been mastered is far more important when you are focusing on assessment of achievement (i.e., reading, writing, and mathematics) than when you are interpreting results from intelligence tests.

Score Tables

Score tables appearing within the body of or at the end of reports are intended for use primarily by other professionals (see Tallent, 1993). Despite our advocacy of the KISS model, which suggests that interpretation be based primarily on the most reliable and general scores yielded by intelligence tests, we encourage you to list all relevant scores in the score tables (e.g., subtest scores, composite scores, and IQs) so that others can access your most basic norm-referenced scores for consideration.

We have always maintained table templates for the tests that we have used most frequently in practice and that we have provided instruction to others in using; such tables can easily be constructed by using the Insert Table function in Microsoft Word. Such tables are far more flexible than using tabs and underscores; narrowing and widening columns and highlighting table borders can be accomplished easily in Microsoft Word. Recently, we have begun using TableMaker for Psychological Evaluation Reports, developed by Schneider and available free online (*http://assessing-psyche.wordpress.com/2012/04/25/tablemaker-for-psychological-evaluation-reports*). This program includes a wide variety of score table templates for intelligence tests (and a variety of other test types). We have found it to be very user-friendly for developing new tables, and some assessors may choose to enter all relevant scores from an assessment into this application and develop and format all the respective tables across instruments at once. These tables from TableMaker can be easily exported to Microsoft Word.

Major Findings: An Alternative to the Traditional Report Sections

In addition to traditional report formats, it is our goal to introduce in this chapter one variant of a traditional report-writing style. It omits the Assessment Results and Summary sections presented in Box 8.1 in favor of integrated paragraphs addressing the important questions raised before the assessment as well as the findings from the assessment; each of these integrated paragraphs is followed by recommendations tailored to them. Below, we describe these Major Findings reports and how to construct them.

Whereas the Summary section in traditional reports typically includes a narrative description of the results, the goal of Major Findings is to integrate the assessment results in a meaningful way (Kamphaus, 2001). We believe that this format makes the report more practical and useful, and there is indirect research support for this conclusion. In many ways, these Major Findings reports are consistent with the organization of the "question-and-answer" format studied by Wiener (1985, 1987) and Wiener and Kohler (1986), which has been shown to be comprehended better and preferred more by elementary teachers and parents than traditional and one-page short-form report formats. They are also consistent with hypothesis-oriented models of report writing, because they address referral concerns so explicitly (see Ownby, 1997).

Preassessment: Preconditions for a Major Findings Report

Of course, the planning of a comprehensive assessment and its implementation are important preconditions for producing a strong, meaningful report. In the preassessment stage, the referral concern should be defined thoroughly so that you are able to determine what specific problem areas to target, what eligibility or diagnostic categories to consider, and what expectations the clients have for the assessment. With this information, you should select assessment instruments carefully, considering both their measurement characteristics and the constructs they target. Your goal is to represent the constructs of interest, using formal and informal assessment instruments and techniques to yield both quantitative and qualitative information. Your constructs may range from general and specific cognitive abilities to reading, writing, and math skills and academic self-efficacy; to internalizing problems (e.g., depressed mood) and externalizing problems (e.g., aggression); to physiological variables and medical problems; and to psychosocial stressors. You may use assessment methods such as intelligence tests; achievement tests; interviews with teachers, parents, and children; observations in naturalistic settings and behaviors during the test session; parent and teacher rating scales; self-report rating scales; review of permanent products; and review of records and prior assessments. The key point in preparing for a comprehensive assessment is to use multiple assessment methods, call on multiple informants, and consider behavior in multiple settings, to promote an understanding of the "whole child."

> In preparing for a comprehensive assessment, use multiple assessment methods, call on multiple informants, and consider behavior in multiple settings, to promote an understanding of the "whole child."

Postassessment: Interpretation and Development of Major Findings

There are at least eight steps to follow in considering your assessment results (see Form 8.2). First, you should evaluate the validity of your quantitative results and evaluate the evidence you have for conclusions drawn from qualitatively based inferences. As discussed in Chapter 4, you should consider the influence of construct-irrelevant influences on test scores, and as discussed in Chapter 6, you should consider that you (like everyone else) are prone to critical thinking errors. Second, you should follow the KISS model and identify deviant scores on measures of interest. In general, obtained scores outside the Average range may be concerning; however, we consider deviant scores as those at least a standard deviation above or below the mean. Deviant scores are markers of exceptionality and may be important in your decision making.

Third, you should consider qualitative idiographic data from the test session that may be relevant. Examples include verbal statements (such as "I am so stupid!" offered during a test session) and behaviors (such as extreme hyperactivity before, during, and after test sessions). Fourth, you should consider all quantitative and qualitative information from other methods that may be relevant. They may include quantitative results from direct behavior observations (e.g., percentage of time on task), errors common across test sessions and permanent products (e.g., spelling errors and letter reversals), and observed speech problems.

Laying out all of these quantitative and qualitative data allows you to engage in bottom-up (i.e., data-driven) analysis while integrating, and these data—be they overlapping or contradictory—should be grouped or clustered into related major findings. The goal of this clustering is to be integrative. We have found the multiaxial system in the *Diagnostic and Statistical Manual of Mental Disorders*, fourth edition, text revision (DSM-IV-TR; American Psychiatric Association, 2000) to be a useful organizing framework. Although the multiaxial system was not retained in the *Diagnostic and Statistical Manual of Mental Disorders*, fifth edition (American Psychiatric Association, 2013), you should first consider how your results relate to known psychological disorders, disabilities, or other conditions that cause academic, social, or occupational impairment (see the DSM-IV-TR's Axis I, Axis II, and Axis V). You should consider medical problems that are related to or distinct from psychological disorders, disabilities, or other conditions (Axis III). Furthermore, you should consider psychosocial and environmental problems that have caused, contributed to, or resulted from the identified problems (Axis IV).

Next, you should consider not only your data from the assessment, but your referral question per se. Sometimes integration based on only the most notable results from your assessment does not directly promote your addressing the referral question. Thus, you must also cluster information to address those concerns if they have not already surfaced. Here you should engage in top-down (i.e., concept-driven) analysis while integrating.

You should also consider information that does not seem to fit into a cluster, but that you believe is important to the prevention or treatment of a problem. This information is often qualitative in nature and obtained through informal assessment techniques. For example, we sometimes address issues related to (1) odd behaviors (e.g., chewing on clothing and picking at dead skin on lips and fingers) observed during the testing section or reported by only a single informant; (2) fatigue and sleep problems; and (3) issues related to promotion decisions (i.e., retention) mentioned by parents and teachers.

Once you have developed clusters of information to address the full range of results and referral concerns, develop a theme for each one. In your mind, consider each one to be like a topic sentence or a conclusion based on your results. Each cluster or group of clusters becomes a Major Finding. Some Major Findings are wide in scope, and others are narrow. Examples of Major Findings focusing on intelligence test results appear in Box 8.4. In some ways, each Major Finding should represent your answer to a question (e.g., "Does Jimmy meet diagnostic criteria for ID?"). You may also think of Major Findings as the brief summaries or points you would like to make if you were given only 5 minutes to present the results. Once you have developed the Major Findings, you should consider all the opportunities to address each one via recommendations. We have found books by Shinn and Walker (2010) and Mather and Jaffe (2002) to be extremely helpful in generating ideas for recommendations, but you should always strive to offer recommendations that are evidence-based.

BOX 8.4. Sample Major Findings Addressing Intelligence Tests Results

Example 1

Major Finding 1

Meredith's general intelligence is extremely high when compared to that of others her age. She obtained a Reynolds Intellectual Assessment Scales (RIAS) Composite Intelligence Index score of 152, which is in the Extremely High range. She scored significantly higher on an RIAS composite representing her vocabulary and world knowledge (Verbal Intelligence Index = 157) than on an RIAS composite representing her ability to reason and process visual information (Nonverbal Intelligence Index = 128), but both scores indicate advanced abilities in these areas.

[Recommendations for this Major Finding are reported in Box 8.1.]

Example 2

Major Finding 1

Bobby was referred for assessment due to his low grades in school and his recent standardized test scores indicating below-basic and below-proficient academic skills; his mother wondered whether he has a learning disability. As part of this assessment, Mrs. Conner rated Bobby on the Behavior Assessment System for Children, Second Edition (BASC-2) Teacher Rating Scale as being in the Clinically Significant range on the Learning Problems (T score = 74) scale. She reported that Bobby almost always has trouble keeping up in class, often complains that lessons go too fast, and obtains failing grades.

Bobby's cognitive abilities were assessed by the measures of general intelligence, IQs, from the Reynolds Intellectual Assessment Scales (RIAS) and the Woodcock–Johnson III Tests of Cognitive Abilities (WJ III COG). Bobby's performance on the four subtests contributing to the RIAS Composite Intelligence Index indicated that his IQ is in the Extremely Low range (standard score [SS] = 67) when compared to children his age. The chances are 9 out of 10 that Bobby's true score falls within the range from 64 to 73. Approximately 99% of other children his age would be expected to receive a score higher than Bobby (percentile rank [PR] = 1). Bobby performed similarly on the WJ III COG. His performance on the seven subtests contributing to the WJ III COG General Intellectual Ability— Standard indicated that his IQ is at the lowest portion of the Low range (SS = 71). The chances are 9 out of 10 that Bobby's true score falls within the range from 67 to 75. These IQs are not significantly different from one another.

Bobby's difficulties at school are likely to stem from deficits associated with his application of higher-order thinking and reasoning skills and acquisition of knowledge. His IQs are notably lower than those typically expected in cases of learning disabilities, and they indicate that Bobby displays significantly below-average intellectual functioning when compared to other children his age. It seems likely that deficits in receptive and expressive language are associated with these deficits in intellectual functioning.

Recommendations

1. Ms. Roberts should submit this report to the eligibility team at Bobby's school, to seek a consultation from a speech–language pathologist.
2. Bobby should participate in a variety of class activities that focus on vocabulary knowledge and language-building skills.

(continued)

3. Bobby's teachers should assess his prior knowledge before introducing new topics and concepts.
4. When adults are presenting directions and discussing concepts at home and in the school setting, they should make a conscious effort to use vocabulary that Bobby can easily understand.

Major Finding 2

The Adaptive Behavior Assessment System, Second Edition (ABAS-II) Parent Rating Scale (PRS) and Teacher Rating Scale (TRS) were used to assess Bobby's adaptive skills. Ms. Roberts's ratings on the ABAS-II PRS place Bobby's Global Adaptive Composite (GAC) in the Low Average range (SS = 81). Her ratings place Bobby in the Low to Low Average range on all other ABAS-II PRS domains. Mrs. Conner's ratings on the ABAS-II TRS place Bobby's GAC in the Very Low range (SS = 61). Her ratings also place Bobby in the Very Low range on all other ABAS-II domains. In addition to deficits associated with Bobby's application of higher-order thinking and reasoning skills, general knowledge, and processing of language (as addressed in Major Finding 1), Bobby lacks some adaptive skills that are needed for a child his age, especially in the school setting. Bobby would benefit from activities in the home and school environment that are geared toward enhancing his adaptive skills.

Recommendations

1. Bobby should be taught to perform more and more activities on his own in his home, and to be encouraged to complete them with minimal assistance or independently.
2. Ms. Roberts should reinforce in the home the academic, daily living, and social skills that Bobby learns at school.
3. Because Bobby has difficulty interacting with peers, he should participate in interventions that teach behavior control and appropriate social skills.
4. Ms. Conner and Bobby's other teachers should ensure that Bobby's assignments are adjusted to his level of language and reading competence.

Major Finding 3

As noted in Major Finding 1, Bobby's IQ was in the Very Low range (SS = 67) on the RIAS and at the lowest end of the Low range (SS = 71) on the WJ III COG when compared to the IQs of his peers. These IQs are not significantly different, and substantial proportions of their confidence intervals fall at 70 and below. They indicate significantly below-average intellectual functioning when compared to that of other children his age. As noted in Major Finding 2, Mrs. Conner and Ms. Roberts reported that some adaptive behavior deficits are evident both at home and at school. In addition, during the parent interview, Ms. Roberts reported that Bobby gets "taken advantage of" because he is "naïve."

Results indicate that Bobby is probably eligible for special education services under the Intellectual Disability (formerly Mental Retardation) category. According to the state guidelines, Intellectual Disability is determined by appropriate assessment of intelligence indicating significantly impaired intellectual functioning, which is an IQ of approximately 70 or below. The state guidelines also convey that there must be a significant impairment in adaptive behavior in the home or community, as well as a significant impairment in adaptive behavior in the school. Although his mother's ratings of adaptive behavior are higher than those of his teacher and do not indicate severe impairment in the home or community setting, the body of evidence seems to indicate that Bobby experiences impairment in communication, social, and practical domains across settings, and that this impairment is probably due in part to his low level of intellectual functioning compared to that of others his age.

(continued)

Recommendations

1. Ms. Roberts should submit this report to the eligibility team at Bobby's school to determine whether Bobby meets eligibility criteria for Intellectual Disability.
2. A behavior management plan should be set up at home and in the classroom, in which Bobby can earn rewards for on-task behavior and completion of work.
3. Ms. Roberts should know that Bobby is capable of developing appropriate social and communication skills, and that he can further advance his academic skills substantially. When he becomes an adult, he can achieve social and vocational skills adequate for self-support and live successfully in the community.

Example 3

Major Finding 1

Consistent with Colin's previous diagnosis of mental retardation, this assessment indicated that Colin's functioning is notably lower than that of his same-age peers in the intellectual and adaptive domains. Previous assessments had yielded IQ scores in the very low range for his age. In 2009, his Differential Ability Scales General Conceptual Ability score was revealed to be 36, and his Leiter International Performance Scale—Revised Full IQ was revealed to be 53. The current assessment results are congruent with the previous findings, as well as with the criteria for mental retardation/intellectual disability. His Wechsler Intelligence Scale for Children—Fourth Edition Full Scale IQ (standard score [SS] = 40) and his Differential Ability Scales, Second Edition General Conceptual Ability score (SS = 33) were similarly low when compared to those for others his age. Colin scored in the Extremely Low range on both tests, and his percentile ranks were <0.1.

The previous adaptive behavior assessment in 2009 revealed that Colin's overall display of adaptive behavior was also well below average for his age. Based on his mother's report in 2009, his Adaptive Behavior Composite score from the Vineland Adaptive Behavior Scale, Survey Interview was 61. Again, the current assessment results are congruent with the previous findings, as well as with the criteria for mental retardation/intellectual disability. Based on his mother's reports on the Vineland-II Survey Interview, his Adaptive Behavior Composite was 66, which is in the Very Low range when compared to that of others his age. The results of this assessment indicate that Colin continues to meet criteria for mental retardation/intellectual disability and should continue to receive intensive intervention services in the school setting.

Recommendations

1. The information in this report should be shared with an Individualized Education Program (IEP) team, to determine whether Colin's current level of services is consistent with his educational needs.
2. Colin should continue receiving special education services, with attention directed toward the development of functional skills through life skills training.
3. Colin's parents are encouraged to review information about transitions programs for students with disabilities, and the IEP team should ensure that a transition plan is developed. Colin's parents may benefit from reviewing information provided about transition programs via the National Down Syndrome Society website (at *www.ndss.org* under "Transition Planning").

Challenges and Benefits in Constructing Major Findings Reports

We see at least two challenges to writing Major Findings reports. First, many professionals are unfamiliar with such reports, and they may seem somehow odd to them. In the same vein, few training resources currently address the development of Major Findings. However, other resources cited in this chapter discuss such integrative methods. Second, it appears to us that developing Major Findings is more intellectually challenging than writing paragraphs devoted to each test used and a summary of results, like those appearing in traditional reports. We suspect, however, that showcasing the case conceptualization skills needed to write Major Findings is the goal of every report writer. We fear that many report writers have insufficient time to complete the process of developing Major Findings, but we know that once they have developed Major Findings to address the most prominent issues surfacing in their practice, tweaking previously written text in Major Findings will be far easier than developing it from scratch. In any case, we believe that the benefits of these reports outweigh potential challenges. Major Findings should provide more meaningful conclusions than summaries included in traditional reports.

THE INFORMING SESSION: PRESENTING THE RESULTS OF YOUR ASSESSMENT

Whereas report writing can be completed in the quiet of your office or a room in a school, clinic, or hospital, you are on stage and in the spotlight when you are asked to describe your findings to the parents or others involved in the assessment (and sometimes to the children and adolescents themselves). In providing this information, you should channel your expertise in test selection, score interpretation, and identification of mental disorders and educational conditions to answer the referral concerns and facilitate the implementation of interventions.

The informing session represents a collaborative process by which you convey the most important findings from your assessment and guide your clients toward effective interventions. We have developed scripts for presenting segments of results and have seen many other assessment professionals do the same. We provide our general outline for presenting results in a university-based psychology clinic in Form 8.3. Below, we offer three broad recommendations when presenting these results: (1) Be prepared, (2) communicate clearly, and (3) promote discussion and use good listening skills.

> **The informing session represents a collaborative process by which you convey the most important findings from your assessment and guide your clients toward effective interventions.**

Preparation

Campbell (2006a) stated that preparation can manifest itself in selecting a setting that is private, quiet, and comfortable for all involved. Although most clinics have conference rooms for such meetings, those working in school settings may need to devote more thought to the setting and the timing of the meeting than those working in other settings may. You should also make sure you have allowed enough time for a parent who needs consultation, consoling, or a referral. In fact, Pope (2010) encourages assessors to anticipate low-probability events (e.g., a parent's anger or revealing of information previously withheld) and develop contingency plans for dealing with them.

We suggest scheduling informing sessions for at least an hour and perhaps more, depending on the level of support needed based on the conclusions from the assessment. In addition, it is wise to be prepared for tears—either of joy or of sorrow. Having a box of tissues nearby reflects that wisdom. Preparation is also needed to determine when to convey the most potentially upsetting results—for instance, a diagnosis of a mental disorder, or the presentation of results indicating sub-optimal performance when there is striving for entrance to programs. We generally recommend saving potentially distressing content for the last segment of the meeting. In addition, you should provide parents with resources (such as handouts, website listings, and the titles of books, and the names of those who can provide interventions) at the informing session. We highly recommend resources such as *Helping Children at Home and School III* (Canter, Paige, & Shaw, 2010), which contains handouts that can be provided to parents or appended to the report.

Communication

Once you are in the session, you should communicate the assessment results clearly. We agree with Kamphaus (2001) that you should be genuine, honest, and forthcoming with information, while also considering the experiences and expectations of those to whom you are reporting the results. To promote clarity, we suggest that you organize your results around Major Findings as previously described and that you supplement your verbal statements with concrete visual aids. For example, we encourage you to consider using a drawing of the normal curve (similar to Form 8.4) when presenting results. This figure will allow you to increase the meaningfulness of descriptions of the norm-referenced scores.

When presenting these results, you may also convey messages orally that you would not necessarily write in your report. For example, we teach students to differentiate standardized scores (especially deviation IQ scores) and percentile ranks from typical scores on school-based exams, which are measured in the *percentage correct* metric. For example, we say,

> "Based on your time in school and from reviewing your child's tests and homework, you are probably accustomed to reviewing 100 as the best score. These scores we will be discussing today include two types. For one type, standard scores, 100 is the perfectly average score—with about 50% of children obtaining higher scores and 50% obtaining lower scores. For the other type, percentile ranks, 100 is an unattainable score, because we are roughly considering where scores fall in ranking your child's performance when it is compared to the performance of 100 typical children her age. I will give these percentile ranks to you as percentages ranging from 1% to 99%."

Finally, it is acceptable to share the responses written on protocols and response booklets to display errors made by the examinees or to generally convey your message more clearly. Such sharing should be done sparingly to protect test security, however.

Discussion

You must not only communicate your messages clearly, but also promote discussion and listen carefully to parents' questions and concerns. We encourage you, early in the informing session, to encourage questions and commenting on findings. We also encourage you to issue "check-ins" throughout. For example, you may ask open-ended questions—such as "Can I clarify any point I made?" and our favorite, "Are those the results you expected?"—after you have presented a Major Finding. When the parents respond, use your best listening skills, such as maintaining eye contact, leaning toward them, summarizing their points, and describing the emotions they must be feeling.

Meetings in which assessment results are presented can be challenging, and we strongly encourage students in training and emerging professionals to practice their communication skills—especially with parents from a variety of backgrounds—and to seek feedback about them from supervisors and others who may be attending the same meeting (e.g., during a school-based team meeting). Recording these sessions with audio or video devices (with approval from all involved) and reviewing them carefully will often reveal many areas to target for improvement.

STAFFING A CASE WITH A SUPERVISOR

For students, interns, and those engaging in postdoctoral supervision, we offer some guidelines for sharing your results with your supervisors during *staffings*. Staffings differ from presentations of assessment results to parents and other caregivers, because you and your supervisors have generally the same knowledge base. As a consequence, you are free to use acronyms and technical terms during your oral presentation, and to move rapidly through your assessment results. We offer the following general recommendations, and an outline is provided in Form 8.5.

Being Organized

When entering the supervision session, you should have all of your assessment results with you and have these materials organized in the order you plan to present the results, so that you can access them easily. In a staffing, you are typically referring to the hard copies of the actual interview forms, protocols, and scoring software output, so striving for completeness and organization of these materials is vital. Furthermore, because a staffing occurs so quickly after the assessment is complete, it is not generally expected that you will have initiated your report writing or will have summarized test results in a written document; however, you should have begun to conceptualize the case and consider prevailing and rival hypotheses.

Presenting Results

As you begin presenting your results, you should strive for brevity and should focus on presenting the test results and your evaluation of them. You should also be prepared to respond to your supervisor's questions and to search for additional information from your notes, test protocols, and scoring software output to answer those questions. We have found that the following sequence of presenting results is common, logical, and consistent with most psychological reports, and we encourage you to adhere to it during initial staffings with your supervisor.

First, present the demographic information about the examinee (such as name, gender, age, race/ethnicity, and grade). Second, describe the referral concern and those involved in it. Third, present background information. You should focus on information directly relevant to the referral concern, but consider addressing the family constellation, developmental history, and academic history. Do not forget to label the source of any information that may not be a verifiable fact. Fourth, present your valid assessment results. Typically, begin with intelligence test results and follow with achievement test results. Consistent with the KISS model of interpretation, focus primarily on the most reliable composite scores, and highlight those that are normatively deviant. Fifth, focus on the results from other forms of assessment. For example, report results of rating scales targeting social–emotional functioning completed by parents and caregivers, teachers, and the child or adolescent. Again, focus on the most reliable composite scores and on scores that are normatively deviant; ignore others if they are irrelevant to the referral concern and not elevated. Finally, integrate the results—perhaps in Major Findings. Consider "rule-outs," engage in steps to make a differential diagnosis, and consider eligibility or diagnostic criteria. Recommendations are not typically developed until after the results have been summarized, so withhold coverage of them until later.

SUMMARY

After you have completed and scored your assessments, your job is not complete. You must make meaning of the results, integrate them, and consider relevant questions brought to you by referral agents. This chapter has highlighted three pathways by which you can address these goals through communicating the results of a psychological assessment in writing and orally. It has also included models and other resources for facilitating completion of these activities.

Narrative Classifications Associated with Varying Standardized Scores and Percentile Ranks Three Standard Deviations above and below the Mean, and Narrative Descriptions of Percentile Ranks

Narrative Classification	Standard Score	*T* Score	Scaled Score	Percentile Rank	Narrative Description of Percentile Ranks
Extremely High	160	90		99.99%	Only about 1 in 10,000 would score as high
	159	89		99.99%	
	158	89		99.99%	
	157	88		99.99%	
	156	87		99.99%	
	155	87		99.99%	
	154	86		99.98%	
	153	85		99.98%	
	152	85		99.97%	
	151	84		99.97%	
	150	83	20	99.96%	
	149	83		99.95%	
	148	82		99.93%	
	147	81		99.91%	Only about 1 in 1,000 would score as high
	146	81		99.89%	
	145	80	19	99.87%	
	144	79		99.83%	
	143	79		99.79%	
	142	78		99.74%	
	141	77		99.69%	
	140	77	18	99.62%	
Very High	139	76		99.53%	
	138	75		99.44%	
	137	75		99.32%	

(continued)

Narrative Classification	Standard Score	*T* Score	Scaled Score	Percentile Rank	Narrative Description of Percentile Ranks
Very High (continued)	136	74		99.18%	Only about 1 in 100 would score as high
	135	73	17	99.02%	
	134	73		98.83%	
	133	72		98.61%	
	132	71		98.36%	
	131	71		98.06%	
	130	70	16	97.72%	
High	129	69		97.34%	
	128	69		96.90%	Obtaining roughly the highest score in a typical class of 25 students
	127	68		96.41%	
	126	67		95.85%	
	125	67	15	95.22%	Obtaining roughly the highest score in a typical class of 20 students
	124	66		94.52%	
	123	65		93.74%	
	122	65		92.88%	
	121	64		91.92%	
	120	63	14	90.88%	Scoring higher than about 9 out of 10 peers; only about 1 out of 10 would score as high
High Average	119	63		89.74%	
	118	62		88.49%	
	117	61		87.15%	
	116	61		85.69%	
	115	60	13	84.13%	
	114	59		82.47%	
	113	59		80.69%	Scoring higher than about 4 out of 5 peers; only about 1 in 5 would score as high
	112	58		78.81%	
	111	57		76.83%	
	110	57	12	74.75%	Scoring higher than about 3 out of 4 peers; only about 1 in 4 would score as high

(continued)

Narrative Classification	Standard Score	T Score	Scaled Score	Percentile Rank	Narrative Description of Percentile Ranks
Average	109	56		72.57%	
	108	55		70.31%	Scoring higher than about 7 out of 10 peers
	107	55		67.96%	
	106	54		65.54%	
	105	53	11	63.06%	
	104	53		60.51%	Scoring higher than about 3 out of 5 peers
	103	52		57.93%	
	102	51		55.30%	
	101	51		52.66%	
	100	50	10	50.00%	Like most other children; perfectly average
	99	49		47.34%	
	98	49		44.70%	
	97	48		42.07%	
	96	47		39.49%	Scoring lower than about 3 out of 5 peers
	95	47	9	36.94%	
	94	46		34.46%	
	93	45		32.04%	
	92	45		29.69%	Scoring lower than about 7 out of 10 peers
	91	44		27.43%	
Low Average	90	43	8	25.25%	Scoring lower than about 3 out of 4 peers; only about 1 in 4 would score as low
	89	43		23.17%	
	88	42		21.19%	
	87	41		19.31%	
	86	41		17.53%	
	85	40	7	15.87%	
	84	39		14.31%	

(continued)

Narrative Classification	Standard Score	T Score	Scaled Score	Percentile Rank	Narrative Description of Percentile Ranks
Low Average *(continued)*	83	39		12.85%	
	82	38		11.51%	
	81	37		10.26%	Scoring lower than about 9 out of 10 peers; only about 1 out of 10 would score as low
Low	80	37	6	9.12%	
	79	36		8.08%	
	78	35		7.12%	
	77	35		6.26%	Obtaining roughly the lowest score in a typical class of 20 students
	76	34		5.48%	
	75	33	5	4.78%	Obtaining roughly the lowest score in a typical class of 25 students
	74	33		4.15%	
	73	32		3.59%	
	72	31		3.10%	
	71	31		2.66%	
Very Low	70	30	4	2.28%	
	69	29		1.94%	
	68	29		1.64%	
	67	28		1.39%	
	66	27		1.17%	Only about 1 in 100 would score as low
	65	27	3	0.98%	
	64	26		0.82%	
	63	25		0.68%	
	62	25		0.56%	
	61	24		0.47%	

(continued)

Narrative Classifications Associated with Varying Standardized Scores and Percentile Ranks *(page 5 of 5)*

Narrative Classification	Standard Score	*T* Score	Scaled Score	Percentile Rank	Narrative Description of Percentile Ranks
	60	23	2	0.38%	
	59	23		0.31%	
	58	22		0.26%	
	57	21		0.21%	
	56	21		0.17%	
	55	20	1	0.13%	
	54	19		0.11%	Only about 1 in 1,000 would score as low
	53	19		0.09%	
	52	18		0.07%	
	51	17		0.05%	
Extremely Low	50	17		0.04%	
	49	16		0.03%	
	48	15		0.03%	
	47	15		0.02%	
	46	14		0.02%	
	45	13		0.01%	
	44	13		0.01%	
	43	12		0.01%	Only about 1 in 10,000 would score as low
	42	11		0.01%	
	41	11		0.01%	
	40	10		0.01%	

Steps for Developing and Writing Major Findings

1. Determine whether quantitative scores are valid. Interpret informal, indirect measures with caution.

2. Identify deviant scores (normatively low or high scores) on valid measures of interest.

3. Identify behaviors or statements during the test session that are clinically relevant.

4. Identify pieces of information from other measures or techniques that are clinically relevant.

5. Cluster the evidence into relevant categories, based on deviant scores and clinically relevant information. Examples of such categories include the following:

   A. Psychological disorders, disabilities, or other conditions that cause academic, social, or occupational impairment (see DSM-IV-TR, Axis I, Axis II, and Axis V).

   B. Medical problems that are related to or distinct from psychological disorders, disabilities, or other conditions (see DSM-IV-TR, Axis III).

   C. Psychosocial and environmental problems that caused, that contributed to, that mediated or moderated display, and/or that resulted from the identified problems (see DSM-IV-TR, Axis IV).

6. Consider the concerns raised in the referral question, and cluster evidence to examine those concerns if they have not already surfaced from data-based clustering.

7. List other evidence that does not seem to fit into a cluster that you believe is important to the prevention or treatment of a problem.

8. Develop the theme of each cluster.

Script for Presentation of Assessment Results to Parents and Other Caregivers

1. Make small talk. Ask for updates about the child or adolescent and family.

2. Explain why you are meeting, and mention upcoming goals.

   "I wanted us to come together to discuss the findings from the assessment. One thing I will do today is summarize all that we have learned about _____ [and his or her school, etc.] during the assessment process. Please know that I will have completed the final written report within 2 weeks, and I will contact you when it is ready for you to pick up."

   "I also wanted to thank you for giving me the opportunity to work with _____."

3. Summarize the assessment process.

   "About __ months ago, we met to discuss your goals for the assessment. We also discussed _____'s history during that meeting. I also gave you some rating scales to complete, and you gave me permission to communicate with _____'s teacher and to ask him or her to complete a rating scale, too. Afterward, I visited _____'s school to observe him or her with peers and in the classroom. Then _____ came to visit the clinic, and he or she completed a number of tests—tests of reading, writing, and math, as well as intellectual abilities. In addition, I chatted some with _____ about home and school life, and asked him or her to complete a rating scale. Finally, you and I met again to complete another interview focusing on what behaviors _____ displays in the home setting. Now we can discuss the results of the entire assessment grouped into the most central concerns for _____, and after each one, I will provide some recommendations. As I am discussing them, please do not hesitate to interrupt me and to ask questions. Do you have any questions before we begin?"

4. Summarize the referral concern.

   "When we first met, you said you were concerned about [referral concern]. Is that correct?"

5. Present results in a structured manner—perhaps organized by Major Findings—and address some recommendations after each set of results.

   "I am going to start by discussing . . . "

   "In particular, you were most concerned about _____," or "You particularly wanted to understand better _____. The results of the assessment indicate . . . "

   "Next, I would like to discuss . . . "

6. Ask for a response, and be prepared to listen.

   "Now that we have reviewed the results, do you have any further questions or concerns or issues I can clarify?" or "Were these findings what you were expecting?"

7. Close the meeting.

   "Thank you again for your time and for meeting with me—and for being helpful and patient throughout this process."

FORM 8.4

Understanding Scores from Testing

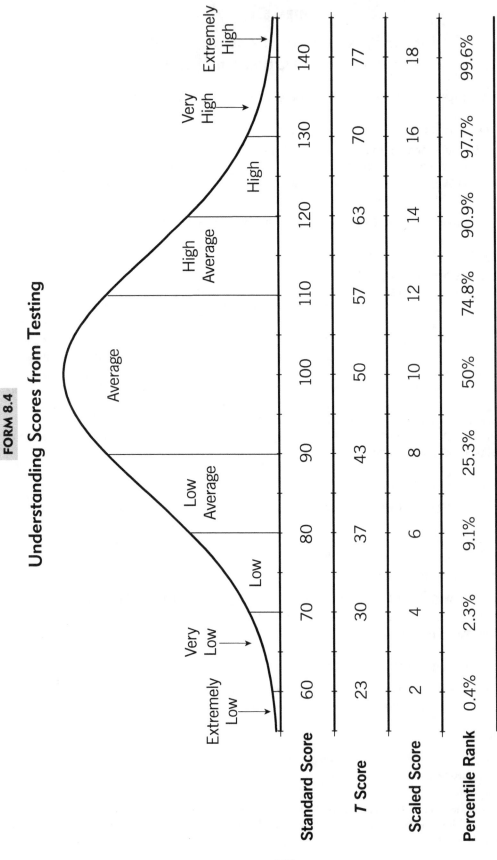

	Extremely Low	Very Low →	Low	Low Average	Average	High Average	High	Very High →	Extremely High →
Standard Score	60	70		80	90	100	110	120	130	140
T Score	23	30		37	43	50	57	63	70	77
Scaled Score	2	4		6	8	10	12	14	16	18
Percentile Rank	0.4%	2.3%		9.1%	25.3%	50%	74.8%	90.9%	97.7%	99.6%

Content to Include When Staffing a Case with a Supervisor

1. Child or adolescent's first name (and last name, if requested): _____

2. Child or adolescent's gender: _____

3. Child or adolescent's age: _____

4. Child or adolescent's race/ethnicity: _____

5. Child or adolescent's grade and school: _____

6. Child or adolescent's referral agent and referral concern: _____

   _____

7. Background information: _____

   _____

   _____

8. Intelligence test results: _____

   _____

   _____

9. Achievement test results: _____

   _____

   _____

10. Behaviors in home and community settings: _____

    _____

    _____

11. Behaviors in school setting: _____

    _____

    _____

12. Child or adolescent's reports: _____

    _____

    _____

13. Summary and diagnostic impressions or Major Findings: _____

    _____

    _____

    _____

    _____

    _____

CHAPTER 9

Response to Intervention and Intellectual Assessment

The assessment of general cognitive ability, or psychometric *g*, was for many years mandated by law for determining eligibility for special education and related services (e.g., for establishing the presence of intellectual disability [ID], specific learning disability [SLD], or intellectual giftedness). In schools, the overall score on standardized tests of intelligence (i.e., an IQ) traditionally has been used as a measure of *concurrent validity*—that is, as a benchmark against which to compare students' current academic achievement, adaptive functioning, or both. For example, the concept of *discrepancy* between general cognitive ability and academic achievement has historically been central to definitions of SLD (see Chapter 12). On the basis of these definitions, children and youth have been identified with SLD when their academic performance falls significantly below what one would expect from their IQ, and when that discrepancy cannot be explained by certain exclusionary criteria (e.g., inadequate educational opportunities and sensory disorders).

The use of intelligence tests, however, has been surrounded by controversy since their inception (e.g., Cronbach, 1975; Gould, 1994, 1996; Siegel, 1989; Snyderman & Rothman, 1987, 1988). In particular, the IQ–achievement discrepancy approach to the identification of SLD has been severely criticized on psychometric grounds (e.g., Francis et al., 2005). Current U.S. special education law—the Individuals with Disabilities Education Improvement Act of 2004 (IDEA, 2004)—allows, but does not require, the determination of a discrepancy between IQ and achievement for the identification of SLD. Less controversial is the use of intelligence tests for the identification of ID (which is still required under IDEA) and for intellectual giftedness.

> **Current United States special education law allows, but does not require, the determination of a discrepancy between IQ and achievement for the identification of SLD.**

In recent years, *response to intervention* (RTI, a.k.a. *multi-tiered systems of support* or MTSS) have received a great deal of attention as a viable model for delivering psychological services in the schools and as an alternative to the IQ–achievement discrepancy method of defining and identifying children with SLD and other disabilities (e.g., Jimerson, Burns, & VanDerHeyden, 2007). A generic model of RTI can be generally described as follows: (1) Students are provided with core instruction by their classroom teachers; (2) universal benchmark screening is conducted three times a year to track their progress; (3) those who do not respond get additional instruction from their classroom teachers or others; (4) their progress is monitored monthly to weekly; and (5) those who still do not respond are referred for a comprehensive assessment (Fuchs, Mock, Morgan, & Young, 2003).

Although RTI is not employed in a uniform manner across all school districts, the problem-solving model is arguably the most widely used approach to its implementation today (e.g., Deno, 1989). Fuchs (1995) has proposed a three-phase process for assessing academic difficulties within the problem-solving model. At Tier 1, the growth rate of all students in the mainstream classroom is monitored to determine the general effectiveness of instruction. Tier 2 involves the identification of students who are performing well below grade-level expectations, despite generally effective instruction. Targeted supplemental services are then provided to such students. Finally, Tier 3 involves planning and monitoring intensive, individualized interventions for children who are at risk for academic failure. In this model, special education and related services are considered only when these educational adaptations fail to improve student academic performance. At Tier 3, comprehensive assessments are conducted to provide information with the goal of designing the most effective intervention.

AIMS OF THIS CHAPTER

There is currently a great deal of debate about the utility of intelligence tests in the problem-solving model. Some argue that intelligence tests are of limited use in the schools, because discrepancy definitions do not effectively discriminate between low-achieving students and those with learning disabilities (Fletcher, Lyons, Fuchs, & Barnes, 2006), and because IQs do not predict response to interventions (e.g., Gresham & Vellutino, 2010). In contrast, others contend that comprehensive assessments must include tests of cognitive ability to measure basic psychological processes in order to be consistent with the definition of SLD in IDEA (e.g., Naglieri & Kaufman, 2008). Given the recent shift in the field of school psychology toward the RTI service delivery model, the focus of this chapter is on the utility of intelligence tests for following the problem-solving model. It is a "downsized" version of a chapter of ours in another book (Floyd & Kranzler, 2013), and it discusses how those engaged in the problem-solving process can apply their understanding of individual differences in general cognitive ability to the practice of school psychology.

Throughout the history of the field, intelligence testing has been one of the cornerstones of training and practice in school psychology (Fagan & Wise, 2007). With the increasing focus on multi-tiered service delivery systems and the use of RTI methods in schools, intelligence testing may occupy a less central role in the delivery of school-based psychological services. Nevertheless, we contend that intelligence testing can contribute to the problem-solving process employed by school psychologists and other professionals. We focus on the interpretation and use of intelligence tests, because we believe that the preponderance of evi-

> **With the increasing focus on multi-tiered service delivery systems and the use of RTI methods in schools, intelligence testing may occupy a less central role in the delivery of school-based psychological services.**

dence supports their use under certain conditions when questions arise about the academic achievement of school-age children.

INTELLIGENCE AND INDIVIDUAL DIFFERENCES

A Brief Review of Research Findings

We first briefly review some of the key research findings discussed in Chapters 1 and 2, to provide a context for discussion of the role of intelligence in schools and schooling; we are assuming that some readers may skip ahead to this chapter, given the timeliness of the topic in the field. Please see these two chapters for more in-depth discussion.

As discussed in Chapter 1, intelligence involves abstract reasoning and thinking, the capacity to acquire knowledge, and problem-solving ability (e.g., Snyderman & Rothman, 1988). Intelligence, in other words, reflects a broader and deeper capability for comprehending that is more than "book learning" or "test-taking skill" (e.g., Eysenck, 1998; Neisser et al., 1996). Individuals differ in their ability to understand complex ideas, to learn from experience, and to engage in various forms of reasoning (e.g., Gottfredson, 2000). As Jensen (1989b) stated, "certain people can acquire particular knowledge and skills that some others cannot acquire at all with any amount of training. Such conspicuous individual differences in learning are most commonly thought of as differences in intelligence" (p. 37). In schools, individual differences in intelligence are manifested in differences among students in the rate at which they acquire academic skills and knowledge, and in their ability to generalize and apply knowledge in new contexts (Braden, 1997).

Regarding the assessment of intelligence, as mentioned in earlier chapters, two things are definitely known beyond dispute. First, the vast majority of intelligence tests measure essentially the same thing (i.e., the same source of individual differences). The degree to which they measure the same source of variance is evident in the high correlations among scores on such tests (i.e., IQs). Second, IQs correlate more highly with assessments of scholastic performance than any other measurable educational or psychological variable that is independent of IQ. These findings do not mean that other ability, personality, and background factors are not importantly related to academic success, or that the inclusion of such variables would not increase predictive validity in addition to IQ.

Nonetheless, aside from direct measures of prior academic achievement (which are also influenced by individual differences in intelligence), no other single item of information that we can presently obtain is as predictive of scholastic performance as IQ. The prediction of real-world criteria from intelligence tests is far from perfect, however. At most, intelligence tests explain approximately 50% of the variance in academic performance, which means that at least half the variance in school grades and achievement test scores is accounted for by other, noncognitive factors. In other words, other things besides intelligence do matter in everyday performance (e.g., Gottfredson, 1997).

On intelligence tests, by far the single largest independent component of individual differences is psychometric g. The general factor usually accounts for more variance than all group factors combined; it is a large superfactor. In addition, psychometric g is a better predictor of performance in school or college, military training programs, and employment in business and industry than any other combination of variables *independent* of g (e.g., Jensen, 1998). Research indicates that g is directly related to the complexity of information processing—and not to specific skills, strategies, or knowledge measured on tests.

Although intelligence tests tend to be excellent measures of psychometric g, the question of how to interpret intelligence test scores when there is significant subtest scatter or variation in composite scores ostensibly measuring more specific abilities is an important issue on which there has long been wide disagreement (e.g., Fiorello et al., 2007; Freberg, Vandiver, Watkins, & Canivez, 2008; McDermott, Fantuzzo, & Glutting, 1990; Watkins, Glutting, & Lei, 2007; see Chapter 6 for further discussion). The preponderance of evidence suggests that on intelligence tests, "profile, scale, and factor score differences do provide opportunities for extensive interpretation of test results; however, despite the long tradition of this practice, empirical support does not exist for the accuracy or utility of these interpretations" (Reschly, 1997, p. 444).

Advances in theory, research, and statistical methodology may lead to exciting breakthroughs in the diagnostic accuracy and treatment utility of intelligence tests, but at the present time, research does not support the analysis of intraindividual patterns of subtest scores or composite scores for group differentiation (e.g., SLD vs. non-SLD; see Flanagan & Harrison, 2012). The only robust aptitude × treatment interaction[*] (ATI) that has been found in the cognitive domain is between psychometric g and method of instruction (for reviews, see Braden & Shaw, 2009; Cronbach & Snow, 1977; Snow, 1977). Instructional methods that yield a beneficial interaction with psychometric g are those that minimize the information-processing demands on students with low general cognitive ability. In contrast, for students with high general cognitive ability, the most effective instructional methods are those that place the burden of information processing on students, encourage self-direction, and utilize discovery or inquiry methods (see Snow, 1977; Snow & Yalow, 1982).

Should We Use Measures of Psychometric g in RTI? If So, When?

As described in the previous section, given the predictiveness of general cognitive ability and the ATI between g and method of instruction for students with lower cognitive ability, there is good reason for school psychologists *not* to abandon the use of intelligence tests in school and related settings. These reasons are evidence-based, reflective of current technologies in psychometrics, and practical in nature.

> **Given the predictiveness of general cognitive ability and the ATI between g and method of instruction for students with lower cognitive ability, there is good reason for school psychologists *not* to abandon the use of intelligence tests.**

Individual Differences in Psychometric g and Their Correlates

Despite the fact that the effects of intelligence, or psychometric g, are probabilistic and not deterministic (e.g., Gottfredson, 1997), scores from intelligence tests do predict academic achievement to a considerable extent. By focusing exclusively on the outcomes of instruction, school psychologists and educators run the risk of assuming that all students will be able to perform at grade level, given the appropriate kind and amount of instruction. Although every student should be encouraged to achieve in school to the best of his or her ability, the reality is that individual differences in psychometric g will be related to individual differences in the rate of learning, and consequently to the ultimate level of learning within the same time frame. Braden (1997) has stated:

---

[*] An aptitude × treatment interaction (ATI) occurs when the effectiveness of interventions varies as a function of the specific abilities of individuals.

> Genuine appreciation of diversity should prompt educators to encourage, rather than eliminate, intellectual and academic differences. However, the real issue is not whether schools will continue intelligence testing. Other than special education, there is nothing to continue. The real issue is whether schools will embrace instructional methods and outcomes assessments that accommodate or promote intellectual differences. (p. 246)

Research Base and Mature Technologies

A number of authors (e.g., Esters, Ittenbach, & Han, 1997; Kamphaus, 2010) have asserted that intelligence tests are *mature technologies*—producing measures representing psychometric g with highly similar reliability and validity, and based on a unifying theory. Consistent with this perspective, Floyd (2010) has noted that

> school psychologists now have access to, more than at any point in history, many well-developed cognitive ability tests that produce reliable and well-validated scores. It appears that these cognitive ability tests have benefited from the incorporation of a larger body of research as well as prominent models of cognitive abilities. (p. 49)

Gone are the days in which practitioners were limited to the Stanford–Binet and the Wechsler intelligence scales. Alfonso, Flanagan, and Radwan (2005) and Floyd, Clark, and Shadish (2008) have described how the most popular intelligence tests are aligned with the three-stratum theory, and how they all produce reliable and valid IQs (as discussed in Chapter 7). To produce measures of psychometric g in their assessments, practitioners may call on (1) full-length, multidimensional intelligence tests, such as the Kaufman Assessment Battery for Children, Second Edition (KABC-2; Kaufman & Kaufman, 2004a), the Differential Ability Scales, Second Edition (DAS-II; Elliott, 2007), and the Woodcock–Johnson III Tests of Cognitive Abilities (WJ III COG; Woodcock, McGrew, & Mather, 2001); or (2) brief intelligence tests, such as the Wechsler Abbreviated Scale of Intelligence—Second Edition (WASI-II; Wechsler, 2011) and the Kaufman Brief Intelligence Test, Second Edition (KBIT-2; Kaufman & Kaufman, 2004b). In addition, several nonverbal tests of intelligence are available for assessing children and youth who are not proficient in English, fully acculturated in mainstream American society, or both; or who have sensory impairments that preclude the administration of a language-loaded test (Braden & Athanasiou, 2005). Widely used nonverbal instruments include the Wechsler Nonverbal Scale of Ability (WNV; Wechsler & Naglieri, 2006) and the Universal Nonverbal Intelligence Test (UNIT; Bracken & McCallum, 1998). All of the tests just mentioned, and many others, are reviewed in Chapter 7.

Legal and Practical Constraints

We believe that intelligence tests should be used in the problem-solving process for both legal and practical reasons. For example, at the present time, all major diagnostic, classification, and eligibility systems require consideration of IQs for at least some educational conditions or disorders. For instance, consider the diagnosis of ID. The American Psychiatric Association (2000, 2013), the World Health Organization (2007), the American Association on Intellectual and Developmental Disabilities (AAIDD, 2010), and IDEA (2004) all define ID in terms of deficits in general ability (often, but not always, as measured by IQs) with concurrent deficits in adaptive functioning and onset during the developmental period (see Chapter 10). In addition, as noted previously, current federal special education law (IDEA, 2004) allows, but does not require, the determination of a discrepancy between IQ and achievement for the identification of SLD (see Chapter 12). Finally, many states define intellectual giftedness in terms of exceptionally high general cognitive ability as measured by intelligence tests, in addition to other criteria (McCoach, Kehle, Bray, & Siegle, 2001; McClain & Pfeiffer, 2012). Because gifted students are not protected under current federal special education law (IDEA, 2004), states must delineate their own definitions of giftedness. The criteria used for the identification of intellectual giftedness, therefore, vary to some degree across states (see Chapter 11).

In addition, intelligence tests may be important to problem solving when psychologists do not have ready access to teachers, school classrooms, or information from school settings in general. It is not infrequent that parents want an assessment of their child conducted outside the school setting (independent educational evaluations) either as a "second opinion" in addition to a school-based assessment, or as a private assessment due to fractured relationships within the school, lack of confidence in the school-based assessment, or other personal reasons (IDEA, 2004). Furthermore, a total of about 1.5 million children (2.9% of the school-age population) in the United States are home-schooled (Institute of Education Sciences, 2008). Based on this statistic, it is possible that school psychologists employed outside school settings might not have access to the teacher interview data, observation data, and curriculum-based measurement (CBM) benchmarking and progress-monitoring data often used in school settings for applying the problem-solving model. As a result, they may need to employ intelligence tests as part of their evaluation procedures, particularly to provide reference points for comparisons to achievement test performance. Thus, the evidence base focusing on the nature and correlates of psychometric *g*, current testing technology, and legal and practical constraints all warrant consideration of intelligence tests during problem-solving activities focused on academic achievement—at least under some circumstances.

USING INTELLIGENCE TEST RESULTS WITHIN AN RTI MODEL

In this section, we focus on using the results from intelligence tests within the problem-solving model. We begin with a general discussion of the match between the central features of problem solving and intelligence test interpretation; we continue with a more detailed analysis of the potential contributions and limitations of intelligence tests when psychologists are engaging in problem solving.

Central Features of Problem Solving

Aligned Features

Given that *intelligence* is defined as the ability to reason abstractly, to solve problems, and to learn new information, IQs share a number of features with other types of information considered to be important during the problem-solving process advocated in the recent school psychology literature (see Merrell, Ervin, & Gimpel Peacock, 2012). For example, IQs are quantitative representations of *observable* "intelligent behaviors," and these quantitative representations are *objectively obtained*. Just as samples of reading behaviors are taken from curriculum-based measurement oral reading probes to produce fluency scores (Derr-Minneci & Shapiro, 1992), IQs stem from samples of behavior in response to standard methods designed to capture the targeted general abilities. Thus, like other standardized assessment procedures, they do so while reducing the influence of many potential confounds that may affect test performance. These samples of intelligent behaviors, when compared to other samples from large groups, produce very reliable indexes with very small standard errors of measurement, and predict a variety of important educational and social outcomes as discussed previously.

Although some judgment is required of examiners in administering and scoring intelligence tests (like that required in completing any other assessment technique), the resulting IQs are objectively obtained. These scores are likely to be far more reliable and valid in predicting outcomes than teacher or parent ratings, especially before the onset of a course of study. Thus intelligence tests are not as susceptible to errant attributions, biases, and context effects as informant ratings and verbal reports from interviews are (see De Los Reyes & Kazdin, 2005).

Features with Weak Alignment

IQs do not readily demonstrate two other features that seem to make them antithetical to the problem-solving process: They do not produce *context-specific* information about specific problem behaviors, and they are not easily linked to specific recommendations for intervening to alter those problem behaviors.

CONTEXT SPECIFICITY

Although intelligence tests are a cost-effective method for obtaining important information about the prediction of general learning outcomes stemming from 1- to 2-hour test sessions (in comparison with a teacher working directly with a student for several weeks to gather the same information), they do not yield much information that is context-specific (Reschly & Grimes, 1995, 2002). That is, they do not sample behaviors that represent the specific concerns of parents and teachers (e.g., reading decoding errors). In addition, they sample behaviors outside the classroom and home settings where these specific problems typically occur.

The criticism that intelligence tests do not produce context-specific information relevant to typical learning environments is not unfounded, but it warrants additional consideration. Psychometric *g* is closely related to *learning ability*, which is correlated with the knowledge and skills that are acquired through learning, but it is important to note that learning ability and the acquisition of knowledge and skills are not the same thing (Jensen, 1998). IQ reflects the cumulative effects of an individual's acquisition of declarative and procedural knowledge in prior informal and formal learning environments, but these effects are general in nature. Thus intelligence tests produce molar explanations for academic difficulties that are not meaningfully linked to specific problem behaviors, whereas other assessment techniques (from systematic direct observations to error analysis of permanent products) provide more molecular explanations for solving specific problems. We acknowledge that these other assessment techniques ultimately produce results that are more conducive to the development of corrective inter-

> **IQ reflects the cumulative effects of an individual's acquisition of declarative and procedural knowledge in prior informal and formal learning environments, but these effects are general in nature.**

ventions than intelligence test results are, but we believe that assessments of general cognitive ability (via IQs) are important, given the difficulties students with low IQs have in learning at a rate comparable to that of the mainstream.

Although it is certainly true that intelligence tests fail to sample all types of intelligent behavior—indeed, this is an impossibility, given that the list of example behaviors is theoretically infinite—we know of no assessment instruments (e.g., reading decoding tests) that sample all components of the targeted construct (e.g., all diphthongs used in English), and no general assessment techniques (e.g., systematic direct observations) that capture all behaviors under consideration and that can be counted on to generalize to most other settings and across time (see Hintze & Matthews, 2004, for discussion of direct behavior observations). Nevertheless, the sampling of intelligent behaviors by intelligence tests is typically so broad and general that the resultant scores predict with significant accuracy the concurrent and long-term outcomes previously described—without apparent content overlap between the predictor and outcome.

It is important to note that because psychometric g is related to processing complexity, intelligence tests will be most predictive of educational outcomes that involve perceiving abstract or conceptual relationships. Those outcomes that primarily consist of rote learning or associative memory, such as the information processes required in reading decoding, will be predicted relatively poorly by intelligence tests and perhaps not at all in highly range-restricted groups of poor readers (e.g., Stuebing, Barth, Molfese, Weiss, & Fletcher, 2009). It is true that as products of this characteristic of generality, IQs provide a benchmark against which to compare achievement now and in the near future, but IQs are not able to explain at a micro level why a child struggles with a specific classroom assignment or to predict small changes in learning rate over the short term.

LINKS TO INTERVENTIONS

Consideration of IQs is not necessarily as outcome-focused as is interpretation of other more narrowly focused, context-specific assessment methods. Research has shown that the malleability of IQ is quite limited, even with dramatic environmental interventions such as adoption (e.g., Locurto, 1990, 1991; Rowe, 1994). Moreover, although certain cognitive skills can be taught, such learning is typically quite context-bound and shows limited general transfer to other domains (e.g., Detterman & Sternberg, 1993). As a result, typical interventions to address varying levels of intelligence are typically general accommodations to increase or decrease the complexity of tasks or instruction; these accommodations are generally taken for granted by those targeting basic skill development, because those interventions already largely consist of rote memory and associative learning (see Gresham & Witt, 1997) — precisely the outcomes that are least well predicted by psychometric g.

Because there is an absence of evidence indicating that IQs (and related scores from intelligence tests targeting more specific abilities) provide direct links to effective academic interventions (a.k.a. treatment utility; Braden & Kratochwill, 1997; Gresham & Witt, 1997), school psychologists must ponder how to apply an understanding of individual differences in psychometric g—a general and relatively stable trait after children reach school age (e.g., Ramey, 1992, 1994)—to their practices, which tend to focus on the assessment of and interventions for specific and alterable behaviors. If psychometric g, with all of its predictive properties, can be measured reliably and validly with intelligence tests, it seems as if it is a *person variable* that is worthwhile to consider during problem solving. In cases of academic problems, according to Bandura's (1978) triadic model of reciprocal determinism, person variables interact with behaviors and the environment (producing mutual effects) throughout development to explain some aspects of both academic accomplishments and academic problems (see Merrell, 2008, for a review). We believe that psychometric g is one such person variable, and that as such, it should not be ignored during problem solving.

Specific Applications to Problem Solving

In the four subsections that follow, we address briefly how IQs can be used, with other assessment techniques, to address achievement problems within the standard stages of problem solving. Of course, when intelligence tests are employed, they should be incorporated in a comprehensive assessment process to ensure that assessment results are cross-validated and contextualized to the maximum extent possible.

Identify the Problem

The first question—"Is there a problem, and if so, what is it?"—guides problem solvers to determine the existence of a perceived problem in academic performance and to clarify its nature (Deno, 2002). Questions such as "Is Evan reading at the level we expect of first-grade students?" and "Is Zoe achieving at the level we expect her to achieve in her geometry class?" are asked at this stage. To answer these questions, information should be gathered from direct assessments of academic performance, teacher interviews, child or adolescent interviews, classroom observations, and review of permanent products to aid in answering these questions. In addition, because children and youth learn at different rates, we believe that expectations for academic performance should be individualized to reflect normal individual differences in the classroom.

Given the substantial correlation between achievement and psychometric g, intelligence tests could be used to predict expected performance for individual students, based on the average achievement of children with the same level of general cognitive ability. Some have suggested that intelligence tests could be used as screening tools to identify children at risk for academic difficulties prior to the onset of instruction, perhaps accompanying the routine vision and hearing tests administered at the beginning of each school year (Brown-Chidsey, 2005). Results of screening measures also would facilitate the identification of intellectually gifted children (see Brown, 2012). In this manner, school psychologists and educators would better understand the normal variability in the classroom and would be able to identify students with above-average cognitive ability who might be meeting expectations for the classroom as a whole but are underachieving in terms of their ability.

Define the Problem

The second step in problem solving, designed to answer the question "Why is the problem happening?", leads problem solvers to develop hypotheses to explain the reason for the problem identified in the first step, and to aid them in formulating interventions. In applications of the problem-solving model, academic expectations are based on the performance of "typical" same-grade peers, without regard to individual differences in learning rate (i.e., intelligence) or subpopulation membership. A common set of local or national norms is used for all students at a particular grade level. When local norms are used, the backgrounds (e.g., learning opportunities) of all children are assumed to be similar. But the backgrounds of all students sometimes differ greatly in schools, particularly when school districts take steps to balance the racial/ethnic or socioeconomic composition of schools (e.g., through busing) or when students change schools often. The use of a common benchmark with heterogeneous populations may not be appropriate for all students, because it will not reflect individual differences in rates of learning.

In typical applications of the RTI model, problem solvers assume, without completing a comprehensive assessment, that the primary cause of any academic problem is insufficient instruction. This narrowing of explanatory variables to those that are relatively easily modified (i.e., environmental variables) is both pragmatic and prudent for many academic problems (especially during the elementary school grades, when typical skill development is rapid). In contrast, as mentioned previously, individual differences in intelligence represent a person variable that is manifested in differences in learning rates among students. Learning rate may be overlooked in a narrowly focused assessment, because it cannot be adequately inferred from measures of concurrent skill development and measures of short-term growth.

Moreover, research indicates that learning problems are also associated with an increased risk for internalizing and externalizing problems (e.g., American Psychiatric Association, 2000; McNamara, Willoughby, & Chalmers, 2005). Learning disabilities may be risk factors for difficulties in other areas of children's lives, but it is also the case that internalizing and externalizing problems can result in difficulties in learning. For these reasons, we believe that more comprehensive assessments—ones that consider a range of variables affecting school success—are needed to inform interventions at the problem definition stage. More comprehensive assessments may range from screening of externalizing and internalizing problems to administration of intelligence tests.

School psychologists operating within the problem-solving model should use a variety of assessment techniques to collect information to test hypotheses regarding the reasons for school problems. These techniques may include interviews, systematic direct observations, rating scales, direct assessment of academic skills, and review of permanent products. The most probable explanations for academic problems, such as specific skill deficits, performance deficits, and problems with generalization of learning, should be assessed with the most reliable, valid, and time- and cost-efficient instruments. Thus, we encourage school psychologists to target malleable academic skills and related behaviors and to engage in assessment of the proximal and distal contexts in which learning occurs (e.g., student instruction, student curricula, and their educational environment during assessment; Howell, Hosp, & Kurns, 2008; Ysseldyke & Elliott, 1999).

We add, however, that person variables should not be ignored at the problem definition stage. In fact, intelligence tests may offer their greatest benefit at this stage (Brown-Chidsey, 2005) in representing general learning ability, as well as contributing to special education eligibility or diagnoses. For example, a nationally normed intelligence test yielding a low IQ for a child with very low letter-naming and number-naming scores on 1-minute probes (when compared to other children in the fall of first grade at this school) would lead an examiner to conclude that the child in question reasons abstractly, solves problems, and learns new information at a slower rate than other children of this age. It is reasonable to conclude that this child's low general ability has had a strong influence on academic behaviors in the classroom, and that these behaviors affect those around the child (e.g., leading the teacher to provide more prompts for academic task completion and to provide more one-on-one instruction). This child's low general ability also has probably led to escape from many academic tasks appropriate for most others at the same grade level, and has limited the generalization of specific academic behaviors to related behaviors and settings beyond those in which instruction occurs. If this child earns an IQ of 70 or below and displays concurrent deficits in adaptive functioning and impairment in the school and home settings, an educational condition warranting special education services and a psychiatric disorder warranting a diagnosis of ID would be apparent.

Explore Alternative Interventions

The third step in problem solving, designed to answer the question "What should be done about the problem?", addresses intervention development and implementation; it logically follows from the conclusions drawn at the second step. As noted previously, there is no strong body of evidence supporting the use of intelligence test results for tailoring academic interventions to students' needs. Of course, it makes good sense to intervene to address children's problem behaviors; such interventions are based on the preliminary assumption that specific skill deficits and performance deficits are the cause of these problem behaviors. For example, a student who has difficulties with correct placement of digits in columns when adding numbers may simply need to be taught how to do it correctly through explanations, modeling, and guided practice. It is intelligence, however, that mediates the student's response to instruction across time, and some students learn mathematics skills more quickly than others. However, learning is more highly correlated with IQ when the material to be learned is hierarchical—that is, when the learning of later concepts depend upon mastery of previously taught concepts, such as mathematics.

We heed Cronbach and Snow's (Cronbach, 1975; Cronbach & Snow, 1977) warnings that attending to ATI and coping with a swarm of ATI hypotheses can be like entering a hall of mirrors, and we recognize that differentiated instruction based on the ipsative (i.e., intraindividual) assessment of specific cognitive abilities (see Good, Vollmer, Katz, Creek, & Chowdhri, 1993; Gresham & Witt, 1997) has not produced positive effects warranting its use. Nevertheless, we contend that a body of evidence is available to support the contention that psychometric *g* is a grand aptitude that necessitates our attention, and that these interaction effects are most evident at very high and very low levels of psychometric *g*. For example, if academic problems identified at earlier stages of problem solving are at least partially due to general normative weaknesses in the ability to reason abstractly, solve problems, and learn new information, expectations can be altered to acknowledge (1) that interventions designed to address the academic problems are likely to be less effective in producing academic achievement consistent with grade-level expectations, and (2) that many academic skills are likely to be acquired at a slower rate than expected across school years.

One challenge that many school psychologists will face when considering psychometric *g* as a grand aptitude is the knowledge that it is a general, relatively stable person variable. Merrell et al. (2012) offer these comments about another human characteristic, visual acuity:

> When developing interventions, it is important to focus on what we can change to enable learning and reduce the discrepancy. For example, knowing that a student has a significant visual impairment is important for instructional planning, but it is unlikely that the cause of the visual impairment will be the focus of the intervention for school personnel. Instead, it is likely that the school will consider instructional accommodations (e.g., modified materials, vocal cues) to enable the student to benefit from instruction, despite the visual impairment. (p. 162)

Consistent with this statement, interventions for children and adolescents with very low and very high levels of psychometric *g* may need to be altered in accordance with their level of cognitive ability.

Apply Selected Interventions

The fourth step in problem solving, designed to answer the question "Did the intervention work?", focuses problem solvers on collecting data to deter-

> **Interventions for children and adolescents with very low and very high levels of *g* will probably need to be altered.**

mine whether the interventions based on the most viable hypotheses lead to reductions in the problem once they are implemented. Instruments that are designed to target specific malleable skills, and that can be administered quickly and repeatedly, will be more useful at this stage than intelligence tests (which were not designed for either purpose). Because of their predictiveness with achievement outcomes, intelligence test results could be helpful in determining the potential of academic interventions, based upon general expectations of learning rate. However, because IQ is less predictive of low-level learning outcomes, the usefulness of these results for predicting basic academic skill growth in the short term will probably be limited.

SUMMARY

This chapter has highlighted the evidence base describing the nature and correlates of psychometric *g*; advances in testing technology; and legal and practical constraints that warrant consideration of intelligence tests during use of the problem-solving model. Although full-length intelligence tests were arguably the "jewel in the crown" of psychologists in the schools for a century or more, they will probably continue to play an important, but narrower, role in the schools related to determining level of general cognitive ability. We believe, though, that intelligence tests produce measures of one of the most explanatory variables in all of the social sciences, psychometric *g*, and that this should be considered when school psychologists are using modern problem-solving methods to seek answers to children's academic problems. The remaining chapters in this book address how to accomplish this goal.

CHAPTER 10

Assessment of Intellectual Disability

The purpose of this chapter is to describe the clinical condition known as *intellectual disability* (ID), and to offer practical guidelines for assessing children and adolescents suspected of having this condition. We begin by presenting varying diagnostic and eligibility criteria for ID, and end by offering recommendations for best practices in assessment.

DEFINITION, DIAGNOSIS, AND ELIGIBILITY

Across both diagnostic and special education eligibility criteria, the general characteristics of ID are consistent. According to the *dual-criterion approach* (American Association on Intellectual and Developmental Disabilities [AAIDD], 2010), deficits in intellectual functioning and deficits in adaptive behaviors must be identified, and these dual criteria must be evident during infancy, childhood, or adolescence. This section outlines the specific criteria for ID as outlined by the AAIDD (2010); the American Psychiatric Association (2000, 2013); and the Individuals with Disabilities Education Improvement Act of 2004 (IDEA; Public Law 108-446, 2004) and Rosa's Law (Public Law 111-256, 2010).

American Association on Intellectual and Developmental Disabilities

> *Intellectual Disability: Definition, Classification, and Systems of Support is arguably the premier text guiding the assesment and identification of individuals with ID.*

The book *Intellectual Disability: Definition, Classification, and Systems of Support* (AAIDD, 2010) is arguably the premier text guiding the assessment and identification of individuals with ID. Its 11th edition contains one of the most striking changes to a diagnostic label in recent memory: labeling the disorder as *intellectual disability* and not *mental retardation*. This change is summarized in the following sentence:

We stipulate, consistent with the President's Committee for People With Intellectual Disabilities (2004), that the term ID covers the same population of individuals who were diagnosed previously with mental retardation in number, kind, level, type, and duration of the disability and the need of people with this disability for individualized services and supports; and every individual who is or was eligible for a diagnosis of mental retardation is eligible for a diagnosis of ID. (AAIDD, 2010, p. xvi)

Consistent with prior definitions of mental retardation offered by the same organization under its previous name (American Association on Mental Retardation, 2002), ID is described as a developmental disorder emerging before age 18 and characterized by "significant limitations both in mental functioning and in adaptive behavior as expressed in conceptual, social, and practical adaptive skills" (p. 1). In the 11th edition, however, the AAIDD has narrowed the focus on intellectual functioning to general mental ability. As described in Chapter 1, this general mental ability is represented by psychometric *g*—which is a representation of abstract reasoning and thinking, the capacity to acquire knowledge, and problem-solving ability—at the construct level, and it is measured by IQs in the practice of psychology. The AAIDD suggests that a significant limitation in intellectual functioning is evident with an IQ of approximately 70 or below, although the effects of random error must also be considered via use of confidence intervals. It recognizes that clinical judgment is required in determining whether this criterion is met. In particular, the AAIDD guidelines focus on both test session behaviors (e.g., display of fatigue or anxiety) and measurement issues (e.g., age of norms)—as discussed in Chapters 4 and 5, respectively—as affecting IQs.

Adaptive behaviors represent the collection of skills that have been learned and are typically performed by people in their everyday lives. The AAIDD focuses on three classes of adaptive behaviors: *conceptual, social,* and *practical.* Conceptual skills are employed when higher-order thinking and achievement-oriented skills are applied to situations; they include expressive and receptive language skills, reading and writing skills, knowledge of money concepts, and self-direction. These skills are most highly related to those measured by intelligence tests. Social skills are displayed when an individual is interacting with others in school and community settings; they include interpersonal skills, personal responsibility, self-esteem, rule following, and engaging in social problem solving to avoid being victimized by others (due to naiveté or gullibility). Finally, practical skills are applied when the individual is engaging independently in activities of daily living, and they include engaging in enriching personal activities and self-care, displaying occupational skills, and maintaining a safe environment.

> *Adaptive behaviors* **represent the collection of skills that have been learned and are typically performed by people in their everyday lives.**

The AAIDD guidelines are explicit in recommending use of formal assessment instruments targeting adaptive behavior skills. They state that "significant limitations in adaptive behavior should be established through the use of standardized measures normed with general populations, including persons with disabilities and people without disabilities" (p. 43). Deficits in adaptive behaviors are operationalized by the following when age-based norms are used: (1) at least one score representing the conceptual domain, social domain, or practical domain that is at least two standard deviations below the mean; or (2) an overall score stemming from items representing the conceptual, social, and practical domains that is at least two standard deviations below the mean. As with the criterion requiring a significant limitation in intellectual functioning, consideration must be given to confidence intervals associated with each of these adaptive behavior scores. More generally, the AAIDD guidelines recommend that assessors focus on typical performance of adaptive behaviors (not their maximum performance) across environments in which such behaviors are normally displayed (e.g., home, school, and community), and on identifying skills in which training and accommodations are most needed.

American Psychiatric Association

The term *mental retardation* was used in the *Diagnostic and Statistical Manual of Mental Disorders*, fourth edition, text revision (DSM-IV-TR; American Psychiatric Association, 2000), but the latest revisions to this diagnostic category recognize the sea change in terminology and refer to both ID and a variant of this term, *intellectual developmental disorder*. We describe both the diagnostic criteria in the DSM-IV-TR and the diagnostic criteria in the new fifth edition of the DSM (DSM-5; American Psychiatric Association, 2013).

Like the AAIDD guidelines for ID, the DSM-IV-TR included three criteria for mental retardation: (1) significantly subaverage intellectual functioning, (2) concurrent deficits or impairments in adaptive functioning in at least two of the adaptive behavior skill areas, and (3) onset before age 18 years. The American Psychiatric Association (2000) defined significantly subaverage intellectual functioning as an IQ of approximately 70 or below on an individually administered intelligence test, and if all other criteria are met for the disorder, the deviation of the IQ from the mean is used to determine the subtypes of mental retardation. Those with IQs from approximately 50–55 to approximately 70 would be labeled as having *mild mental retardation*; those with IQs from approximately 35–40 to approximately 50–55 would be labeled as having *moderate mental retardation*; those with IQs from approximately 20–25 to approximately 35–40 would be labeled as having *severe mental retardation*, and those with IQs below approximately 20-25 would be labeled as having *profound mental retardation*. Because all recently published individually administered intelligence tests yield IQs with a standard deviation of 15, the boundaries for these subtypes are roughly represented as the IQs being three, four, and five standard deviation units below the mean; it is notable, however, that very few intelligence tests produce IQs lower than 40 (see Chapter 7). About 85% of those with ID can be said to have mild mental retardation, 10% moderate mental retardation, 3–4% severe mental retardation, and 1–2% profound mental retardation.

Like the AAIDD (2010), the American Psychiatric Association (2000) defined adaptive behaviors as effectiveness in meeting age-based standards as established by an individual's cultural group, and it focuses on typical and not maximum performance. The DSM-IV-TR, however, did not highlight deficits in or across the conceptual, social, and practical domains described by the AAIDD (2010). Instead, it highlighted deficits in 11 *skill areas*: communication, use of community resources, functional academics, home living, health, safety, leisure, self-care, self-direction, social and interpersonal skills, and work. For diagnosis, deficits must have been evident in at least two of the skill areas. Unlike the AAIDD criteria, the DSM-IV-TR criteria did not prescribe the types of techniques (e.g., norm-referenced rating scales or interviews) required to identify adaptive behavior deficits; did not include the specific thresholds needed to meet these criteria (e.g., scores two standard deviations below the mean); and do not encourage the assessor to consider measurement error when interpreting scores from adaptive behavior assessment instruments.

The diagnostic criteria in the DSM-5 (American Psychiatric Association, 2013) are generally similar to those from the DSM-IV-TR (American Psychiatric Association, 2000). Perhaps the biggest difference between these two editions is the transition from *mental retardation* to *intel-*

lectual disability. (The term *intellectual developmental disorder* is also considered a viable alternative term in the DSM-5 in order to align it more closely with the *International Classification of Diseases*.) Recent conceptualizations of symptoms of the disorder are also evident in the DSM-5 criteria. The first criterion refers to "deficits in intellectual functions, such as reasoning, problem solving, planning, abstract thinking, judgment, academic learning, and learning from experience" (American Psychiatric Association, 2013, p. 33) in a manner consistent with AAIDD's focus on psychometric *g*. Although there is reference to *intellectual functions* rather than *intellectual functioning* in the DSM-5 diagnostic criteria—which may indicate that there should be increased focus on assessment of specific cognitive abilities rather than psychometric *g*—and there is no explicit reference to IQs in the diagnostic criteria, the frequent references to *general mental abilities*, occasional references to *intellectual capacity* (a somewhat outdated term), and discussion of IQs in the text supporting the diagnostic criteria indicate that the focus of the assessment should remain psychometric *g*. It is implied that the IQ threshold to demonstrate deficits in intellectual functions should be two standard deviations below the mean (i.e., 70), considering random error via confidence intervals. The 11 adaptive behavior skill areas described in the DSM-IV-TR are no longer listed in the second criterion for ID; areas of impairment in adaptive functioning are now closely aligned with the AAIDD's (2010) conceptual, social, and practical domains. Impairment in at least one of these domains must be evident. There are no subtypes of ID based on IQ level; however, four severity levels (*mild, moderate, severe*, and *profound*) can be specified based on a match between an individual's adaptive behaviors and the DSM-5's qualitative descriptions of the levels of severity. Thus, score thresholds needed to meet the adaptive behavior impairment criterion are not articulated. In contrast to the DSM-IV-TR, however, the DSM-5 seems to place additional emphasis on the types of techniques required to identify adaptive behavior impairment.

Individuals with Disabilities Education Improvement Act and Rosa's Law

In 2004, the federal definition of *mental retardation* characterized the condition as follows: "significantly subaverage general intellectual functioning, existing concurrently with deficits in adaptive behavior and manifested during the developmental period, that adversely affects a child's educational performance" (IDEA, 2004). In October 2010, a bill introduced by U.S. Senator Barbara Mikulski in November 2009, Rosa's Law, was signed. Rosa's Law (2010) eliminated the terms *mental retardation* and *mentally retarded* from the federal legal code; it was named after a child with Down syndrome who, with her family, worked to have these terms removed from the Maryland health and education code. Consistent with the recommendations of the AAIDD (2010), the official term for this condition in the United States became *intellectual disability*.

> **Rosa's Law (2010) eliminated the terms *mental retardation* and *mentally retarded* from the federal legal code.**

Although mental retardation and, currently, ID are included in federal special education legislation, each individual state has autonomy in labeling this condition as well as determining the specific eligibility criteria. Bergeron, Floyd, and Shands (2008) extended prior research examining these criteria across states. In 2005 and 2006, they obtained the state-level guidelines for identification of *mental retardation* from the Departments of Education of the 50 United States and the District of Columbia. The results were startling. At that time, 53% of states used the term *mental retardation*, and approximately 14% used the term *mental disability*. In stark contrast to the diagnostic guidelines offered by the AAIDD (2010), the DSM-5 (American Psychiatric

Association, 2013), and the current use of ID in the federal law, only 6% of states used this term. In addition, various other terms were used: *cognitive impairment, cognitive disability, cognitive delay,* and *severely limited intellectual capacity.* Most states did not differentiate subtypes of mental retardation based on severity or impairment. In the 35% of states that did so, children and adolescents were classified as displaying *mild, moderate,* and *severe/profound* mental retardation based on IQ levels (cf. American Psychiatric Association, 2000).

About one-quarter of states did not provide specific guidelines for identification of mental retardation or ID beyond reproducing the federal definition, and those states that did so varied somewhat in their markers of significantly subaverage intellectual functioning. Slightly more than three-fifths of states used an IQ cutoff of at least two standard deviations below the normative mean (or standard scores of 70 or below), whereas only approximately 1 in 20 required the IQs to be *below* two standard deviations (or standard scores below 70). Only about two-fifths of states specified consideration of measurement error using either an IQ range (e.g., 70–75) or confidence intervals. Based on these findings, you should be well informed about your state's and neighboring states' special education eligibility criteria for ID because they are likely to differ at least somewhat.

ASSESSMENT CONSIDERATIONS

Psychologists and others working with children and adolescents who have or are suspected of having ID should engage in best practices by becoming knowledgeable about recently revised diagnostic criteria and eligibility guidelines affecting their decision making during the assessment and identification process. Sound clinical judgment is also needed, as the AAIDD (2010) emphasizes:

> Clinical judgment is essential, and a higher level of clinical judgment is frequently required in complex diagnostic and classification situations in which the complexity of the person's functioning precludes standardized assessment alone, legal restrictions significantly reduce opportunities to observe and assess the person, historical information is missing and cannot be obtained, or there are serious questions about the validity of the data. Clinical judgment is defined as a special type of judgment rooted in a high level of clinical expertise and experience and judgment that emerges directly from extensive training, experience with the person, and extensive data. The purpose of clinical judgment and the use of clinical judgment strategies is *[sic]* to enhance the quality, validity, and precision of the clinician's decision or recommendation in a particular case. (p. 29)

To promote application of research-based knowledge, professional ethics, and professional standards to clinical judgments, we offer a brief checklist to consult during the process of assessing a child or adolescent suspected of having ID (see Form 10.1), and we elaborate on its components below.

Intelligence Testing

Test Selection

Because normatively low IQs have marked (and continue to mark) the key feature of the condition now known as ID, the first three questions in our checklist target the selection of at least one intelligence test and the interpretation of its primary score, the IQ. Consistent with the descriptions of the criteria for selecting intelligence tests described in Chapter 5, those involved in assessment of

ID should select intelligence tests (1) that have been recently normed (preferably during the past 10 years); (2) that produce IQs with high internal consistency (.95 or higher) and high short-term test–retest reliability (.90 or higher); and (3) that have validity evidence supporting their use for children and adolescents with ID. In general, you should consider administering two intelligence tests in cases of suspected ID, due to the likelihood that the different intelligence tests will yield different IQs and to the stigma associated with ID.

It is important that you pay particular attention to inadequate subtest floors and to subtest requirements that may interfere with accurate measurement of psychometric *g*. As noted in Chapter 5, Bracken (1987) and others have asserted that an adequate floor for a subtest would be indicated by a raw score of 1 producing a standardized score at least two standard deviations below the mean. Our review of the intelligence tests described in Chapter 7 suggests that inadequate floors are not problems for IQs, but that inadequate floors sometimes exist at the subtest level for the youngest age groups. Without adequate subtest floors, the truest estimate of psychometric *g* will be unattainable; you should ensure that every subtest has an adequate floor before initiating testing, and monitor floor effects if they cannot be avoided in selection.

Due to the common co-occurrence of sensory and motor disabilities with ID in children and adolescents (American Psychiatric Association, 2000), you should select intelligence tests that minimize the influence of *access skills* (Braden & Elliott, 2003; Phillips, 1994). Access skills are irrelevant to the targeted construct and might preclude the accurate measurement of psychometric *g*. For example, a child with cerebral palsy and minor fine motor problems who is suspected of having ID should not be administered a test including subtests that require quick and facile movement of manipulatives or drawing of intricate symbols with a pencil during a speeded administration. Furthermore, tests should be selected that will reflect psychometric *g* without undermining effects from a child or adolescent's linguistic background or ethnic/cultural differences (see Chapter 13). It is possible that accommodations will be needed during test administrations to reduce or eliminate the effects of these influences (Braden & Elliott, 2003, and Chapter 4, this volume). When any modification to standardized administration (e.g., use of a reinforcement system, inclusion of a caregiver in the room, or use of an interpreter) is made, this modification should be noted in both oral and written reports (see Chapter 8).

Score Interpretation

In order to meet the primary diagnostic or eligibility criterion for ID, the resulting IQ must be approximately two standard deviations below the mean (i.e., a standard score of 70) or lower, according to age-based norms (see Form 10.1). Confidence intervals around the IQs should be considered and reported. In our opinion (although it is speculative), if any portion of the 95% confidence interval band is in the range of 70 or below, we believe that this diagnostic or eligibility criterion for ID has been met. Thus IQs as high as 75 may produce confidence interval bands that enter this range.

Of course, a score of 70 or below is not sufficient to meet this criterion; the IQ's validity must also be verified. You should have considered—*before you obtained the norm-based scores*—whether or not all of the subtests (or even more narrowly, their items) contributing to the IQ appear to have yielded reasonably accurate results. As discussed just above and in Chapter 4, the child's or adolescent's engagement during the testing (a.k.a. motivation) and access to the subtests' content (even if the subtests were well selected) should have been ensured, and any anomalies during testing should have been evaluated. Consistent with our KISS model described in Chapter 6, we cannot support the practice of disregarding the IQs from wisely selected and validly completed intelligence tests when the norm-referenced subtest scores or composite scores stemming from those subtests (e.g., factor indexes) are substantially varied. There is a long history of recommendations from prominent scholars (e.g., Kaufman, 1979, 1994; Mervis & John, 2010) to engage in such practices, and the DSM-IV-TR (American Psychiatric Association, 2000) included the following statement: "When there is significant scatter in the subtest scores, the profile of strengths and weaknesses, rather than the mathematically derived full-scale IQ, will more accurately reflect the person's learning abilities. When there is a marked discrepancy across verbal and performance scores, averaging [them] to obtain a full-scale IQ score can be misleading" (p. 42). In order to avoid a failure to identify children or adolescents with ID, we believe that this practice is not a prudent one. Research (e.g., Freberg, Vandiver, Watkins, & Canivez, 2008; Watkins, Glutting, & Lei, 2007)

> **The practice of invalidating the IQ because of variability in the subtests contributing to it when it was obtained under reasonably ideal conditions appears to be outdated.**

has shown that the predictive power of IQ is not undermined when there are substantial differences across subtests or index scores contributing to the IQ. The practice of invalidating the IQ because of variability in the subtests contributing to it (or associated composites) when it was obtained under reasonably ideal conditions appears to be outdated.

You should also know that measurement issues, such as *regression toward the mean* and *combinatorial probabilities*, make it highly probable that children and adolescents with ID who obtain IQs of 70 or below will have subtest scores or composite scores above this criterion and far closer to the mean, except in the most extreme cases of ID (Bergeron & Floyd, 2005, 2013). Regression toward the mean is the general statistical phenomenon by which repeated measurement produces scores that are less extreme and closer to average due to chance occurrence alone (Nesselroade, Stigler, & Baltes, 1980). Because of regression toward the mean, we would expect (1) that children and adolescents with very low IQs will exhibit some subtest or composite scores that are closer to the population mean than their IQs; and (2) that the subtests and composite scores demonstrating the lowest correlations with the others will be most affected. In addition, when ID cannot be linked to biological causes (i.e., single-gene defects or chromosomal abnormalities), IQs for those falling in this group will rise over time due to regression toward the mean of the general population (Humphreys, 1989). In contrast, when ID is due to biological causes, the prognosis is for regression toward the mean of the population with that condition (e.g., Turner syndrome or Down syndrome).

When children and adolescents obtain scores indicating extreme normative weaknesses across the vast majority of subtests or composite scores—in many ways, going against the expectations of regression toward the mean—the relations between these scores and the IQ can be explained by combinatorial probabilities. Just as it is increasingly improbable that a person will roll a 5 on each consecutive roll of a die, it is increasingly improbable that an examinee will score consistently lower than his or her peers across subtests and composite scores. As a result of combinatorial probabilities, IQs will be more deviant (i.e., further away from the mean) than the average of the scores that contribute to them, representing this increasing improbability (see the excellent instructional video by Schneider, 2011a). Accordingly, for individuals with very low IQs, subtest scores and composite scores will be higher than expected from their IQs. The effects of regression toward the mean and combinatorial probabilities on these scores may result in errors in decision making when considering ID.

Adaptive Behavior Assessment

It is insufficient to rely only on IQs when determining ID. It is explicitly stated in recent diagnostic and eligibility guidelines (e.g., AAIDD, 2010) that the presumption is that low general mental ability will lead to adaptive behavior deficits in cases of ID, but these constructs are somewhat loosely associated. In fact, the correlations between IQs and adaptive behavior scores are modest at best—typically ranging from .30 to .50 on such instruments as the Adaptive Behavior Assessment System—Second Edition (ABAS-II) and the Vineland Adaptive Behavior Scales, Second Edition (Vineland-II) (see Harrison & Oakland, 2003; Sparrow, Cicchetti, & Balla, 2005). Consistent with best practices (e.g., AAIDD, 2010), we encourage assessors to consider adaptive behaviors from an ecological perspective; thus, we support collection of adaptive behavior assessment data from multiple informants who observe the children and adolescents in different settings. At a minimum, these practices prevent the identification of the "6-hour retarded child" (President's Committee on Mental Retardation, 1969)—that is, a child who is perceived as being impaired only in the school setting—and they promote identification of patterns of relative strengths and weaknesses in adaptive behaviors that children and adolescents display across settings.

> **We encourage assessors to consider adaptive behaviors from an ecological perspective; thus, we support collection of adaptive behavior assessment data from multiple informants who observe the children and adolescents in different settings.**

To identify potential adaptive behavior deficits, you should draw on the most well-developed norm-referenced assessment instruments, and should interpret those scores that are the most reliable and that are supported by the most validity evidence. Consistent with the AAIDD (2010) guidelines, we encourage you (1) to consider adaptive behavior composite scores (e.g., the Global Adaptive Composite score from the ABAS-II [Harrison & Oakland, 2003] and the Adaptive Behavior Composite from the Vineland-II [Sparrow et al., 2005]), and (2) to follow the same guidelines presented previously for interpretation of IQs. In other words, these adaptive behavior composite scores must be at least two standard deviations below the mean, and the confidence intervals around them should be considered. Current diagnostic criteria recommend consideration of conceptual, social, and practical domain scores, but scores addressing these more specific domains tend to be lower in reliability and to be supported by weaker bodies of validity evidence than total composite scores.

In addition to the use of norm-referenced adaptive behavior assessment instruments, we encourage consideration of other, more qualitative evidence of deficits in important conceptual, practical, and social domains. This evidence may surface from reports of parents and teachers, review of records, and observations in the home setting or in preschool or classroom settings. Examples of such evidence includes perceptions of parents when contrasting a child's development to that of siblings or other relatives, documentation of language delays and related services, and low scores on academic skill benchmark assessments (e.g., early literacy probes).

Consideration of Other Conditions

When you are engaged in decision making about diagnosis or eligibility for ID, it is important (1) to consider other conditions that may lead to the symptoms of ID (i.e., to make a differential diagnosis), and (2) to consider other conditions that co-occur with ID (i.e., to determine comorbidities). The last three questions in Form 10.1 address these issues.

Differential Diagnosis

You should ensure that sensory and motor disorders are eliminated as the primary causes of the symptoms of ID. Despite the fact that sensory and motor disorders would be expected to lower scores on most adaptive behavior assessment instruments, considering the child's characteristics when you are selecting an intelligence test (see Chapters 4 and 5) should allow for these effects to be eliminated as causes of low IQs. Similarly, wisely selected intelligence tests can also eliminate the influence of limited English proficiency (LEP) and lack of acculturation to U.S. mainstream culture on IQs. In many cases, screening for LEP should be conducted before testing, but even after testing, it could be conducted to confirm the hypothesis that LEP did not confound test results.

Other learning or psychiatric disorders should also be eliminated as the primary cause of the ID symptoms. We have seen that severe language problems—such as the DSM-IV-TR's (American Psychiatric Association, 2000) expressive–receptive language disorder, now referred to as *language disorder* in the DSM-5 (American Psychiatric Association, 2013)—can lead to low IQs and adaptive behavior deficits in communication and social skills, and as such may indicate ID. In such cases, we suggest consulting a speech–language therapist for advice and completing additional assessment to make a differential diagnosis. Furthermore, children with attention-deficit/ hyperactivity disorder (ADHD) and oppositional defiant disorder (ODD) may obtain low IQs due to interfering factors and fail to demonstrate adaptive behaviors at the expected level; under ideal testing conditions, however, they tend to score in or near the Average range on intelligence tests and to function only slightly below their peers on adaptive behavior measures.

When learning disabilities are considered in the era of response to intervention (RTI), it is likely that a child with ID (especially with a mild form of the condition) would be identified first as being at risk for reading problems, based on performance on early literacy benchmarking assessments. This child might be moved through the multiple levels of support and be determined eligible for special education services as having a learning disability (see Chapters 9 and 12). Teachers should be on the lookout for more general deficits across academic content areas and areas of adaptive functioning among such children. Psychologists and other assessment professionals should consider administering well-validated brief or abbreviated intelligence tests (see Chapter 7) and having teachers complete adaptive behavior rating scales in such cases, in order either to rule out ID as a cause of the academic problems or to facilitate a comprehensive assessment.

Comorbidity with Medical Disorders

One simple way to conceptualize the causes of ID is to group them into two categories: (1) those stemming from biological causes (including genetic disorders and environmental agents affecting brain development), and (2) those stemming primarily from psychosocial (cultural and familial) causes. Typically, the more severe symptoms of ID are, the more likely it is that identifiable biological causes have produced them. Approximately two-thirds of cases of ID will have identifiable causes (American Psychiatric Association, 2000), such as genetic disorders and other hereditary components; early alterations in embryonic development due to environmental influences (e.g., teratogens such as alcohol exposure or lead poisoning); pregnancy and perinatal problems (e.g., hypoxia); and general medical conditions acquired in infancy or childhood. Often these biological causes can be identified, but if they cannot be identified, cultural–familial influences, including normal variations in intelligence (see Chapter 2), are identified as the primary reasons for the ID.

Consistent with these conceptualizations of the causes of ID, the AAIDD (2010) guidelines for diagnosis recommend that greater consideration be given to the health of children and adolescents suspected of having ID. We encourage you to incorporate medical examinations into your multidisciplinary assessments, or to route parents and caregivers to medical professionals to complete a thorough medical examination. A medical examination may identify possible biological causes for the ID in order to eliminate or treat them. Although the effects of most biological causes cannot be reversed, some may be treatable through medical interventions (e.g., through use of dietary restrictions for a child with phenylketonuria); or, once they are identified, their effects on yet-unborn children or infants can be prevented through interventions with parents (e.g., substance use treatment and parental education). In addition, a medical evaluation, including genetic testing, can identify and facilitate treatment of medical conditions associated with ID (e.g., heart conditions and epilepsy).

Comorbidity with Mental Disorders

Children and adolescents with ID are likely to demonstrate comorbid mental disorders at a rate that is three or four times greater than in the general population. This high incidence of comorbid disorders may lead to two challenges during completion of a comprehensive assessment. First, you may find it difficult to identify other mental disorders in children and adolescents with ID, because these other disorders may have "atypical" clinical presentations (American Psychiatric Association, 2000). For example, you may be asked to make the judgment about whether ADHD symptoms displayed by a child with ID are more severe than would be expected from the child's cognitive developmental level. Cognitive developmental level has traditionally been synonymous with *mental age* (MA), which has its roots in early intelligence testing metrics (see Chapter 2), but MA is often represented by age equivalent scores from modern developmental screening and intelligence tests (see Chapters 6 and 7). A child with an IQ associated with an age equivalent score of 3.4 might be expected to display the same levels of inattention and impulsivity as an average 3-year-old—which is a rather low expectation for sustained attention and self-control. In light of the challenges posed by atypical clinical presentations of these other disorders, rating scales targeting common behavior problems in the general population of children and adolescents (e.g., Reynolds & Kamphaus, 2004) may not be appropriate for children and adolescents with ID. Campbell (2006b) has offered a worthwhile review of rating scales designed to assess the social–emotional functioning of children and adolescents with ID.

Second, comorbid disorders may overshadow the deficits associated with ID to such an extent that ID goes undiagnosed. For example, the qualitative differences in communication and social interactions and behavioral excesses associated with severe autism spectrum disorder, and the aggressive and defiant behavior associated with ODD, may be incredibly problematic to parents and teachers seeking your services; in such cases, general intellectual functioning may be largely ignored. In light of this challenge, we recommend routine screening for deficits in intellectual functioning and deficits in adaptive behaviors during comprehensive assessments.

Consideration of Levels of Needed Support

The final consideration during assessment is to determine how the child or adolescent's independent functioning could be improved with additional supports. The AAIDD (2010) defines *supports* as "resources and strategies that aim to promote the development, education, interests, and personal well-being of a person and that enhance individual functioning" (p. 18). In considering these supports, you should identify not only the current absolute limitations that the child or adolescent may be displaying, but also his or her absolute and relative strengths across domains. For example, despite meeting criteria for ID, a child may have strong social skills, display adequate attention to assignments in class, and engage in sporting activities. With a personalized support plan targeting areas of deficits for intervention while building existing strengths, it is likely that the child or adolescent's long-term functioning will be vastly improved across development.

SUMMARY

ID is a developmental disorder that is characterized by significant limitations in both mental functioning and display of adaptive behavior and that emerges early in development. Assessing a child or adolescent with ID presents some unique challenges, but proper training in the administration of intelligence tests, broad understanding of ecological and multidisciplinary assessment standards, knowledge of consensus-based definitions of ID, consideration of psychometric standards and anomalies that may surface from testing, and clinical sensitivity will go a long way in allowing you to provide the ideal services for these children and adolescents and their families.

Questions to Consider
during Diagnostic and Eligibility Assessment for ID

INTELLIGENCE

1. Was at least one intelligence test administered under conditions that should ensure valid results?
   a. Was it recently normed?
   b. Does the IQ demonstrate internal consistency reliability of .95 or higher and test–retest reliability of .90 or higher?
   c. Is the IQ supported by sufficient validity evidence (ideally, studies of those with ID)?
   d. Do the test's subtests have sufficiently low floors?
   e. Was the child or adolescent sufficiently motivated to respond, and was there an absence of interfering factors?

2. Was an IQ obtained that is approximately 70 or below?

3. Was a 95% confidence interval considered when the IQ was interpreted?

ADAPTIVE BEHAVIOR

4. Were adaptive behavior assessment instruments completed by multiple informants who observed the child or adolescent in distinct settings (e.g., teachers in school classrooms and on playgrounds, and parents or other caregivers at home and in the community)?

5. Does an adaptive behavior composite score or domain scores (especially in the areas of conceptual, practical, and social skills) indicate development deviance (e.g., as indicated in scores that are at least two standard deviations below the mean)?

6. Were 95% confidence intervals considered when the adaptive behavior composite score or domain scores were interpreted?

7. Is there other evidence that the child or adolescent is developmentally delayed in important conceptual, practical, and social domains?

OTHER ISSUES

8. Have other explanations for the symptoms of ID been eliminated?
   a. Have severe sensory disorders (e.g., visual impairment and hearing impairment) or motor disorders been eliminated as the primary causes of the low IQ and deficits in adaptive behavior evident from the assessment?
   b. Have LEP and lack of acculturation been eliminated as the primary causes of the low IQ and deficits in adaptive behavior evident from the assessment?
   c. Have other learning or psychiatric disorders (e.g., expressive–receptive language disorder, learning disability, and ADHD) been eliminated as the primary causes of the low IQ and deficits in adaptive behavior evident from the assessment?

9. Has a thorough medical evaluation been completed?
   a. Have medical causes for the ID been investigated?
   b. Have comorbid medical conditions associated with ID been investigated?

10. Does the child or adolescent need increased levels of support from teachers and caregivers to function in a general education setting or to prepare him or her to function independently as a young adult?

CHAPTER 11

Assessment of Intellectual Giftedness

Sir Francis Galton (1822–1911) is widely regarded as the founder of *differential psychology*, the scientific study of the ways in which individuals and groups differ in their psychological traits (Jensen, 2002). Galton (1869) defined *genius* as exceptionally high mental ability that is largely attributable to heredity (p. viii). Because practical tests of intelligence did not yet exist, Galton examined the family trees of individuals who were famous for their intellectual accomplishments. He found that eminence tended to run in families (which is consistent with the genetic basis of genius), but not always in the same field of accomplishment. Galton (1869) conceptualized intelligence as a very broad, general ability:

> In statesmanship, generalship, literature, science, poetry, art, just the same enormous differences are found between man and man; and numerous instances recorded in this book, will show in how small degree, eminence, either in these or any other class of intellectual powers, can be considered as due to purely special powers. They are rather to be considered in those instances as the result of concentrated efforts, made by men who are widely gifted. People lay too much stress on apparent specialties, thinking over-rashly that, because a man is devoted to some particular pursuit, he could not possibly have succeeded in anything else. They might just as well say that, because a youth had fallen desperately in love with a brunette, he could not possibly have fallen in love with a blonde. He may or may not have more natural liking for the former type of beauty than the latter, but it is more probably as not the affair was mainly or wholly due to a general amorousness of disposition. (p. 64, as quoted by Jensen, 2002, pp. 146–147)

> **Galton believed that "special abilities" or talents in particular fields were not sufficient for outstanding accomplishment; a high level of general intelligence was also necessary.**

Although Galton recognized the importance of "special abilities" or talents in particular fields (e.g., mathematics, music, art), he believed that they were not sufficient for outstanding accomplishment; a high level of general intelligence was also necessary. He did not equate genius with high general ability, however. According to Galton (1865),

Success of this kind implies the simultaneous inheritance of many points of character, in addition to mere intellectual capacity. A man must inherit good health, a love of mental work, a strong purpose, and considerable ambition, in order to achieve successes of the high order of which we are speaking. (p. 318)

Nevertheless, with Galton's work the conceptualization of giftedness as hereditary was clearly established (Subotnik, Olszewski-Kubilius, & Worrell, 2011). His assertion that genius results from some combination of a number of interacting inherited characteristics is quite consistent with the contemporary *emergenic* models of greatness (e.g., Simonton, 2001).

In the United States, the scientific study of intellectual giftedness began with the work of Lewis Terman (1877–1956). In 1916, Terman published a revision of the Binet–Simon intelligence test, which he named the Stanford–Binet Scale of Intelligence. He translated the test into English and expanded the number of items administered at each age, to facilitate the assessment of children and youth at all levels of intellectual ability. He also standardized test administration and provided norms for score interpretation. Last, he adopted and popularized the concept of the intelligence quotient, or IQ, developed several years earlier by Stern (1912). For the next two decades, the Stanford–Binet was the most widely used individually administered test of intelligence in the United States and a major part of the measurement movement in education (Chapman, 1988).

Terman was greatly influenced by Galton's theory of genius; he conceptualized intellectual giftedness as primarily determined by high IQ. He classified those with scores above 135 as *moderately* gifted, those with scores above 150 as *exceptionally* gifted, and those with scores greater than 180 as *profoundly* gifted. Terman (1916) argued for the use of intelligence tests to identify and place intellectually gifted students in special classes in schools. Thus, although Terman believed that intellectual giftedness is largely inherited, he nevertheless advocated for early identification and special services or programs for the intellectually gifted so that they could reach their full potential. He thereby recognized the important roles played by both nature and nurture in the development of giftedness.

Prior to the advent of intelligence tests, research on intellectual giftedness consisted largely of retrospective studies. In these studies, researchers first identified adults who were considered geniuses, and then looked back at events that took place in their childhood to shed light on the nature and development of giftedness (e.g., Cox, 1926). With the availability of intelligence tests, however, it became possible to conduct prospective studies in which samples of intellectually gifted children and youth could be followed over time.

In 1921, Terman initiated the famous *Genetic Studies of Genius* (Terman, 1925; Terman & Oden, 1947, 1959), the first longitudinal study of over 1,500 intellectually gifted children and youth with IQs of 140 or above. Terman and his colleagues gathered an extensive amount of data on these individuals for over 50 years. The "twofold purpose of the project was, first of all, to find what traits characterize children of high IQ, and secondly, to follow them for as many years as possible to see what kind of adults they might become" (Terman, 1954, p. 223).

It is noteworthy that he first attempted to identify children and youth who showed exceptional talent in any of the following areas, regardless of level of IQ: music, art, mechanical inventiveness, and ingenuity. However, he quickly became aware that the available instruments for measuring specific talents were lacking in reliability and validity. Furthermore, he found a high degree of overlap between those identified with exceptional talent and those identified with high general intelligence (Zigler & Farber, 1985).

Results of Terman's seminal study indicated that as adults, in general, the intellectually gifted sample was happier, healthier, and more successful than their average-IQ peers (Terman, 1925, 1954; Terman & Oden, 1947, 1959). Moreover, his results contradicted the then-prevailing stereotype that the intellectually gifted tended to have poor social skills and were more prone to emotional maladjustment. Nevertheless, despite the fact that the gifted participants in Terman's study were generally very successful in life, some did not achieve to their full potential, and very few were recognized for eminence in their field as adults. These results, therefore, indicated that high general intelligence is necessary but not sufficient for the highest levels of performance and productivity in society. In other words, in addition to a sufficiently high level of general intelligence, other domain-specific or noncognitive factors (e.g., motivation, creativity, task commitment) are required. Terman (1954) stated:

> The follow-up of these gifted subjects has proved beyond question that tests of "general intelligence," given as early as six, eight, or ten years, tell a great deal about the ability to achieve either presently or 30 years hence. Such tests do not, however, enable us to predict what direction the achievement will take, and least of all do they tell us what personality factors or what accidents of fortune will affect the fruition of exceptional ability. Granting that both interest patterns and special aptitudes play important roles in the making of a gifted scientist, mathematician, mechanic, artist, poet, or musical composer, I am convinced that to achieve greatly in almost any field, the special talents have to be backed up by a lot of Spearman's g, by which is meant the kind of general intelligence that requires ability to form many sharply defined concepts, to manipulate them, and to perceive subtle relationships between them; in other words, the ability to engage in abstract thinking. (p. 224)

CONTEMPORARY THEORIES OF GIFTEDNESS

Over the past 40 years, many different theories of intellectual giftedness have been proposed. Almost all of these expand upon the historical conception of giftedness as an all-purpose, inherited quality of the individual that is identified primarily by an intelligence test (see Sternberg & Davidson, 1986, 2005). Contemporary conceptions of giftedness have expanded beyond an emphasis on general intelligence to include domain-specific cognitive and other abilities related to leadership, creativity, and the arts. In this section, we provide examples of a few prominent contemporary theories of intellectual giftedness.

> **Over the past 40 years, almost all theories of intellectual giftedness have expanded upon the historical conception of giftedness as an all-purpose, inherited quality of the individual that is identified primarily by an intelligence test.**

Domain-Specific Models

Domain-specific models of giftedness focus on different areas of aptitude and the development of capacity within those areas. Gardner's (1983, 1993, 1999, 2006) theory of *multiple intelligences* (MI) is perhaps the most widely recognized domain-specific conceptualization of giftedness (cf. Brody & Stanley, 2005). In Gardner's theory, intelligence is viewed as a complex system stemming from the interaction of many cognitive and noncognitive variables. Cognitive ability is described by a distinct set of mental abilities, or *intelligences*, not as a single thing. Although these intelligences are held to be independent, they often interact. Gardner defined an intelligence as "an ability or set of abilities that permits an individual to solve problems or fashion products that are of consequence in a particular cultural setting" (Walters & Gardner, 1986, p. 165).

According to MI theory, bona fide intelligences must be universal to humans and rooted in biology; they must also have (1) an identifiable set of core operations, and (2) the capability of being represented in a symbol system (Walters & Gardner, 1986). Based upon his results, Gardner (1999) asserted that there are eight different kinds of intelligence: linguistic, logical–mathematical, spatial, musical, bodily–kinesthetic, interpersonal, intrapersonal, and naturalist.

Gardner's MI theory has helped broaden conceptions of giftedness to include beyond general intelligence domains in which giftedness can be recognized. Gardner (1983) argued that intelligence tests measure only those intelligences that are valued in formal schooling—namely, the logical–mathematical and linguistic intelligences. He maintained that all eight intelligences should be assessed in a contextually relevant way, and that the focus of assessment should be on the natural products of each kind of intelligence. To date, however, Gardner and his colleagues have not developed reliable and valid measures of these intelligences. Moreover, so much empirical evidence has been gathered in support of a general factor of cognitive ability (see Chapters 1 and 2) that the notion of distinct logical–mathematical and linguistic intelligences, at least, is untenable. Gardner (2006) himself recently conceded that the general factor underlying individual differences on all tests of cognitive ability, psychometric *g*, may account for some (but not all) of his proposed intelligences.

Systems Models

In *systems* models, giftedness is conceptualized as an integrated system in which "the total operation is dependent on a confluence of psychological processes operating together" (Kaufman & Sternberg, 2008, p. 76). One of the initial and most influential systems models is Renzulli's (1978, 1986) *three-ring* model of giftedness. As shown in Figure 11.1, in this model giftedness is viewed as resulting from an interaction of three characteristics: above-average cognitive ability, exceptional creativity, and a very high level of task commitment. According to the three-ring model, "individuals capable of developing gifted behavior are those possessing or capable of developing this composite set of traits and applying them to any potentially valuable area of human performance" (Reis & Renzulli, 2011, p. 242).

Renzulli distinguished between the so-called "schoolhouse" gifted, or those who only excel in school (e.g., test taking and academic assignments) and are identified as gifted but do not distinguish themselves during their professional careers, and the "creative–productive" gifted, or those who make creative contributions to society as adults. The former group is considered to have high ability but to be lacking in either creativity, task commitment, or both, whereas the latter group possesses all three important characteristics.

In the three-ring model, above-average ability is defined as either general or domain-specific. In this model, general ability appears to consist not only of psychometric *g*, but also of the broad abilities at stratum II of Carroll's (1993) three-stratum model (see Chapter 1). According to Renzulli, general ability primarily reflects abstract thinking that is mostly applicable in academic contexts and in novel situations, and is measured well by standardized tests of IQ and aptitude. Domain-specific abilities, in contrast, are reflected in the ways in which individuals perform in specialized

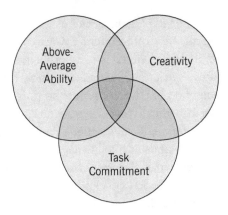

FIGURE 11.1. Renzulli's three-ring model of giftedness. From Reis and Renzulli (2011).

real-world situations, such as mathematics, musical performance, dance, and art (e.g., sculpture, photography). According to him, domain-specific abilities that are closely related to academic achievement (e.g., mathematics, creative writing) can be measured adequately with standardized achievement tests and tests of specific aptitudes, but others require the use of performance-based or portfolio assessments (e.g., dance and art).

In the three-ring model, general ability is viewed as a "threshold variable" below which socially significant accomplishment is highly unlikely. Renzulli estimated this minimum level of requisite IQ to be approximately 120, which is more than one standard deviation above the mean and is demonstrated by approximately the top 10% of the population. This is considerably higher than the 2–3% typically identified by intelligence tests using a score of 130 or above (McClain & Pfeiffer, 2012). In addition, research suggests that this threshold may be different across various fields and subjects (e.g., Barron, 1968). Thus, after one's IQ surpasses this threshold, other factors become more important in the prediction of real-world success, such as creativity and task commitment.

Recent research, however, has questioned the cognitive ability threshold as a component of the model (e.g., Park, Lubinski, & Benbow, 2007, 2008; Robertson, Smeets, Lubinski, & Benbow, 2010). Robertson et al. (2010), for example, found that individual differences in general cognitive ability among the top 1% of adolescents were significantly related to educational, occupational, and creative outcomes many years later. Other criticisms of the three-ring model include the lack of measures with psychometric support for the assessment of creativity and a number of domain-specific abilities (e.g., Zigler & Farber, 1985; Worrell, 2009). Others have argued that creativity may be better used as an outcome variable than as a predictor of giftedness; that is, outstanding creative products usually result from the persistent pursuit of goals in a specific talent domain (e.g., Winner, 1996). Thus, although the three-ring model broadens the definition of giftedness and criteria for identification, it is not without its detractors (e.g., see Delisle, 2003; VanTassel-Baska, 2005).

Developmental Models

In *developmental* models of giftedness, emphasis is placed on "the constantly changing nature of these so-called 'gifts,' and [these models] broaden the net even wider than the systems model by including various *external* factors that might interact with the *internal* factors of the individual to produce gifted behavior" (Kaufman & Sternberg, 2008, p. 77; emphasis in original). In other words, these models attempt to identify the underlying factors that lead to the manifestation of gifted potential. Tannenbaum's (2003) model of talent development was one of the first attempts to explain the development of natural abilities into specific expert skills or talents. Tannenbaum (1986) defined giftedness as follows:

> Keeping in mind that developed talent exists only in adults, a proposed definition of giftedness in children is that it denotes their potential for becoming critically acclaimed performers or exemplary producers of ideas in spheres of activity that enhance the moral, physical, emotional, social, intellectual, or aesthetic life of humanity. (p. 33)

In Tannenbaum's theory, the environment plays a central role in the manifestation and development of giftedness. According to him, five factors must be present: (1) superior general ability, (2) special or domain-specific aptitude, (3) psychosocial abilities (e.g., motivation, perseverance), (4) external support, and (5) chance. Tannenbaum asserted that the amount of general ability required for high performance varies by domain. In addition to sufficiently high general cognitive ability, or *g*, the gifted individual also possesses other domain-specific aptitudes or psychosocial abilities associated with that domain (Subotnik et al., 2011).

One component of developmental models such as Tannenbaum's is that intellectual giftedness requires a special environment to develop fully (Subotnik et al., 2011). This includes the presence of significant others who are interested in and supportive of the developing gifted child. It is also important to note the important role that chance can play in the development of giftedness. Children do not select the environments into which they are born. Environments that are favorable or unfavorable to the development of particular traits are often imposed upon them. An example is when a child with superior musical ability is born to and raised by parents who provide a musically stimulating environment. Environments can also be selected or created by others in reaction to an individual's predisposition, such as when teachers nominate children who have demonstrated academic promise for special programs for the intellectually gifted. Of course, gifted individuals also often select or create environments that are correlated with their natural abilities. For example, children with superior musical ability may spend more time listening to, thinking about, and practicing music than other children, regardless of whether anyone wants them to or not.

Another important aspect of developmental models is the emphasis on "giftedness" as an outcome reflecting advanced performance in a specific domain that is attained through a combination of cognitive and noncognitive factors over time. According to this model, giftedness is not an enduring characteristic of an individual (i.e., it is not the case that someone either is or is not gifted). Research within talent development models also emphasizes the facts that there are different developmental trajectories in different domains, and that exceptional talents may not be stable over time (e.g., Simonton, 1999, 2001). Thus, as Simonton (2001) has stated, some "early bloomers" may demonstrate relative declines over time, and so-called "late bloomers" may overtake them. According to Worrell and Erwin (2011), the field is gradually moving toward the realization that "(a) giftedness involves more than just ability or potential in a domain and (b) the classification of giftedness may shift across developmental periods" (pp. 319–320). The developmental models also underscore the fact that giftedness is a culture-bound conceptualization, which means that what is considered gifted in one culture may not be in another (e.g., Nicpon & Pfeiffer, 2011).

Summary of Contemporary Models

As we hope this brief review makes clear, many diverse conceptions of giftedness can be found in the current literature. Nonetheless, as Kaufman and Sternberg (2008) have asserted, "no serious giftedness researcher today believes that general intelligence is the whole picture, or believes that gifted abilities are solely the result of innate, genetic endowment" (p. 79). Reis and Renzulli (2011) add that "despite decades of attempts to study and identify a standard pattern of intellectual giftedness among high-potential children and individuals, no clear pathway has been identified and no specific formula exists regarding the 'right' combination of genes, personality, and environment

> **Despite decades of attempts to study and identify a standard pattern of intellectual giftedness, no clear pathway has been identified and no specific formula exists regarding the "right" combination of genes, personality, and environment.**

needed to produce intellectual giftedness" (p. 237). Despite the progress made over the past century, none of these contemporary models is considered the predominant models of giftedness—and all have had minimal impact on the process of identifying giftedness in the schools. In the next section, we examine current definitions of giftedness in the schools.

IDENTIFICATION OF GIFTED CHILDREN AND ADOLESCENTS

Federal and State Definitions of Giftedness

In 1972, U.S. Commissioner of Education Sydney Marland presented the first national report on gifted education to Congress. The purpose of the Marland Report was to examine the degree to which intellectually gifted students were being served in schools across the nation. This report is widely viewed as ground-breaking, insofar as it recognized the following six different types of giftedness: general intellectual ability, specific academic aptitude, creative or productive thinking, leadership ability, ability in visual and performing arts, and psychomotor ability. The Marland Report also encouraged states to identify a minimum of 3–5% of the school population as gifted and to provide these children and youth with appropriate educational programs.

In 1978, the federal definition of gifted and talented was revised to include "children and, whenever applicable, youth who are identified at the pre-school, elementary, or secondary level as possessing demonstrated or potential abilities that give evidence of high performance capability in areas such as intellectual, creative, specific academic, or leadership ability or in the performing and visual arts, and who by reason thereof require services or activities not ordinarily provided by the school" (Purcell, 1978, Public Law 95-561). The main difference between the 1972 and 1978 definitions was the elimination of psychomotor ability as a domain of giftedness.

The Marland Report also led to the enactment of legislation such as the Jacob K. Javits Gifted and Talented Students Education Act, which was passed as part of the Elementary and Secondary Education Act of 1988 and reauthorized in 1994. The Javits Act is the only federal legislation that specifically supports the development of gifted and talented students in the United States. In contrast with the Individuals with Disabilities Education Improvement Act of 2004 (IDEA, 2004), however, the Javits Act does not afford any federal protections for the gifted and talented (such as due process and equal protection rights; Stephens, 2011).

The current federal definition of giftedness is part of the No Child Left Behind (NCLB) Act of 2001 (2002), which is based on the Javits Act:

Children and youth with outstanding talent perform or show the potential for performing at remarkable high levels of accomplishment when compared with others of their age, experience, or environment. These children and youth exhibit high performance capability in intellectual, creative, and/or artistic areas, possess an unusual leadership capacity, or excel in specific academic fields. They require services or activities not ordinarily provided by the schools. Outstanding talents are present in children and youth from all cultural groups, across all economic strata, and in all areas of human endeavor.

It is important to note that the emphasis in the NCLB Act is on minimum proficiency or competency, and not on excellence. As a result, the primary emphasis in schools today is on the remediation of students performing below grade level and not on the highest achievers. Not surprisingly, most states report that NCLB has had a negative impact on gifted education (National Association for Gifted Children [NAGC], 2009). Moreover, federal funding for the National Resource Center on the Gifted and Talented has declined steadily since 2002, and funds for the program were eliminated in the fiscal year 2012 federal budget (Stephens, 2011).

Given the absence of a federal mandate related to identification of and educational services for the gifted, states and school districts are left to their own devices. According to the most recent report from the NAGC, in 2008–2009 only 32 states indicated that they had mandates for gifted education, and gifted education was fully funded in only 6 of those 32 states. Perhaps needless to say, insufficient funding was listed as the primary area of need by state directors of gifted programs (NAGC, 2009).

Historically, most states' definitions of giftedness were based on the 1978 federal definition of giftedness (McClain & Pfeiffer, 2011). Nevertheless, until only recently the majority of states identified giftedness predominantly in terms of high general intelligence. Over 20 years ago, most state definitions were closely aligned with the 1978 definition and defined giftedness according to a single criterion (i.e., IQ; Cassidy & Hossler, 1992).

Since then, substantial changes have been made in both the definition and categories of giftedness in many states (cf. McClain & Pfeiffer, 2012; Stephens & Karnes, 2000). In a recent national survey of coordinators of state gifted programs, McClain and Pfeiffer found that all but two states (South Dakota and Massachusetts) currently have established definitions of giftedness. Half of the states with definitions of giftedness had revised their definition of giftedness during the 10 years preceding the survey. All but three states use *gifted and talented*, or simply *gifted*, as the terminology for this category of exceptional students. The other three states (Indiana, Nebraska, and Washington) use the term *high-ability student* in their definition. Thus, as McClain and Pfeiffer's results show, there continues to be a lack of consensus among educators on how to define giftedness.

Figure 11.2 shows the changes in categories/types of giftedness recognized in state definitions from 2000 to 2010. As can be seen here, intelligence is the most widely recognized category of giftedness, followed by academic achievement. Moreover, changes in these categories over the past decade suggest an increasing emphasis on intelligence and achievement in state definitions. According to Worrell and Erwin (2011), the sustained focus on general intelligence and/or academic domains is likely to result from (1) the fact that educational programming is predominantly focused on core academic subjects (i.e., reading, writing, arithmetic, and science); and (2) the lack of resources to provide educational services in other areas of talent. Kaufman and Sternberg (2008) have stated that intelligence tests are probably widely used not only because they are relatively cheap and have demonstrated construct validity, but also because they are known to be predictive of general achievement outcomes, which constitute the primary emphasis of many gifted education programs.

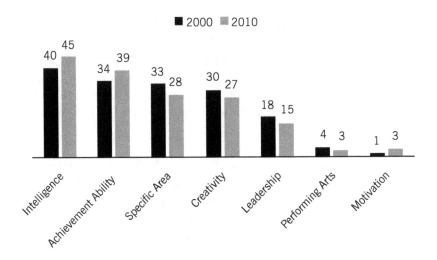

FIGURE 11.2. Change in categories/types of giftedness recognized in state definitions from 2000 to 2010. From McClain and Pfeiffer (2012).

McClain and Pfeiffer (2012) also examined the following decision-making models used by states to determine eligibility for gifted services:

1. *Single-cutoff.* A single cutoff score on an intelligence test (e.g., IQ > 130) is used to determine eligibility.
2. *Single-cutoff, flexible-criterion.* Only one test score is used, but flexibility is allowed in selecting the type of test (e.g., intelligence test or test of creativity) and the specific cutoff score used.
3. *Multiple-cutoff.* Cutoff scores on more than one measure are used (e.g., IQ and achievement tests).
4. *Averaging.* Scores on multiple measures are averaged across domains (e.g., IQ, achievement, creativity).
5. *Dynamic.* One or more measures are used to measure the amount of growth over time.

McClain and Pfeiffer found that 27 states reported using a multiple-cutoff or averaging decision-making model. None of the states used the single-cutoff model, but 7 used the single-cutoff, flexible-criterion model. A total of 16 states reported that they do not require a specific decision-making model for gifted eligibility determination. Table 11.1 shows the states that do and do not use specific cutoff scores and the scores used. When cutoff scores are used for gifted identification, they typically correspond to selection of 3–5% of all students (McClain & Pfeiffer, 2012).

ISSUES IN ASSESSMENT OF GIFTEDNESS

Figure 11.3 displays the assessment methods that are required by states for determining eligibility for gifted programs. As this figure shows, standardized intelligence and achievement tests are the two most widely required assessments, followed by teacher and/or parent nominations. It is beyond

TABLE 11.1. States Using Specific Models for the Selection and Identification of Gifted Students

State	Single-cutoff	Single-cutoff, flexible-criterion	Multiple-cutoff or averaging	Dynamic	No model
Alabama		×			
Alaska					×
Arizona		×			
Arkansas			×		
California			×		
Colorado		×			
Connecticut			×		
Delaware					×
Florida			×		
Georgia			×		
Hawaii			×		
Idaho			×		
Illinois					×
Indiana					×
Iowa					×
Kansas			×		
Kentucky			×		
Louisiana		×			
Maine					×
Maryland					×
Massachusetts					×
Michigan					×
Minnesota					×
Mississippi			×		
Missouri			×		
Montana			×		
Nebraska			×		
Nevada			×		
New Hampshire					×
New Jersey			×		
New Mexico			×		
North Dakota					×
Ohio		×			
Oklahoma		×			
Oregon			×		
Pennsylvania		×			
Rhode Island					×
South Carolina			×		
South Dakota					×
Tennessee			×		
Texas			×		
Utah			×		
Vermont					×
Virginia			×		
Washington			×		
West Virginia			×		
Wisconsin			×		
Total	0	7	27	0	16
%	0%	14%	54%	0%	32%

Note. Adapted from McClain and Pfeiffer (2012).

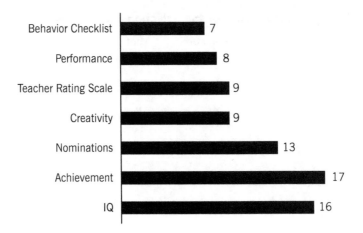

FIGURE 11.3. Required assessment methods for identification of giftedness. From McClain and Pfeiffer (2012).

the scope of this chapter to describe each of these methods and their advantages and limitations (for reviews, see Pfeiffer & Blei, 2008; Worrell & Erwin, 2011). Rather, here we discuss several important issues pertaining to the use of intelligence tests for determining giftedness and eligibility for gifted services.

Who Is Intellectually Gifted?

If we agree with Humphreys (1985) that "the fundamental basis for intellectual giftedness is a high level of general intelligence" (p. 332), then what level of intelligence constitutes giftedness? Should it be an IQ of 120, 130, 140, or above? Wherever one draws the line, it is completely arbitrary. As mentioned in Chapter 2, the distribution of intelligence in the population is approximately normal. Above the mean, the distribution of intelligence is continuous, not discrete. Qualitative differences do not exist between those at the high end of the intelligence distribution, as they do at the extreme low end (e.g., below IQs of 55), where intellectual disability (ID) tends to result from single-gene defects or chromosomal abnormalities and not from normal variability. Given that the differences among those at the high end of the intelligence distribution are quantitative and not qualitative, the label of *giftedness* is nothing more than a social construction indicating high aptitude in one or more domains (Pfeiffer, 2003).

> Given that the differences among those at the high end of the intelligence distribution are quantitative and not qualitative, the label of *giftedness* is nothing more than a social construction indicating high aptitude in one or more domains.

As one moves from the mean toward the extremely high end of the distribution, however, the number of cases becomes increasingly rare. If a cutoff score of 130 is used, then about 20 out of every 1,000 students would be eligible. If a cutoff score of 140 is used, then only about 4 out of every 1,000 could meet the criterion. The belief that 3–5% of the school-age population is gifted is a long-standing myth, most likely resulting from Marland's recommendations in 1972 (Borland, 2009). The percentage of students identified for gifted and talented programs, therefore, depends wholly on the needs of aims of educators for some desired social purpose and on the availability of funding for special programs and services for the gifted.

Use of Cutoff Scores

The reliability of test scores provides an estimate of the degree to which differences in true scores are reflected in differences in observed scores. A reliability coefficient of .90, for example, indicates that 90% of the observed differences in test scores are due to differences in true scores and 10% to error (error = 1.00 – reliability). As all measurement contains error, the reliability of test scores is always less than 1.00. No test is likely to provide perfectly consistent scores for individuals tested on more than one occasion or across alternate forms of the same test.

When an estimate of the accuracy of measurement for an individual is desired, the standard error of measurement (SE_m) is often used (see Chapter 6). In contrast to reliability, which provides information regarding the consistency of a test's scores, the SE_m estimates how widely different measures of the same person tend to be distributed around his or her true score. The SE_m is a kind of standard deviation of a set of measurements of the same construct. The SE_m is used to describe a *confidence interval* for an individual's obtained score. A confidence interval is defined as an interval within which a true score has a certain probability of being found.

Confidence intervals are employed to take into account the fact that all tests have less than perfect reliability. Because errors are assumed to be randomly distributed around the true score, the normal curve is used to estimate the size of the interval. As the obtained score is the best estimate of an individual's true score, that person's true score has a 68% chance of falling within ± 1 SE_m of the obtained score, a 95% chance of falling within ± 2 SE_m of the obtained score, and so on. For example, for an obtained score of 130 with a SE_m of 3, the 68% confidence interval is 130 ± 3, or 127–133. The 95% confidence interval for this obtained score is 100 ± 6, or 124–136. Note that the size of the interval corresponds to the degree of confidence that the true score is between the upper and lower limit of the interval. Confidence intervals therefore "reflect the accuracy and inaccuracy of scores and help in understanding the relative verity and utility of those scores in decision making" (Glutting, McDermott, & Stanley, 1987, p. 608). The existence of measurement error on all tests underscores the importance of not using the results of a single test and strict cutoff scores to identify intellectual giftedness.

Different types of confidence intervals are used for different situations. One common confidence interval is based on the SE_m. This method, however, does not take into account the effects of regression toward the mean. This is particularly important when one desires a relatively stable estimate of an examinee's intellectual functioning over time. In their classic work, Campbell and Stanley (1963) stated:

> Regression toward the mean is a ubiquitous phenomenon, not confined to pretesting and posttesting with the same test or comparable forms of a test. The principal who observes that his highest-IQ students tend to have less than the highest achievement-test score . . . would be guilty of the regression fallacy if he declared that his school is understimulating the brightest pupils. (p. 11)

In other words, some degree of "underachievement" is predictable with the gifted population. The opposite is true for individuals scoring near the bottom of the IQ distribution.

The fact that individuals at the extreme ends of the distribution are measured with less accuracy than individuals near the middle is related to regression. Hence, their confidence intervals should reflect this fact. Unfortunately, the SE_m does not take regression into account because it uses the obtained score. The *standard error of estimated true scores* (SE_E) does, however. In this method, the estimated true score is first determined, derived from regression of the obtained score toward the mean. A confidence interval is then built around the estimated true score in much the same way as that for the SE_m, except that regression is taken into account here as well. The obtained score will be within this interval. It is important to note that for obtained scores at the extreme ends of the distributions, the resulting confidence interval will be asymmetrical around the obtained score. However, symmetrical confidence intervals will be found (1) for all obtained scores when the reliability is perfect, which is virtually impossible to attain; and (2) for those obtained scores at the mean of the distribution, regardless of the test's reliability. Lastly, it is important to note that the SE_E should not be confused with standard error of the estimate, which is a different statistical test that is often used in hypothesis testing.

Giftedness as a Developmental Construct

Historically, children and youth were identified early in the primary grades on the basis of a high score on an intelligence test and placed in a program for the gifted for their entire educational careers, regardless of their future performance in school. As Nicpon and Pfeiffer (2011) have recently observed, however,

> Many students identified as gifted in kindergarten, for any number of reasons, do not distinguish themselves academically in the later years. And many students who are not identified as high IQ, intellectually precocious, or academically advanced in the early years are late bloomers and prove to have extraordinary potential and excel in their later years. (p. 296)

The categorical approach—wherein children are determined to be either eligible or ineligible for gifted programs and services, once and forever—is presumably based on the incorrect notion that intelligence tests measure something that is innate and therefore fixed. The presumed constancy of IQs has resulted in policies and practices based on long-term predictions of students' cognitive abilities that are not justified.

Scores on intelligence tests reflect the repertoire of knowledge and skills that an individual has developed at a particular point in time. They do not reflect something "bred in the bone." Indeed, the size of an individual's repertoire is a function of both his or her genetic endowment and the environments to which the person has been exposed. Although scores on intelligence tests are highly reliable after children reach school age, an individual's IQ can change considerably over time (e.g., Neisser et al., 1996).

The stability of IQs is related to the interval between test occasions: The longer the interval, the lower the stability. If we assume a stability coefficient of .70 over a 10-year period, "gifted" students with an IQ of 140 will obtain, on the average, a score of 125 on retesting a decade later. This change in scores results simply from the ubiquitous measurement phenomenon of regression toward the mean; it does not indicate that schools have failed to develop the cognitive abilities of these children.

The instability of IQs over development implies that the "educational system should be forgiving of early performance that is less than illustrious and should not give undue weight to early illustrious performance" (Humphreys, 1989, p. 203). It further implies that determining eligibility for gifted programs and services should be an ongoing process. Students classified for gifted on the basis of high potential (i.e., IQ > some cutoff score) should be held to high standards of domain-based performance to retain the gifted label (Worrell & Erwin, 2011). This perspective is consistent with developmental models of giftedness (e.g., Subotnik et al., 2011), as well as response-to-intervention (RTI) service delivery models (e.g., Jimerson, Burns, & VanDerHeyden, 2007).

Fairness in Assessment of Giftedness

Most experts agree that a sufficiently high level of general intelligence is a necessary but not sufficient condition for giftedness (e.g., see Sternberg & Davidson, 2005). Although intelligence tests are better predictors of outcomes in educational than any other measureable human characteristic (e.g., Gottfredson, 2002), the prediction of real-world criteria by intelligence tests is not perfect. In schools, at most *half* of the variance in school grades and on achievement tests is explained by intelligence tests; this indicates that other cognitive and noncognitive variables are also important (e.g., Gottfredson, 1997). It also means that the identification of giftedness should never rely upon the result of one test, including intelligence tests.

In addition, research clearly indicates that the most widely used intelligence tests are not significantly biased against English-speaking children born and raised in the United States (see Chapter 13). These findings, however, do not generalize to children and youth who are not native-born or who have limited English proficiency (LEP). The results of verbally loaded tests with this population should be interpreted carefully, if at all, and should be supplemented by nonverbal intelligence tests. Several standardized nonverbal tests of intelligence with adequate psychometric properties and norms are available for use with children and youth from diverse linguistic and cultural backgrounds (for a review, see Braden & Athanasiou, 2005). Recent research has found that use of nonverbal tests is an important component of eligibility determination for gifted and talented programs with diverse populations (e.g., Lohman, Korb, & Lakin, 2008; Lohman & Lakin, 2007).

According to the Ethical Principles of Psychologists and Code of Conduct of the American Psychological Association (APA, 2002, 2010a),

> When interpreting assessment results, including automated interpretations, psychologists take into account the purpose of the assessment as well as the various test factors, test-taking abilities, and other characteristics of the person being assessed, such as situational, personal, linguistic, and cultural differences, that might affect psychologists' judgments or reduce the accuracy of their interpretations. They indicate any significant limitations of their interpretations. (Standard 9.06)

When interpreting their results, therefore, assessors must always consider the potential impact of cultural and linguistic background on test performance.

Twice-Exceptionality

Twice-exceptional is a term used for any student who simultaneously is gifted and has a diagnosed disability. In other words, despite above-average general intelligence, the student experiences learning difficulties as a result of a disability, such as specific learning disability (SLD), obsessive–compulsive disorder, or attention-deficit/hyperactivity disorder (ADHD) (Assouline & Whiteman, 2011). Estimates of the prevalence of twice-exceptional students range from 2% to 5% of the gifted population, although it is possible that this is a conservative estimate (Delisle & Galbraith, 2002). Given the number of potential concomitant disabilities, no consistent profile of these students is possible. Children who are twice-exceptional tend to exhibit a marked pattern of talents or strengths on the one hand, and areas of weaknesses in others (Baum & Owen, 1988; Fox, Brody, & Tobin, 1983; Whitmore & Maker, 1985).

According to Assouline and Whiteman (2011), gifted students with SLD are among the most underserved in the schools today. These students generally fall into three groups: (1) students identified as gifted who have learning difficulties in specific domains; (2) students with identified SLD who are also gifted; and (3) students who are intellectually gifted and have a disability but are not identified because their academic achievement falls in the average range.

Controversy currently surrounds the identification of this third group, given that an IQ–achievement discrepancy is no longer required for the identification of SLD. In an RTI service delivery model, which many districts are adopting across the nation, the focus is on the identifica-

> **Gifted students with SLD are among the most under-served in the schools today.**

tion of students who do not meet minimum expectations. In an RTI model, this latter group of students may not be identified unless their academic performance falls below expected benchmarks. Without the administration of intelligence tests, it is unclear how these students can be identified when their performance falls within normal expectations. Assouline and Whiteman (2011), therefore, recommend a comprehensive assessment, including an individually administered intelligence test, to identify achievement discrepancies and areas of strengths and disability. At the present time, however, there is a paucity of empirical research on twice-exceptional children and youth. Over the past 20 years, only 43 empirical articles have been published on this population (Assouline & Whiteman, 2011). Further research is needed, therefore, particularly within RTI models, to determine whether this approach is effective with this population or whether other intervention strategies are required.

SHARING RESULTS AND RESOURCES

Consistent with other chapters, we have provided a basic checklist of considerations for assessment of intellectual giftedness. (Chapter 8 provides text for psychoeducational assessment reports that describe the results of assessments targeting giftedness and its associated features.) Table 11.2 lists questions to consider during the assessment of students for intellectual giftedness. These questions address not only good assessment practices (e.g., using instruments with established validity and from multiple sources), but other important considerations, such as the state or district definition of giftedness.

SUMMARY

Over the past 20 years, much has changed in the field of gifted education. New theories have been proposed that expand the conception of giftedness beyond the traditional definition of high general intelligence and attempt to explain the factors related to the development of outstanding accomplishment. This chapter has reviewed a number of contemporary theories and current assessment practices. Although the assessment of intelligence currently plays an important role in determining eligibility for gifted and talented programs in many states, intelligence tests are rarely the sole determinant of eligibility; if the present trend continues, even less emphasis may be placed on their results in the future.

TABLE 11.2. Questions to Consider during Diagnostic and Eligibility Assessment for Intellectual Giftedness

Preassessment considerations

1. Is the goal of the gifted program (a) to allow students to examine concepts in greater depth or in an earlier grade than they might in a typical classroom (acceleration), or (b) to allow students to move through the curriculum at a faster pace than peers (acceleration)?
2. What academic and other domains (e.g., mathematics, language arts, and science) is the gifted program planning to target?
3. What domain-specific skills are important to measure alongside general intelligence?
4. Are the individuals being identified likely to have well-developed skills in the domain, or do preskills need to be assessed?
5. Is the level of exposure to the domain likely to vary widely among individuals being assessed on the basis of background variables, such as socioeconomic status or first language? If yes, how are these concerns addressed in your identification protocol?

Intelligence assessment considerations

6. Was at least one intelligence test administered under conditions that should ensure valid results?
   a. Was it recently normed?
   b. Does the IQ demonstrate internal consistency reliability of .95 or higher and test–retest reliability of .90 or higher?
   c. Is the IQ supported by sufficient validity evidence (ideally, studies of children with intellectual giftedness)?
   d. Do the test's subtests have sufficiently high ceilings?
   e. Was the child sufficiently motivated to respond, and was there an absence of interfering factors?
7. Was an IQ obtained that indicates a high level of general intelligence?
8. Were 90% or 95% confidence intervals considered when the IQ was interpreted?
9. If measures targeting more specific cognitive abilities are targeted in the assessment, do they meet psychometric standards for assessment of students with giftedness?
   a. Does the measure demonstrate internal consistency reliability of .90 or higher and test–retest reliability of .90 or higher?
   b. Is the measure supported by sufficient validity evidence (ideally, studies of children with intellectual giftedness)?
   c. Do the test's subtests contributing to the measures (and the measure itself) have sufficiently high ceilings?

Other assessment considerations

10. Has a comprehensive achievement test been administered, and does it meet psychometric standards for assessment of students with giftedness?
11. Has screening for mental health disorders (e.g., obsessive–compulsive disorder or ADHD) been conducted?

Note. Adapted from Worrell and Erwin (2011).

CHAPTER 12

Assessment of Learning Disabilities

Almost 2.5 million children and youth in the United States, or more than 5% of the entire school-age population, are classified as having a specific learning disability (SLD). SLD is also by far the largest disability category in special education (National Center for Education Statistics [NCES], 2011). Almost 40% of all students receiving special education services under the Individuals with Disabilities Education Improvement Act of 2004 (IDEA, 2004) have SLD as their primary disability category; this exceeds the percentages of children with the second and third most prevalent disability categories (viz., Speech or Language Impairment and Other Health Impairment) *combined*. Moreover, the number of children and youth identified as having SLD has increased over 100% since the passage of the Education for All Handicapped Children Act of 1975 (i.e., Public Law 94-142, the original version of IDEA).

Despite the prevalence of SLD in the schools, a heated debate has long surrounded the definition and diagnosis of SLD. Many of the contemporary issues in SLD theory and research stem from the reauthorization of IDEA in 2004, which allows the use of response to intervention (RTI) as an approach for identifying SLD, rather than sole reliance on the traditional IQ–achievement discrepancy approach.

In this chapter, we first review the various definitions of SLD, followed by research on the nature of SLD. Next, we discuss the three main methods for identifying SLD, and the role played by intelligence tests within each. We conclude with a discussion of best practices for the identification of SLD.

WHAT IS A LEARNING DISABILITY?

The term *learning disability* can be conceptualized in either a broad or narrow sense. In the broad sense, it refers to a general difficulty in learning that does not meet the criteria for intellectual disability (ID) (i.e., IQ < 70). Individuals with learning disabilities in this sense are often referred to as *slow learners*, because they have difficulty grasping concepts at the same rate and depth of understanding as their same-age peers do. Although the term *slow learner* is not a diagnostic category, because it represents the low end of the normal range in intelligence, it has traditionally been defined as someone with an IQ between 70 and 85 (e.g., Shaw, 2010). Given the approximately normal distribution of intelligence, this means that about 16% of the school-age population has an IQ below 85. As the name implies, slow learners do indeed learn. However, they tend to benefit from very explicit, hands-on instruction, and they often need more time and repetition to be successful in school than their peers need.

> **The term *learning disability* can be conceptualized in either a broad or narrow sense.**

In contrast to the broad-sense conceptualization of learning disability, this term in the narrow sense refers to *unexpected underachievement*. That is, individuals experience difficulty with learning in some, but not all, areas of academic achievement (e.g., reading or mathematics), despite adequate educational opportunity, motivation, and cognitive ability. At the heart of this conceptualization is the concept of *discrepancy* in cognitive functioning, traditionally defined by the difference between IQ and achievement. The narrow-sense conceptualization of learning disability is the traditional definition of SLD and is what most people mean when they refer to SLD. According to IDEA (2004), a child may be determined to have SLD in the following areas: (1) oral expression, (2) listening comprehension, (3) written expression, (4) basic reading skill, (5) reading fluency skills, (6) reading comprehension, (7) mathematics calculation, and (8) mathematics problem solving.

The term *learning disability* was first introduced in 1962 in a textbook by Samuel Kirk titled *Educating Exceptional Children*. According to Kirk,

> A learning disability refers to a retardation, disorder, or delayed development in one or more of the processes of speech, language, reading, spelling, writing, or arithmetic resulting from a possible cerebral dysfunction and/or emotional or behavioral disturbance and not from mental retardation, sensory deprivation, or cultural or instructional factors. (1962, p. 263)

Kirk later stated that a learning disability refers to "a discrepancy between a child's achievement and his apparent capacity to learn as indicated by aptitude tests, verbal understanding, and arithmetic computation" (Kirk & Kirk, 1983, p. 20). In this *IQ–achievement discrepancy approach*, SLD is identified when an individual's level of performance or rate of skill acquisition in a particular academic area falls substantially below the level one would predict from his or her intelligence. Although multiple exclusionary criteria exist in this definition (i.e., ID, sensory deprivation, cultural or instructional factors), the IQ–achievement discrepancy is the primary inclusionary criterion for SLD diagnosis.

Consistent with Kirk's (1962) definition of SLD, the Education for All Handicapped Children Act of 1975, the first federal legislation mandating a free and appropriate education for all children, required the identification of a "severe discrepancy between achievement and intellectual ability in one or more of the following areas: oral expression, listening comprehension, written expression, basic reading skill, reading comprehension, mathematics calculation or mathematics reasoning" (U.S. Office of Education, 1977). Shortly after the passage of the 1975 Act, the vast majority of state regulations for special education involved some type of an IQ–achievement discrepancy formula for the identification of SLD (e.g., Mercer, Jordan, Allsopp, & Mercer, 1996).

The *Diagnostic and Statistical Manual of Mental Disorders*, fourth edition, text revision (DSM-IV-TR; American Psychiatric Association, 2000), which uses the term *learning disorders (formerly academic skills disorders)*, is also consistent with the IQ–achievement discrepancy approach:

> Learning Disorders are diagnosed when the individual's achievement on individually administered, standardized tests in reading, mathematics, or written expression is substantially below that expected for age, schooling, and level of intelligence. The learning problems significantly interfere with academic achievement or activities of daily living that require reading, mathematical, or writing skills. A variety of statistical approaches can be used to establish that a discrepancy is significant. *Substantially below* is usually defined as a discrepancy of more than 2 standard deviations between achievement and IQ. A smaller discrepancy between achievement and IQ (i.e., between 1 and 2 standard deviations) is sometimes used, especially in cases where an individual's performance on an IQ test may have been compromised by an associated disorder in cognitive processing, a comorbid mental disorder or a general medical condition, or the individual's ethnic or cultural background. If a sensory deficit is present, the learning difficulties must be in excess of those usually associated with the deficit. Learning Disorders may persist into adulthood. . . . There may be underlying abnormalities in cognitive processing (e.g., deficits in visual perception, linguistic processes, attention or memory, or a combination of these) that often precede or are associated with Learning Disorders. (American Psychiatric Association, 2000, pp. 49–50)

The DSM-IV-TR recognizes the following learning disorders: *reading disorder, mathematics disorder, disorder of written expression*, and *learning disorder not otherwise specified*.

In the recently published DSM-5 (American Psychiatric Association, 2013), in contrast, the identification of SLD does not specifically mention in IQ–achievement discrepancy. Instead, "specific learning disorder" is defined as academic performance in reading, writing, or mathematics that is "substantially and quantifiably" below expectations for individuals of the same chronological age, as indicated by comprehensive clinical assessment that includes scores on individually administered standardized tests of academic achievement. Although the use of IQ tests is not specifically mentioned, according to the exclusionary criteria in the DSM-5 one must rule out ID as an explanatory factor for underachievement.

The definition of *learning disabilities* by the National Joint Committee on Learning Disabilities (NJCLD, 1994) also clearly avoids the IQ–achievement discrepancy approach:

> Learning disabilities is a general term that refers to a heterogeneous group of disorders manifested by significant difficulties in the acquisition and use of listening, speaking, reading, writing, reasoning, or mathematical abilities. These disorders are intrinsic to the individual, presumed to be due to central nervous system dysfunction, and may occur across the life span. Problems in self-regulatory behaviors, social perception, and social interaction may exist with learning disabilities but do not by themselves constitute a learning disability. Although learning disabilities may occur concomitantly with other handicapping conditions (for example, sensory impairment, mental retardation, serious emotional disturbance), or with extrinsic influences (such as cultural differences, insufficient or inappropriate instruction), they are not the result of those conditions or influences.

Furthermore, the NJCLD (1994) stated that "cognitive ability/achievement discrepancies should be used cautiously because a learning disability can exist when a numerical discrepancy does not." Therefore, two different views have emerged over the years: one that defines SLD in terms of an IQ–achievement discrepancy, and another that does not.

The definition of SLD in IDEA (2004) is particularly important. Although it applies only to schools, virtually all individuals are diagnosed with SLD while in school. The following is the IDEA definition of SLD:

> *Specific learning disability* means a disorder in one or more of the basic psychological processes involved in understanding or in using language, spoken or written, which may manifest itself in the imperfect ability to listen, think, speak, read, write, spell, or do mathematical calculations. Such term includes such conditions as perceptual disabilities, brain injury, minimal brain dysfunction, dyslexia, and developmental aphasia. Such term does not include a learning problem that is primarily the result of visual, hearing, or motor disabilities, of mental retardation, of emotional disturbance, or of environmental, cultural, or economic disadvantage. (IDEA, 2004)

This definition resembles that of the DSM-5 and the NJCLD, in that it does not refer to intelligence or aptitude and does not mention an IQ–achievement discrepancy. It is important to note that although there was no change in the definition of SLD in the reauthorization of this law in 2004, determination of a discrepancy between IQ and achievement for the identification of SLD is allowed, *but no longer required*. As an alternative identification method, IDEA (2004) allows the use of RTI, or "a process that determines if the child responds to scientific, research-based intervention as a part of the evaluation procedures" (IDEA, 2004), in determining whether a child has SLD (see Chapter 9). In 2011, for the identification of SLD, five states required the use of RTI only, and eight states required RTI and some other method (O'Connor et al., 2012).

Florida is an example of a state that has adopted an RTI approach to SLD identification and does not require determination of a discrepancy between IQ and achievement. According to the Florida rules and regulations for exceptional student education (Florida Department of Education, 2011):

> A specific learning disability is defined as a disorder in one or more of the *basic learning processes* involved in understanding or in using language, spoken or written, that may manifest in significant difficulties affecting the ability to listen, speak, read, write, spell, or do mathematics. Associated conditions may include, but are not limited to, dyslexia, dyscalculia, dysgraphia, or developmental aphasia. A specific learning disability does not include learning problems that are primarily the result of a visual, hearing, motor, intellectual, or emotional/behavioral disability, limited English proficiency, or environmental, cultural, or economic factors. (p. 258, emphasis added)

Note that the Florida regulations have replaced the term *basic psychological processes* with *basic learning processes*, presumably to emphasize the assessment of academic achievement and to deemphasize the assessment of intelligence or psychological processing.

In Florida, in addition to the usual exclusionary criteria, determination of SLD is based on an academic performance discrepancy and inadequate rate of progress:

1. *Performance discrepancy.* The student's academic performance is significantly discrepant for the chronological age or grade level in which the student is enrolled, based on multiple

sources of data when compared to multiple groups, which include the peer subgroup, classroom, school, district, and state level comparison groups.

2. *Rate of progress.* When provided with well-delivered scientific, appropriate research-based general education . . . instruction and interventions of reasonable intensity and duration with evidence of implementation fidelity, the student's rate of progress is insufficient or requires sustained and substantial effort to close the achievement gap with typical peers or academic expectations for the chronological age or grade level in which the student is currently enrolled . . . (Florida Department of Education, 2011, pp. 268–269)

Thus, in a dual-discrepancy model such as Florida's RTI approach, SLD is identified when an individual's level of performance or rate of skill acquisition in a particular academic area falls substantially below the level one would predict from his or her age or grade peer group, rather than the level of achievement one would predict from the individual's cognitive ability.

At present, no consensus-based definition of SLD exists. Nevertheless, the most prevalent definitions of SLD are similar in a number of ways: (1) All individuals with SLD share a difficulty with school learning; (2) certain factors must be ruled out before SLD can be identified (e.g., inadequate educational or language background, sensory impairment, ID); and (3) discrepancy in achievement is a fundamental aspect of identification. Clearly, the biggest point of disagreement among the most widely used definitions of SLD is the need for assessment of intelligence for SLD diagnosis (see Fletcher-Janzen & Reynolds, 2009).

> **The most prevalent definitions of SLD are similar in a number of ways: (1) All individuals with SLD share a difficulty with school learning; (2) certain factors must be ruled out before SLD can be identified; and (3) discrepancy in achievement is a fundamental aspect of identification.**

THE NATURE OF SLD

According to the recent position statement on SLD by the National Association of School Psychologists (NASP, 2010b), there is widespread agreement among researchers on the following:

- Specific learning disabilities are endogenous in nature and are characterized by neurologically based deficits in cognitive processes.
- These deficits are specific; that is, they impact particular cognitive processes that interfere with the acquisition of academic skills.
- Specific learning disabilities are heterogeneous—there are various types of learning disabilities, and there is no single defining academic or cognitive deficit or characteristic common to all types of specific learning disabilities.
- Specific learning disabilities may coexist with other disabling conditions (e.g., sensory deficits, language impairment, behavior problems), but are not primarily due to these conditions.
- Of children identified as having specific learning disabilities, the great majority (over 80%) have a disability in the area of reading.
- The manifestation of a specific learning disability is contingent to some extent upon the type of instruction, supports, and accommodations provided, and the demands of the learning situation.
- Early intervention can reduce the impact of many specific learning disabilities.

- Specific learning disabilities vary in their degree of severity, and moderate to severe learning disabilities can be expected to impact performance throughout the life span.
- Multi-tiered systems of student support have been effective as part of comprehensive approaches to meet students' academic needs. (p. 1)

In a recent review of the SLD literature, Brown, Daly, and Stafanatos (2009) concluded that "while no single biological marker has been implicated among individuals with learning disabilities, there is evidence from genetics, neuroimaging studies, and studies of the neurotransmitters to suggest that this disorder is firmly rooted in the brain" (p. 166).

Results of behavior genetic research strongly indicate that SLD has a substantial heritable component and is therefore related to the functioning of the brain (e.g., Berninger, 2008). For example, family studies indicate that siblings and parents of children with reading disabilities (RD) have more reading difficulties than control families. LaBuda, Vogler, DeFries, and Fulker (1986) examined 125 families with at least one child with RD and 125 matched-control families. Consistent with a genetic hypothesis, the families of the children with RD obtained significantly lower scores on measures of reading than did the control families. The rates of reading problems among children who have parents with RD are estimated to be as high as 30–60% (Breiger & Majovski, 2009).

Results of twin studies also have found substantially higher concordance rates for monozygotic (MZ) twins than for dizygotic (DZ) twins for RD (e.g., DeFries & Gillis, 1993; Stevenson, Graham, Fredman, & McLoughlin, 1987). Differences in the criteria used to define RD are one likely cause of at least some of the variability in the results of these studies. Although less is known about the heritability of SLD in other academic areas (e.g., mathematics, spelling, and written expression), behavior genetic research clearly shows that SLD has a sizeable genetic component. This underscores the need to consider characteristics of the individual and of his or her interaction with the environment when one is diagnosing SLD.

At the current time, the majority of behavior genetic and neurocognitive research that has been conducted has focused on RD. Several neurological and biological theories of RD have been postulated, including those related to biochemical and electrophysiological functioning of the brain, as well as its neurological structure. Although it is difficult to summarize the results of this research, the evidence suggests that disruption of the language-processing system in specific brain regions results in difficulty with phonological processing for individuals with RD (e.g., see Shaywitz & Shaywitz, 2003, for a review).

Phonological processing involves the ability to associate the letters of words with discrete sounds. Phonological processing includes three components that are important for reading: (1) phonological awareness (i.e., knowledge that letters represent certain sounds), (2) rapid naming/word retrieval, and (3) working memory. Most individuals with RD experience difficulty with phonological awareness. Although less is presently known about the cognitive processing deficits underlying other types of SLD (e.g., mathematics), recent research has revealed that the heritability of math disabilities and of RD overlaps, suggesting that the same genes are related to both types of SLD (for a review, see Plomin & Kovas, 2005).

Despite the considerable progress made by neuroscience in clarifying the biological basis of SLD, the application of the results of this research to educational intervention has been limited (Therrien, Zaman, & Banda, 2011). As Swanson (2009) has stated, "although brain studies linking neurological underpinnings to behavioral function are necessary to provide a theoretical context to understanding [S]LD, altering instruction as a function of this knowledge base has not been clearly formulated" (p. 30). Nevertheless, Vaughn and Fuchs (2003) asserted that "although there is little doubt that many individuals with SLD have neurological deficits, the field simply has been unsuccess-

> **Despite the considerable progress made by neuroscience in clarifying the biological basis of SLD, the application of the results of this research to educational intervention has been limited.**

ful at reliably identifying those deficits and, more importantly, in linking the assessment of processing deficits to effective instructions" (p. 140). Indeed, some have summarized what is known about SLD as "a rather arbitrarily defined class of unclearly differentiated deficits in cognitive functions broadly conceived, but less behaviorally pervasive than would be implied by mental retardation" (Jensen, 1987, p. 68).

One potential explanation for the unsuccessful identification of the processing deficits hypothesized to underlie SLD concerns the use of traditional psychometric tests. Elsewhere (Floyd & Kranzler, 2012), we have argued that these instruments are far too complex for the assessment of underlying processing disorders. Not only do individual differences on these tests reflect various factors of human cognitive ability, but the test scores involve many distinct lower-order cognitive processes and reflect only the results of mental activity and not the cognitive processes themselves. Given the complexity of psychometric tests, advances in the assessment of SLD are likely to depend on the development of new assessment instruments, such as ones related to the techniques of mental chronometry (e.g., see Jensen, 2006, for a review), that are closer to the interface between brain and behavior.

METHODS FOR DETERMINING ACHIEVEMENT DISCREPANCY

Despite the fact that no consensus definition of SLD exists, at the core of each of these definitions is the concept of discrepancy in academic functioning. Figure 12.1 presents a scatterplot of the correlation between the overall scores for intelligence and reading achievement for 1,485 children and youth on the Woodcock–Johnson III (WJ III) Tests of Cognitive Abilities and Tests of Achievement (Woodcock, McGrew, & Mather, 2001). As shown here, there is a strong positive correlation between intelligence and reading achievement of +.68. This correlation means that on average, the higher one's intelligence, the better one is at reading, and vice versa. If we exclude those with ID (i.e., IQ < 75), who has SLD? The child with an above-average IQ who is reading in the average range? Or the child who is reading in the lowest quartile, regardless of IQ?

In this section, we address this question by briefly reviewing the most prevalent methods for identifying an achievement discrepancy, and therefore determining whether an individual has SLD: (1) the traditional IQ–achievement discrepancy method, and (2) the need-based or RTI discrepancy method now allowed under IDEA (2004). As we will see, the method one chooses for identifying SLD will result in largely different groups of individuals.

IQ–Achievement Discrepancy

In the IQ–achievement discrepancy approach, SLD is identified when an individual's level of performance or rate of skill acquisition in a particular academic area falls substantially below the level one would predict from his or her intelligence. In this approach, IQ is used as a benchmark

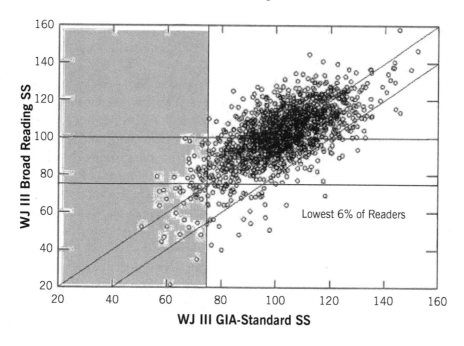

FIGURE 12.1. Correlation between reading and intelligence ($r = +.68$; $N = 1,485$). SS, standard score. Data from the Woodcock–Muñoz Foundation.

against which to compare achievement, and students' achievement is assumed to be commensurate with their IQ.

The simplest and most straightforward way to determine the presence of IQ–achievement discrepancy is to determine whether a large difference (D) exists between scores on IQ and achievement tests, when scores are expressed in the same metric, such as standard-score (z-score) units, as in this formula:

$$D = Z_{IQ} - Z_{ach}$$

A significant discrepancy exists if

$$D > Z_{critical}$$

where $Z_{critical}$ is some predetermined cutoff score, such as a z score of 1.0 or 1.5.

Figure 12.1 shows the individuals who would qualify for a diagnosis of SLD when this simple discrepancy approach is used. The diagonal line in the middle of the scatterplot is the expected level of achievement across intelligence. Achievement scores below the diagonal line that is parallel to but lower than the line in the middle of the scatterplot are significantly lower than the level of performance expected on the basis of intelligence. These are the students who are potentially eligible for a diagnosis of SLD in the IQ–achievement discrepancy approach. As can be seen here, within this approach, the group with SLD consists of individuals with IQs in the average to above-average range. Children and youth with IQs in the below-average range who do not have ID are generally not eligible for special education services, despite the fact that their reading achievement is among the lowest in mainstream classes. Because their IQ and reading achievement scores are comparably low, the discrepancy between them is not of a significant magnitude to qualify for special education.

One criticism of the use of the IQ–achievement discrepancy approach is that it precludes the identification of low-performing students (without ID) who have serious educational needs for special education and related services. Because it is often difficult to determine a severe discrepancy until as late as the third grade, the IQ–achievement discrepancy model is often referred to as a "wait-to-fail" model (e.g., Vaughn & Fuchs, 2003). The simple discrepancy model, however, has also been criticized on psychometric grounds, because it does not account for regression toward the mean and measurement error. Regression models, therefore, are generally seen as an improvement over the simple model for determining significant intelligence–achievement discrepancies, because they take into account the phenomenon of regression toward the mean.

As noted in earlier chapters, *regression toward the mean* refers to the fact that when two variables are correlated (imperfectly), as intelligence and achievement are, an individual's score on the predicted variable tends to be not as extreme as his or her score on the predictor. Also, the more extreme the score on the predictor is, the more that score is subject to regression. Campbell and Stanley (1963) stated 50 years ago:

> The more deviant the score, the larger the error of measurement it probably contains. Thus, in a sense, the typical extremely high scorer has had unusually good "luck" (large positive error) and the extremely low scorer bad luck (large negative error). Luck is capricious, however, so on a posttest we expect the high scorers to decline somewhat on the other average, the low scorers to improve their average. . . . Regression toward the mean is a ubiquitous phenomenon, not confined to pre-testing and post-testing with the same test or comparable forms of a test. (p. 11)

In other words, some degree of academic "underachievement" is predictable for students with high IQs. The opposite is true for individuals scoring near the bottom of the IQ distribution. When regression to the mean is *not* taken into account in the identification of SLD, this results in the *overidentification* of children with above-average IQs and the *underidentification* of children with below-average IQs.

Simple regression models, therefore, compare the difference between the *obtained* achievement score and the *predicted* achievement score, which is determined by the regression of IQ on achievement. In this way, "real" underachievement is compared with "expected" underachievement. If the obtained achievement score is significantly below what one would predict from that child's level of intelligence, then a discrepancy is said to exist. Thus, this model is actually an expected–actual achievement model and not an IQ–achievement discrepancy model. Although the simple regression model adequately takes regression toward the mean into account, it does not control for errors of measurement that creep into assessment as a function of unreliability.

To correct for measurement error, the full regression model was developed to "evaluate the difference between regressed achievement and aptitude scores (but regressed as a function of the unreliability of the scores)" (Reynolds, 1984–1985, p. 462). In other words, the full regression model examines the difference between the *obtained* IQ and achievement scores that have been independently regressed to their respective means on the basis of measurement error, as estimated by the internal consistency reliability of each instrument. Unlike the simple regression model, this model takes errors of measurement into account. Unfortunately, this model does not actually correct for the problem of regression. It can therefore be criticized on the same grounds as the *z*-score discrepancy model.

Reynolds (1984–1985) and Shepard (1989) argued that the full regression model is not only (according to Reynolds) "mathematically unacceptable," but "conceptually flawed" as well. Reynolds (1984–1985) stated that the full regression model is appropriate for use only when measures of low reliability are available. Of course, virtually every standardized IQ and achievement test in use today has more than adequate reliability, so there is little or no need for the full regression formula. Shepard (1989) concurred, pointing out that the full regression model does not consider the well-established empirical relationship between measures of IQ and achievement. According to Shepard, this model is inappropriate because it treats intelligence and achievement tests "as if they were estimators of the same underlying ability" (p. 560). This is problematic, she added, because it "contradicts our understanding of SLD as specific learning deficits that are distinct from general intellectual functioning" (p. 560). Neither Reynolds nor Shepard, therefore, recommended the use of the full regression model.

In addition to these concerns, critics have argued that intelligence tests are irrelevant to the identification of SLD (e.g., Siegel, 1989, 1992; Stanovich & Siegel, 1994). As Francis et al. (2005) have stated, "these arguments are supported by studies demonstrating that IQ-discrepant and low achieving groups overlap and are difficult to differentiate on cognitive and behavioral characteristics, response to intervention, prognosis, and other areas" (p. 98). Consequently, they have argued for the identification of SLD simply on the basis of significant low achievement (e.g., see Shinn, 2005). At the current time, the IQ–achievement discrepancy approach has few proponents; even the American Psychiatric Association (2013) has moved away from it in the DSM-5.

Problem-Solving/RTI Achievement Discrepancy Method

Fuchs (1995) has proposed a problem-solving model within which the assessment of disabilities occurs in three phases (see Chapter 9). Tier 1 involves tracking the academic performance of all students in general education classes to determine whether instruction is adequate. Progress in RTI models is typically tracked in elementary schools with curriculum-based measurement (CBM) of basic academic skills. Most CBM approaches involve administering a set of short-duration fluency measures to assess basic skills in such academic areas as reading, spelling, written expression, and mathematics computation (e.g., Shinn & Bamonto, 1998). In Tier 2, students who are performing well below grade-level expectations are identified and given more intensive instruction. The academic progress of students identified at Tier 2 is then monitored. Special education and related services at Tier 3 are considered only when these educational adaptations fail to improve student academic performance. Thus, in the RTI achievement discrepancy approach, students with SLD are defined as those who are performing below expectations in comparison to their age or grade peers.

Differentiating among those students who do not respond to academic interventions is the key question in determining eligibility for special education services. In the RTI model, "CBM-guided decision making relies primarily on a norm-referenced approach" (Shinn & Habedank, 1992, p. 12). Academic progress is monitored during instructional intervention by examining change in CBM performance within students (i.e., rate of growth on CBM). In contrast, screening and determination of eligibility for special education and related services depend upon norm-referenced interpretation (i.e., comparison of a student's CBM performance with that of peers).

At the current time, there are at least three different ways to categorize responders and non-responders in the RTI literature (see Fuchs & Deshler, 2007): (1) examination of academic growth rate, as measured by the slope of CBM scores over time; (2) comparison of academic achievement to a final benchmark, as measured either by a standardized achievement test or CBM; or (3) a dual-discrepancy approach, as measured by both the slope of CBM scores over time and a comparison of final performance on fluency CBM to a benchmark at the end of instruction. In each of these methods, nonresponders are defined by performance that falls below a predetermined cutoff point, in comparison to either school, district, or national norms. For example, nonresponders have been alternatively defined as having a CBM slope that is below the median in comparison with same-grade peers (Christ, Zopluoglu, Long, & Monaghen, 2012; Vellutino et al., 1996); a standardized achievement test score that is below the 25th percentile (Torgesen et al., 2001); or a CBM slope and final CBM score that are one standard deviation below those of classroom peers (Fuchs & Fuchs, 1998). In Figure 12.1, the two horizontal lines show the average level of achievement for all students and the cut-off for those whose level of achievement is in the lowest 6% of all readers. In RTI achievement discrepancy approach, those falling below the lower of the two horizontal lines would be considered to have SLD.

Shinn (2007) has opined that "using a RTI model, it is not expected that different students will be identified as SLD than those identified historically" (p. 601). In actuality, however, very little is known about whether the different RTI identification methods will yield students with profiles of disability similar to those produced via the IQ–achievement discrepancy method (Fuchs & Deshler, 2007). Reynolds (2009) has predicted that because of the strong positive correlation between intelligence and achievement, use of the RTI achievement discrepancy approach will inevitably lead to the overrepresentation of children and youth with IQs < 85. As shown in Figure 12.1, regardless of where one sets the cutoff point for a significant achievement discrepancy, it seems highly likely that there will be an overrepresentation of slow learners among those identified as having SLD. In fact, the results of recent research by Fletcher et al. (2011) support Reynolds's contention. In a study of the cognitive correlates of inadequate response to reading intervention, Fletcher et al. found that the mean IQ for groups of nonresponders was below 90, in comparison to mean IQs of responders and typically achieving children in the average range (see also Brown Waesche, Schatschneider, Maner, Ahmed, & Wagner, 2011; Fuchs, Fuchs, & Compton, 2004).

If Reynolds (2009) is correct, then the RTI achievement discrepancy approach to identification represents a fundamental shift in the concept of SLD from the narrow-sense definition of unexpected underachievement to the broad-sense definition of being a slow learner. As he has argued, individuals with above-average IQs and academic achievement in the average range will not receive individualized or special education services, because their performance compares favorably to the mean performance of their peers. We agree with Reynolds (2009) that although one might argue that this is consistent with the principles of social justice, it is in the best interests of society to promote the optimal academic achievement of all children and not just the lowest-performing ones.

Moreover, the RTI achievement discrepancy approach has been found to be susceptible to psychometric criticisms similar to those leveled at the IQ–achievement discrepancy approach. For example, Francis et al. (2005) examined the stability of diagnoses of SLD based on the IQ–achievement and RTI achievement discrepancy (e.g., Shinn, 2007) approaches. Results of their study, using both simulated and actual longitudinal data, revealed that both methods were relatively unstable in terms of diagnosis over time. Thus, a major criticism of the IQ–achievement discrepancy method of identification—that is, the unreliability of SLD diagnosis—also applies to the RTI achievement discrepancy method. Francis et al. (2005) concluded that neither approach is viable by itself, because both essentially use a single indicator (viz., IQ–achievement discrepancy or low achievement) as the inclusionary criterion to identify SLD. They concluded that this criticism does not invalidate the concept of SLD in the narrow sense (i.e., unexpected underachievement); it only means that other factors need to be considered, such as exclusionary criteria and responsiveness to intervention, in making a diagnosis of SLD.

Figure 12.1 shows the proportions of children and youth who will be identified with SLD under the different diagnostic approaches. As can be seen, the groups of students identified with SLD will differ in largely predictable ways according to identification method. The IQ–achievement discrepancy method will tend to identify a greater number of students with above-average IQs, depending on the method of discrepancy used (e.g., simple or regression), whereas the RTI achievement discrepancy approach will tend to result in more students with below-average IQs, many of whom will fall in the slow-learner range of intellectual functioning (i.e., IQ < 85).

> **The groups of students identified with SLD will differ in largely predictable ways according to identification method.**

BEST PRACTICES IN SLD DIAGNOSIS

General Recommendations

The diagnosis of SLD is made by multidisciplinary teams in schools and by private practitioners in other settings (e.g., Reschly & Hosp, 2004). In schools, IDEA (2004) provides a definition of SLD and the legal underpinnings for the identification process. Rules and regulations at the state and district levels, however, define the required steps in the assessment process within individual schools. Because the federal law defines SLD primarily in terms of exclusionary criteria—that is, by what SLD is not, not by what it is—conceptual definitions of SLD and their accompanying classification criteria are generally consistent with federal law but tend to vary from state to state (e.g., Reschly & Hosp, 2004). The implication of this variability is that eligibility determination for SLD for special education and related services in schools depends to some degree upon an individual's state of residence. Outside schools, private practitioners may adopt the definition of SLD and identification criteria of the state educational agency or use another classification approach, such as that of the American Psychiatric Association (2013).

Regardless of the regulations used to diagnose SLD, it important to follow best-practice recommendations, such as those by the NASP (2010b) and NJCLD (2010). Because the identification of SLD occurs primarily in schools, we focus on best-practice guidelines within the educational context. And given the variability in conceptual definitions of SLD and their classification criteria, we provide general best-practice guidelines for SLD diagnosis. The rules and regulations of every state education agency specify the requirements for a comprehensive assessment of SLD, according to IDEA (2004).

Table 12.1 provides recommendations by the NJCLD (2010) for conducting a comprehensive assessment for the identification of SLD by multidisciplinary teams for IDEA purposes. As indicated here, the identification of SLD cannot be based only on any single assessment method or measure. In other words, SLD diagnosis cannot be based on the identification of a significant IQ–achievement discrepancy; nor can it be based only on level and rate of achievement data in an RTI service delivery model. Data from RTI can be an important component of SLD identification, however. In fact, RTI can be seen as a primary means of eliminating the instructional context as a viable explanation of academic failure, and thereby of suggesting that the cause is a disabling condition within the individual (Fuchs, Fuchs, & Compton, 2004). Also important is the consideration of information gathered from both formal methods (e.g., norm-referenced tests) and informal methods (e.g., interviews and observations).

TABLE 12.1. Procedures for Comprehensive Assessment and Evaluation of SLD under IDEA

A comprehensive assessment should:

1. Use a valid and the most current version of any standardized assessment.
2. Use multiple measures, including both standardized and nonstandardized assessments, and other data sources, such as the following:
   - Case history and interviews with parents, educators, related professionals, and the student (if appropriate).
   - Prior test results and information provided by parents.
   - Direct observations that yield informal (e.g., anecdotal reports) or data-based information (e.g., frequency recordings) in multiple settings and on more than one occasion.
   - Standardized tests that are not only reliable and valid, but culturally, linguistically, and developmentally appropriate, as well as age-appropriate.
   - Curriculum-based assessments, task and error pattern analysis (e.g., miscue analysis), portfolios, diagnostic teaching, and other nonstandardized approaches.
   - Continuous progress monitoring repeated during instruction and over time.
3. Consider all components of the definition of SLD in IDEA 2004 and/or its regulations, including the following:
   - Exclusionary factors.
   - Inclusionary factors.
   - The eight areas of SLD (i.e., oral expression, listening comprehension, written expression, basic reading skill, reading comprehension, reading fluency, mathematics calculation, mathematics problem solving).
   - The intraindividual differences in a student, as demonstrated by "a pattern of strengths and weaknesses in performance, achievement, or both relative to age, State-approved grade level standards or intellectual development" [34 CFR 300.309(a)(2)(ii)].
4. Examine functioning and/or ability levels across motor, sensory, cognitive, communication, and behavior domains, including specific areas of cognitive and integrative difficulties in perception; memory; attention; sequencing; motor planning and coordination; and thinking, reasoning, and organization.
5. Adhere to the accepted and recommended procedures for administration, scoring, and reporting of standardized measures. Express results that maximize comparability across measures (i.e., standard scores). Age or grade equivalents are not appropriate to report.
6. Provide confidence interval and standard error of measurement, if available.
7. Integrate the standardized and informal data collected.
8. Balance and discuss the information gathered from both standardized and nonstandardized data, which describes the student's current level of academic performance and functional skills, and informs decisions about identification, eligibility, services, and instructional planning.

Note. Adapted from NJCLD (2010, pp. 8–9).

Each state's eligibility criteria must guide the multidisciplinary team. The team must carefully consider all components of the definition of SLD. This includes close examination of inclusionary (e.g., RTI achievement discrepancy) and exclusionary criteria. As stated by the NJCLD (2010), "underachievement is common among students with learning disabilities, but it is not synonymous with learning disabilities" (p. 7). Underachievement is a necessary but not sufficient condition for SLD identification.

In addition to determining that achievement deficits are evident, competing explanations of underachievement must be eliminated before an individual can be diagnosed with SLD. Factors that must be ruled out before a diagnosis of SLD can be made include ID, sensory impairments, problems in social–emotional functioning, cultural and linguistic background (e.g., limited English proficiency [LEP]), and inadequate educational opportunity.

The NJCLD guidelines also call for comprehensive assessment across multiple domains of behavior, including motor, sensory, cognitive, communication, and behavioral functioning. This is important for two reasons. First, SLD is often comorbid with other disabilities (e.g., attention-deficit/hyperactivity disorder [ADHD]). Although these disabilities may not cause SLD, their identification is important for appropriate intervention planning. Second, as stated by the NJCLD (2010), "learning disabilities can occur in students who are also gifted and/or talented. These 'twice exceptional' students often [demonstrate] achievement at age and grade expectations and are thus not considered to be struggling in school" (p. 9). Examination of intraindividual differences in skills and performance across domains can suggest SLD.

Table 12.2 presents critical decision points in the determination of SLD within an RTI model. It can be seen that important decisions about diagnosis of SLD occur at all stages, from prereferral to eligibility determination. The administration of intelligence tests is an important component of the comprehensive assessment process, usually occurring at Tier 3 in an RTI model.

Intelligence Tests and SLD Diagnosis

At the current time, there is a great deal of disagreement about the usefulness of intelligence tests in the SLD identification process (e.g., Reynolds & Shaywitz, 2009). Given that there is little connection between the results of intelligence tests and the design of effective instructional interventions, some argue that there is little use in administering intelligence tests in the SLD identification process (e.g., Shinn, 2005). Although the evidence does not at present support the treatment utility of intelligence test results for children with SLD, they are necessary for differentiating between SLD and ID. As Wodrich, Spencer, and Daly (2006) have argued, not only are SLD and ID different disability categories in IDEA, but they have different etiologies and prognoses in schools. In addition, Fuchs and Young (2006) found IQ to be significantly related to educational outcomes for individuals with reading difficulties. Thus, inclusion of intelligence tests is an important component of any comprehensive assessment for SLD. Caution must be used in selecting and interpreting intelligence tests during a comprehensive assessment for SLD, however. On heavily English-language-loaded tests, for example, the results for individuals with language impairment or LEP may not be valid. In these cases, it is advisable to select an appropriate intelligence test that will yield an estimate of psychometric *g* while avoiding the assessment of such construct-irrelevant variance (see Chapter 5).

> **Inclusion of intelligence tests is an important component of any comprehensive assessment for SLD.**

TABLE 12.2. Critical Decision Points in Determination of SLD

Stage	Methods	Critical decision points
Prereferral	Student may be designated as at risk during screening and progress monitoring; student may be identified through child study teams; parent may note concern for a student's progress.	Current performance identifies student as at risk. Data collected do not indicate positive response to interventions.
Referral	Failure to progress even with Tier 2 level intervention in an RTI model; failure to progress given substantial, research-based accommodations and modifications.	Data collected do not indicate positive response to interventions.
Evaluation	List your components in order of evaluation—for example: 1. Interindividual academic ability analysis. 2. Evaluation of exclusionary factors. 3. Interindividual cognitive ability analysis. 4. Reevaluation of exclusionary factors. 5. Integrated ability analysis (evaluation of underachievement)—in what areas does the underachievement occur? 6. Evaluation of interference with functioning—why is it occurring? 7. Related considerations—limitations in social skills, motor, vision, hearing. 8. Other.	Patterns or level of evidence; criteria for evidence of a component.
Eligibility	Individualized, comprehensive assessment.	Criteria and patterns indicate presence of SLD.

Note. Adapted from National Research Center on Learning Disabilities (NRCLD, 2007). Adapted by permission of the NRCLD.

SUMMARY

Controversy has long surrounded the definition and diagnosis of SLD. At present, no consensus definition of SLD exists. SLD can either be viewed as a disability in learning in general (i.e., slow learner) or as unexpected underachievement in some, but not all, areas of academic achievement (e.g., reading or mathematics). Nonetheless, contemporary definitions of SLD are similar insofar as they refer to individuals who share a common difficulty with school learning. In addition, ruling out certain exclusionary criteria (e.g., inadequate educational or language background, intellectual disability) and determining a significant discrepancy in achievement are important components of SLD identification regardless of definition. Although the use of intelligence tests may not be required for determining a discrepancy in achievement, they are necessary for ruling out intellectual disabilities.

CHAPTER 13

Assessment of Children and Adolescents from Diverse Cultural and Linguistic Backgrounds

The demographic composition of the public schools in the United States has changed dramatically over the past 40 years. Between 1972 and 2007, the percentage of students from diverse racial/ethnic backgrounds increased from 22% to 44% (National Center for Education Statistics [NCES], 2007). In 2005, 3.8 million students received English as a second language (ESL) services (NCES, 2009), and approximately 20% did not speak English fluently (Crawford, 2009). Given the trend toward increasing diversity in U.S. schools, the validity of cognitive assessment of children and youth from diverse backgrounds is an important concern.

Intelligence tests are routinely administered in the schools as part of the process of identification for special education and related services, despite the fact that some view them as biased against children and youth from diverse backgrounds (e.g., see Vazquez-Nuttal et al., 2007). Critics argue that the overrepresentation of certain racial/ethnic groups in programs for students with intellectual disability (ID), and their underrepresentation in programs for the gifted and talented, both stem from the use of biased intelligence tests (e.g., see Rhodes, Ochoa, & Ortiz, 2005). The fact that many students from racial/ethnic minority groups do not have the same experiential backgrounds as the European American majority is seen as one probable cause of test bias. Attempts to reduce the cultural loading of intelligence tests, most often by using abstract figural material as a basis for relation eduction (e.g., Cattell, 1971), however, have not eliminated group differences in intelligence test performance (see Reynolds & Carson, 2005). This finding has been interpreted by some to indicate that performance on intelligence tests is not influenced by cultural or linguistic background.

Given this disagreement, it may come as a surprise to know that no one today seriously questions whether socioeconomic and racial/ethnic groups differ, on average, in the scores obtained on standardized intelligence tests. There is simply too much empirical evidence for anyone to argue convincingly otherwise (e.g., see Nisbett et al., 2012), although the mean group differences appear to be declining over time. Nevertheless, a prolonged and heated debate has raged on the *meaning* of these differences. Do they reflect real differences in intelligence? Or do they result from test bias or possibly invalid tests? What, then, are best practices for school psychologists and other professionals assessing children from diverse backgrounds? Before reviewing the recommended best practices, in this chapter we briefly discuss fundamental issues and research on test bias.

CONCEPTUALIZATIONS OF TEST BIAS

What is *test bias?* Unfortunately, "discussions" of test bias are often conducted in a metaphorical Tower of Babel, where productive discourse is unfortunately rare. Due to the conflicting assumptions and theoretical orientations of researchers on opposing sides of the debate, a consensus-based definition of test bias does not exist. Moreover, the various conceptualizations of test bias that have been articulated in the literature vary considerably, especially in terms of their scientific merit. The following is a review of the most common definitions of test bias (cf. Jensen, 1980, 1981).

> The various conceptualizations of test bias that have been articulated in the literature vary considerably, especially in terms of their scientific merit.

The Egalitarian Definition

Perhaps the simplest definition of test bias is based on the widespread belief that all people are created equal. Underlying this notion of bias is the postulate that the genotypic intelligence of all socioeconomic and racial/ethnic groups is the same. According to the egalitarian definition, an unbiased test reveals differences among individuals in intelligence, but not among groups. Any test on which group differences are found, therefore, must be a biased test. If this definition of bias is accepted, then yardsticks are biased, because men are taller on average, than women.

The main reason that the egalitarian definition of test bias is fallacious, however, is not that it leads to clearly untenable conclusions such as this. The main reason is that it is based on the a priori assumption of group equality. The fallacy of this definition is that it assumes the answer to the question in point. There is simply no way to empirically prove or disprove the postulate of group equality in intelligence; by definition, any observed difference in test scores between groups is taken as evidence of bias. Because the egalitarian definition of bias is unfalsifiable, it is a pseudoscientific definition of bias and should be rejected.

The Standardization Definition

According to the standardization definition of bias, intelligence tests that are standardized using certain racial/ethnic groups are ipso facto biased against all groups that are omitted from the standardization sample. This definition is based on the a priori assumption that racial/ethnic groups are inherently different, which of course is exactly the opposite of that assumed by the egalitarian definition of bias. (Interestingly, critics of intelligence tests sometimes use both of these fallacious definitions simultaneously as evidence of bias, despite the fact that they are based on contradictory assumptions.) Although also based on an a priori assumption, standardization bias on tests can be proven or disproven.

Test standardization involves two main steps: the selection of items and the norming of scores (see Chapter 5). Test items are selected on the basis of difficulty level and ability to discriminate between high and low test scores. Norming involves the development of standard scores. Standardization bias exists when the test items that meet rigorous criteria for selection for the racial/ ethnic groups included in the test norming sample differ from those items selected for groups not included. Norming itself does not lead to bias, because it involves the linear transformation of raw scores into standardized scores and does not affect item selection or change the shape of the distribution.

Contemporary intelligence test developers, however, routinely analyze items for evidence of standardization bias by applying state-of-the-art item selection procedures (e.g., item response theory) to each racial/ethnic group included in the standardization sample separately and retaining only those items meeting similar standards of item selection across groups (see Reynolds & Carson, 2005). The important thing to remember here is that a test is not ipso facto biased against the racial/ethnic groups that are omitted from the standardization sample. Such a test might very well be biased against those groups, but it might not be. The only way to identify standardization bias is to analyze empirical data with objective statistical methods. The fallacy in this definition is the argument that a test is biased against certain groups simply because they are not represented in the standardization sample.

The Culture-Bound Definition

Another common definition of test bias concerns the fact that most standardized intelligence tests include a significant number of *culture-loaded* items. Culture loading is defined as the

> specificity or generality of the informational content of a test item, as contrasted with the item's demands for educing relationships, reasoning, and mental manipulations of its elements. Test items can be ordered along a continuum of culture loading in terms of the range of cultural backgrounds in which the item's informational content could be acquired. The answer to an item may depend on knowledge that could only be acquired within a particular culture, or locality, or time period. The opportunity for acquiring the requisite bit of knowledge might be greatly less in some cultures, localities, or time periods than in others. (Jensen, 1981, p. 130)

According to this definition, intelligence tests with items that are culturally loaded are biased against racial/ethnic minority groups, because their backgrounds are presumed to be significantly different from the majority.

Figure 13.1 shows example items with differing degrees of culture loading. Item 1 is an item with a high degree of culture loading, because the correct answer (David) is only known to the family members and close friends of one of us (JHK). Carolyn is JHK's mother and Jerry is his father, whereas Koko is his mother-in-law and David is his father-in-law. Because this item involves the simple relation eduction of husband to wife, this is a very easy item for members of his family, but a difficult one for others, because they do not have the relevant background information to answer the item correctly. Item 2 is an example of the kind of item commonly thought to be biased, because it possibly requires information that may be more prevalent or easily accessible in some cultures than in others. Items 3 and 4 have decreasing degrees of culture loading. One involves knowledge of basic mathematics, whereas the other involves only abstract symbols. As can be seen

1. Carolyn is to Jerry as Koko is to (a) Steve, (b) David, (c) Bill, or (d) Fred.

2. Romeo is to Juliet as Tristan is to: (a) Carmen, (b) Elizabeth, (c) Isolde, or (d) Marguerite.

3. 60 is to 30 is to 15, as 20 is to 10 is to _____ .

4. Continue the series: X OOOO XX OOO XXX OO _____ .

FIGURE 13.1. Test items reflecting different degrees of culture loading. Based on Jensen (1981).

in these examples, culture loading is not related to item difficulty per se, but to the opportunity to acquire the necessary information to respond correctly. Culture loading and complexity of processing are entirely different things.

It is also important not to equate culture loading with test bias. Test items can be arranged on a continuum, with *culture-reduced* (one cannot have a *culture-free* test, because testing itself is a cultural activity) at one end of the continuum and *culture-saturated* at the other. Items typically thought to be biased are those near the culture-saturated end of the continuum. These items typically involve esoteric kinds of knowledge (e.g., the fine arts, literature, and history of science). Although panels of racial/ethnic majority and minority psychologists tend to agree on the degree of culture loading of specific items, research has shown that they are unable to reliably identify items that are in fact biased (e.g., Frisby & Braden, 1999; Jensen, 1980; Reynolds & Kaiser, 1990). Hence, test bias cannot be identified by subjective judgments of an item's culture loading (e.g., Cormier, McGrew, & Evans, 2011; Kranzler, Flores, & Coady, 2010). The only way to identify test bias related to culture loading is to analyze actual data with objective statistical methods. The fallacy in this definition is the argument that a test is biased against certain groups simply because it contains items that are culture-loaded.

The Statistical Definition

Psychometricians widely agree that test bias is best defined in a strictly mathematical sense (e.g., see Frisby & Braden, 1999; Jensen, 1980, Reynolds & Carson, 2005; Reynolds & Kaiser, 1990). According to this definition, test bias is *systematic* measurement error (Reynolds, Lowe, & Saenz, 1999). According to Jensen (1980), "in psychometrics, bias refers to systematic errors in the predictive validity or the construct validity of tests scores of individuals that are associated with the individual's group membership" (p. 375). Bias does not refer to *random* error, of which there are two kinds: *measurement* error and *sampling* error.

> Psychometricians widely agree that test bias is best defined in a strictly mathematical sense. According to this definition, test bias is *systematic* measurement error.

No measurement for any group of individuals is perfect—there is always some degree of error—and the different kinds of measurement error on psychological tests can be estimated by reliability coefficients (r_{xx}; e.g., internal consistency and stability), where $1 - r_{xx}$ = error. Sampling error refers to the variability in the values of a statistic that is observed whenever one selects a portion of the population (i.e., a sample) for study. Systematic measurement error, in contrast to these two types of error, occurs when the test (1) measures one thing for one group and another thing for another group, or (2) predicts performance on some external criterion (e.g., academic achievement) well for one group but not for another. For example, if a verbally loaded intelligence test is administered to individuals with limited English proficiency (LEP), test scores no doubt would be reflective of their LEP and not of their intelligence. Thus, the test would be biased against those individuals, and the results would be invalid.

Statistical indicators of bias fall into two main categories: *internal* and *predictive*. Internal criteria of bias concern statistical properties of the test and its items (e.g., reliability, rank order of item difficulty, and factor structure). Bias is detected by comparing these and other internal indicators across socioeconomic or racial/ethnic groups. If any of these indicators differs significantly across groups, then bias is objectively determined to exist. Bias in predictive validity involves the comparison of regression parameters (slopes, intercepts, and standard errors) across groups. Basically, predictive bias is detected if, on average, persons with the same test score from different groups perform differently on a relevant external criterion, such as academic performance or job success. Tests that are biased against certain groups would tend to underpredict performance on the criterion. Test bias can also be favorable, however, resulting in the overprediction of certain groups' performance on the external criterion (i.e., performance is worse in the "real world" than predicted by test scores). Therefore, the focus of research on test bias is squarely on the validity (i.e., inferences and actions based on test scores) of intelligence tests across groups—not on reliability, as some have suggested (cf. Rhodes et al., 2005; Vazquez-Nuttall et al., 2007), although internal indicators of bias are one important aspect of bias research.

RESEARCH ON TEST BIAS

A great many empirical research studies have been conducted on test bias over the years, all of them reaching essentially the same conclusion (for reviews, see Brown, Reynolds, & Whitaker, 1999; Frisby & Braden, 1999; Gordon, 1987; Jensen, 1980; Neisser et al., 1996; Reynolds & Carson, 2005; Reynolds et al., 1999; Wigdor & Garner, 1982).

The research literature on test bias is robust and clear: For native-born, English-speaking children in the United States, regardless of socioeconomic status or racial/ethnic group, standardized tests of intelligence are not substantially biased according to the statistical definition of bias. As Reynolds and Kaiser (1990) have stated,

no consistent evidence of bias in construct validity has been found with any of the many tests investigated. This leads to the conclusion that psychological tests (especially aptitude tests) function in essentially the same manner, that tests measure the same construct with equivalent accuracy for blacks, whites, Mexican-Americans, and other American minorities of both sexes and at all levels of SES. (p. 638)

> **For native-born, English-speaking children in the United States, standardized tests of intelligence are not substantially biased according to the statistical definition of bias.**

When bias is detected, it is usually on predictive criteria and in favor of—not against—the racial/ethnic groups that tend to obtain the lowest average scores on intelligence tests (e.g., Reynolds &

Carson, 2005). Furthermore, often overlooked in discussions of test bias is the fact that the highest-scoring racial/ethnic group on average is not Whites, but Asians/Pacific Islanders, particularly on tests that measure spatial and numerical reasoning (e.g., Suzuki, Short, & Lee, 2011). This simple fact alone demonstrates that standardized intelligence tests are therefore not biased against all racial/ethnic minority groups. The relatively high performance of Asians/Pacific Islanders is often overlooked by critics of intelligence tests (e.g., see Rhodes et al., 2005).

It is important to note, however, that not all agree with the conclusion that standardized tests of intelligence are not biased. Scheuneman (1987) noted, for example, that "the evidence . . . clearly and strongly supports the existence of at least some degree of bias in mental tests" (p. 161), usually in the neighborhood of 2–3% of the variance. Sternberg (1988a) hypothesized that mean racial/ethnic group differences might be explained by differences in familiarity with the specific processes (or with the higher-order strategies that facilitate those processes) required for the solution of certain test items, although we are not aware of any substantiating empirical research supporting this hypothesis. In any case, standardized tests that control for hypothesized disparities in underlying cognitive processes across groups currently do not exist, nor may they ever (see Floyd & Kranzler, 2012).

Again, for native-born, English-speaking children in the United States, regardless of socio-economic status or racial/ethnic group, the empirical research indicates that the major tests of intelligence are *not* significantly biased. It is, however, extremely important to note that these results are not clearly generalizable to children and youth who do not speak English well or were not reared in the United States. As Jensen (1981) stated, "the fact that all these groups obtain lower scores on verbal than nonverbal tests, and on reading tests than on arithmetic tests, strongly suggests that their different language background may handicap their performance on verbal or language-loaded tests" (pp. 138–139).

What, then, are best practices for assessing the intellectual ability of children and youth who have recently immigrated to the United States, or who have LEP, or both? In the next section, we address this question by discussing best practices in the assessment of children and youth from diverse backgrounds.

BEST PRACTICES
IN ASSESSMENT OF DIVERSE CHILDREN AND YOUTH

Reschly and Grimes (1990) stated that "best practices considerations require careful judgments about *when* intellectual assessments are used, *how* they are used, the selection, administration, and interpretation of tests, and efforts to protect children and youth from misuses and misconceptions" (p. 436; emphases in the original). Although written more than two decades ago, the following recommendations for best practices still apply to all assessment situations, including the assessment of children from culturally and linguistically diverse backgrounds:

1. Appropriate use requires a context that emphasizes prevention and early intervention rather than eligibility determination as the initial phase in services to students with learning and behavior problems. . . .
2. Intellectual assessment should be used when the results are directly relevant to well defined referral questions, and other available information does not address those questions. . . .

3. Mandatory use of intellectual measures for all referrals, multi-factored evaluations, or reevaluations is not consistent with best practices. . . .

4. Intellectual assessment must be part of a multi-factored approach, individualized to a child's characteristics and the referral problems. . . .

5. Intellectual assessment procedures must be carefully matched to characteristics of children and youth. . . .

6. Score reporting and interpretations must reflect the known limitations of tests, including technical adequacy, inherent error in measurement, and general categories of performance. . . .

7. Interpretation of performance and decisions concerning classification must reflect consideration of overall strengths and weaknesses in intellectual performance, performance on other relevant dimensions of behavior, age, family characteristics, and cultural background. . . .

8. Users should implement assertive procedures to protect students from misconceptions and misuses of intellectual test results. . . . (Reschly & Grimes, 1990, pp. 436–438)

These are excellent recommendations for practice that should never be compromised. We emphasize several of these points within the context of assessment with children from culturally and linguistically diverse backgrounds before discussing the pros and cons of the main assessment alternatives with these populations.

Cultural and Linguistic Background

In assessing children and youth from diverse backgrounds, it is important to consider their *cultural* background (e.g., Rhodes et al., 2005; Ryan-Arredondo & Sandoval, 2005). Valencia and Lopez (1992) have defined culture as "the particular traditions, values, norms, and practices of any people who share a common ancestry" (p. 400). As they have stated,

> it is widely acknowledged that tests and other assessment tools measure samples of behavior. Furthermore, it is well known that culture influences behavior. Thus, in the context of psychoeducational assessment, the connection between measurement instruments and culture is clear: Assessment information, especially test data, gathered by school psychologists and other practitioners is—[to] varying degrees—culturally shaped. (p. 400)

Indeed, as we have noted in Chapter 1, the behavior measured on intelligence tests is not only related to biological functioning, but also to one's experiences during development, which includes the cultural environment in which one is raised.

According to Rhodes et al. (2005), school psychologists must familiarize themselves with the diverse cultural backgrounds of their local student population and understand that such diversity could influence all phases of assessment—from the collection of data to the interpretation and use of results. They recommend caution, however, in generalizing from cultural groups as a whole to individuals within cultures, because individual differences within cultural groups are generally greater than the differences between groups. In assessment, therefore, a nomothetic perspective is best complemented by an idiographic one (see Chapter 6). Valencia and Lopez (1992) have also recommended that (1) information about cultural background should be gathered from as many sources, particularly parents and teachers, as possible; and (2) the focus of assessment should be on the child's demonstrated skills and actual school and home experiences.

parameters.

Level of *acculturation* is another variable that many believe is important to consider when assessing children and youth from diverse backgrounds. Acculturation is defined as "those phenomena, which result when groups of individuals having different cultures come into continuous first-hand contact, with subsequent changes in the original cultural patterns of either or both groups" (Redfield, Linton, & Herskovitz, 1936, p. 149, as cited in Ryan-Arredondo & Sandoval, 2005, pp. 861–862). According to Marín (1992), acculturation involves "changes in individuals that are produced by contact with one or more cultural groups" (p. 237), and it is best viewed "as a fluid process (probably a lifelong event) that involves many dimensions of an individual's life (e.g., behaviors, attitudes, norms, and values) and that does not typically follow a deficit model, but rather implies growth across a variety of continua" (p. 242).

In a more recent literature review, however, Ryan-Arredondo and Sandoval (2005) concluded that "there is little agreement among researchers as to which cultural aspects, behaviors, and constructs accurately comprise acculturation" (p. 865). Moreover, given that the vast majority of research in this area has been conducted with college students and adults, little is known about the process of acculturation among school-age children and youth. Finally, at present, the acculturation scales that have been developed are limited in their psychometric support and the quality of their norms. These measures also do not include children and youth of all age ranges in their standardization samples and are limited to one or two ethnic groups (for more details, see Ryan-Arredondo & Sandoval, 2005).

Linguistic background is another important consideration in the psychological assessment of children and youth from diverse backgrounds. For children with academic problems who have LEP, assessment of the home language and development in English is essential. Unfortunately, as Rhodes et al. (2005) have noted, language assessment of Spanish-speaking and other children and youth with LEP is limited. Consequently, standardized tests of languages other than English often yield equivocal results—or they simply do not exist at all—for many children and youth with LEP living in the United States. Determining whether a child's academic problems result from LEP or from a language disorder is therefore difficult. Qualitative measures can be useful, but they can be counted on to provide only a rough estimate of a child's level of native-language functioning. The best practice is therefore to use multiple sources of information gathered from a variety of sources, including standardized tests, qualitative measures, interviews, and observations.

In addition to assessing the primary language of children with LEP, evaluators should gather information on their English-language development. This is done most effectively with a single-subject (time-series) research design (see Kazdin, 2010). According to Cummins (1984), one of the most common errors in evaluating children with LEP is to equate basic communication skills in English with competence in using English in decontextualized academic settings. He has stated that it takes about 1–2 years for most children to learn to communicate effectively in English, but that it may take 5 years on average for them to learn to use English in academic contexts as effectively as native speakers do.

For these reasons, informal approaches to gathering information about the cultural and linguistic background of diverse children and youth are arguably best (e.g., Rhodes et al., 2005). Indeed, the formal assessment of acculturation is apparently quite rare (Ryan-Arredondo & Sandoval, 2005). Including questions that address these areas during a comprehensive interview, therefore, is one

The information gathered from interviews should be used to inform the decision about the degree to which culture or language attenuates the results of intelligence test scores.

TABLE 13.1. Questions on Linguistic Background and Acculturation for Parents

Language history

1. What language(s) did _____ [the child] first speak?
2. What language(s) does _____ prefer to speak now?
3. What language(s) do parents, grandparents, siblings, other family members, family friends, and _____'s friends speak at home?
4. What language(s) do you usually use at home when you speak to _____?
5. Is _____ able to hold a conversation in your home language?
6. Does _____ speak to persons outside the family in your home language?
7. Does _____ ever help interpret for other family members?
8. In what language is _____ usually disciplined?
9. In what language does _____ speak to you when _____ is hurt or upset?
10. In what language does _____ speak to his or her brother(s) or sister(s)?

Acculturation status

11. What are _____'s favorite television shows and movies?
12. In what language?
13. What kind of music does _____ enjoy listening to?
14. In what language?
15. Where has _____ lived?
16. What holidays do you celebrate as a family?

Note. Adapted from Rhodes, Ochoa, and Ortiz (2005). Copyright 2005 by The Guilford Press. Adapted by permission.

approach for gathering this information. Table 13.1 is a list of questions for parent interviews that could be used as part of a comprehensive assessment to gather information pertaining to linguistic and cultural background (see Chapter 4). The information gathered from interviews should be used to inform the decision about the degree to which culture or language attenuates the results of intelligence test scores (Vazquez-Nuttall et al, 2007).

Selecting Acceptable Tests

When evaluating the appropriateness of a test for *any* assessment situation, one should *always* consider the nature and purpose of the test, the quality of its norms, the available reliability and validity data, and the examinee's particular capabilities and limitations, among other criteria. (See Chapter 5 for guidelines for test evaluation and selection.) Because of the wide cultural and linguistic backgrounds of children in the schools, we next discuss the characteristics of acceptable tests in general terms.

Quality of Test Norms

As we have mentioned above, tests that have been standardized in certain racial/ethnic groups are *not* ipso facto biased against all groups omitted from the standardization sample. The best-case scenario is when the minority group of the child being assessed is included in the standardization sample, but the absence or disproportionately low representation of that child's group does not necessarily imply that the test is biased against him or her. It may be biased, but it may not be. Valencia (1988), for example, found that the average performance of English-speaking Mexican American children was at the mean of 100 on the McCarthy Scales, despite their virtual absence from the standardization sample. Tests that do not include a particular child's racial/ethnic group should therefore be considered, but additional information about the norms and how they were developed should always be examined too. Such information can usually be found in the test manual, but one should be sure to consult the published scholarly literature to get a balanced opinion of the test's advantages and limitations.

Reliability and Validity

Valencia and Lopez (1992) have stated that "racial and ethnic minority populations, given their cultural and linguistic diversity, present challenges to test measurement specialists in the establishment of adequate reliability and validity of tests" (p. 409). This is an understatement. Unfortunately, for many minority groups this information is simply nonexistent. Validity, of course, refers to the soundness with which test scores can be interpreted for a particular purpose. Tests are therefore *not* unconditionally valid (or invalid) for every socioeconomic or racial/ethnic group and for all psychoeducational purposes. For tests to be used with confidence, information on a test's reliability and validity should be available.

Four Alternative Assessment Practices

Four main alternatives are available for assessing the intelligence of children from diverse backgrounds when no tests with demonstrated validity for those backgrounds are available.

Nonverbal Tests of Intelligence

The first and, in our opinion, best option is to administer a multidimensional nonverbal intelligence test (see Chapter 7). Level of acculturation and LEP are construct-irrelevant sources of variance in the assessment of intelligence. When test performance primarily reflects these two factors and not cognitive ability, then the interpretation of test scores is invalid. The language of the test is important, especially for those who speak a foreign language or are bilingual (with English as their second language). Interpretation of the results of verbally loaded tests for children with LEP, therefore, should be supplemented with non-language-based tests and other assessment data. When using non-verbal intelligence tests, assessors should take care to ensure that the examinees completely understand the instructions, because the administration of all tests requires communication of some kind between examiner and examinee, and some nonverbal tests do in fact have English instructions.

> **The first and, in our opinion, best option is to use a nonverbal test.**

In a recent review of the most widely used contemporary nonverbal measures of cognitive ability, Braden and Athanasiou (2005) concluded that a number of these instruments are appropriate for use with diverse populations. Many of these tests—such as the Universal Nonverbal Intelligence Test (UNIT; Bracken & McCallum, 1998), the Leiter International Performance Scale—

Third Edition (Leiter-3; Roid, Miller, Pomplun, & Koch, 2013), and the Wechsler Nonverbal Scale of Ability (WNV; Wechsler & Naglieri, 2006)—have strong psychometric properties, are based upon well-articulated theoretical frameworks, and are excellent measures of psychometric *g* (see Chapter 7). Moreover, a number of studies support the use of nonverbal intelligence tests with children and youth from diverse backgrounds (e.g., Lohman, Korb, & Lakin, 2008; Lohman & Lakin, 2008; Naglieri, Booth, & Winsler, 2004).

When using nonverbal intelligence tests, examiners must note that, as a whole, they tend not to predict academic achievement as well as verbal tests—for all groups. This is because the content of verbal tests overlaps to a greater extent with past academic achievement. Although the predictive validity of these instruments is generally acceptable, recommendations and interventions based on the results of nonverbal tests for children with LEP should *always* be tentative and short-term (no longer than 1 year at most). In addition, as Flanagan, Ortiz, and Alfonso (2007) have noted, "nonverbal tasks may actually carry as much if not more cultural content than that found in verbal tests" (p. 165). Given that testing is itself a cultural activity, all tests have some degree of cultural loading.

Culture–Language Interpretive Matrices

A new direction for the assessment of diverse populations involves the interpretation of standardized intelligence tests within *culture–language interpretive matrices* (C-LIMs). Flanagan et al. (2007) created C-LIMs for each of the most widely used standardized intelligence tests. Each C-LIM consists of a 3 × 3 table in which the test's subtests are categorized according to whether they are judged to have a Low, Medium, or High degree of linguistic demand and cultural loading. According to this approach, analysis of the pattern of test scores in the C-LIM can facilitate identification of students whose academic difficulties stem from language or cultural differences and those whose difficulties are attributable to other causes (e.g., specific learning disability [SLD]).

Figure 13.2 shows the general pattern of expected results in a generic C-LIM for individuals from diverse cultural and linguistic backgrounds. When test scores are lowest on subtests with the highest degree of cultural loading and linguistic demand, and highest on subtests with the lowest degree of cultural loading and linguistic demand, this is interpreted as evidence that LEP and acculturation have invalidated the test results. In contrast, when subtest scores do not follow this pattern in the C-LIM, then it is believed that LEP and acculturation can be ruled out as the cause of a student's learning difficulties.

At the current time, however, research on the use of C-LIMs has only just begun, and the empirical support for this approach is rather limited (see Dhaniram-Beharry, 2008; Nieves-Brull, 2006; Tychanska, 2009; Verderosa, 2007). Furthermore, several recent studies have raised issues about the validity of this interpretive approach and the need to refine it (Cormier et al., 2011; Kranzler et al., 2010). Kranzler et al. (2010) have concluded:

> Despite the fact that our results do not substantiate the use of C-LIMs, our findings should *not* be interpreted to suggest that cultural and linguistic background do not have an impact on cognitive ability test performance. Nothing could be further from the truth—language and cultural background matter on tests—especially for English language learners who were not born and raised in the USA. Nonetheless, our results do suggest that revision of the theory underlying the use of the C-LIMs, the test-specific matrices (at least for the WJ-III), or perhaps both, is needed. (p. 443)

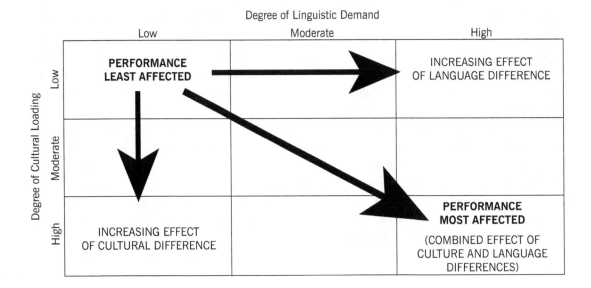

FIGURE 13.2. Predicted test performance for individuals from culturally and linguistically diverse backgrounds within a generic culture–language interpretive matrix (C-LIM). From *Essentials of Cross-Battery Assessment* (2nd ed.) by D. P. Flanagan, S. O. Ortiz, and V. C. Alfonso. Copyright 2007 by John Wiley & Sons, Inc. Reprinted by permission.

At present, until further research has been conducted substantiating their utility, we cannot recommend use of the C-LIMs for the assessment of children and youth from diverse backgrounds (cf. Ortiz, Ochoa, & Dynda, 2012).

Use of a Translated Test or a Translator

One logical solution to the issue of assessing the intelligence of a student with LEP is to translate a test with a moderate to high degree of linguistic demand in English into the student's dominant language. Translation of a verbal test is problematic, however, because some English words do not have exact equivalents in other languages. In addition, common words in English may be unusual in another language, and vice versa. As a result, the difficulty level for a translated word could be quite different than the difficulty level for its English counterpart. Advances have been made in research on the translation and adaptation of educational and psychological tests in recent years, however (for a review, see Hambleton & Li, 2005).

Administration of verbal tests with the assistance of a translator is also problematic, even though translators may have received training. The literature offers no real guidelines based on empirical research on how to train and use an interpreter (Vazquez-Nuttal et al., 2007). Moreover, little, if anything, is known about the validity of measuring a bilingual child's intelligence when an interpreter is used. As Rhodes et al. (2005) have stated, "very little information is available . . . regarding how to best incorporate interpreters into daily practice" (p. 91). If an interpreter is used, it is recommended that he or she be well prepared; this preparation should include instructions on the patterns of communication (viz., who talks to whom and when), seating arrangements, and the like. Care should also be taken in instructing translators on whether to employ a literal, word-for-word translation without regard for context, or a free translation in which an interpreter attempts to communicate the exact meaning of the original communication (Hambleton & Li, 2005). Rhodes et al. (2005) provide further guidelines for the selection and use of translators in intellectual assessment.

Test–Teach–Test Approaches

The fourth and final assessment alternative is to use the "test–teach–test" paradigm derived from Vygotsky's notions of the *zones of proximal and distal development*. Such assessment is often called *dynamic assessment*. Some have viewed Feuerstein's Learning Potential Assessment Device (LPAD; see Feuerstein, Rand, & Hoffman, 1979), for example, as a promising alternative for the assessment of children from culturally and linguistically diverse backgrounds (e.g., Oades-Ses, Esquivel, & Añon, 2007). Although Kirschenbaum (1998) has argued that dynamic assessment may be a promising approach for assessing the intelligence of children and youth with LEP for gifted and talented programs, little is known about the use of the LPAD for children and youth with LEP. Frisby and Braden (1992), however, have asserted that dynamic assessment amounts to "little more than ideological philosophy in search of empirical support" (p. 283). In a more recent review, Vazquez-Nuttall (2007) stated that "what advantages such approaches might hold [with linguistically and culturally diverse individuals] are not entirely clear and yet to be demonstrated" (p. 280). Regardless of the specific method of dynamic assessment chosen for assessment, the important thing to keep in mind is that all approaches should be based on sound theory *and* should be supported by the results of empirical research. At present, many of these assessment approaches simply do not have sufficient empirical support for their use in the schools today.

SUMMARY

In summary, test bias is best defined in the statistical sense, as *systematic* measurement error or estimation. Research on test bias has shown that the major standardized tests of intelligence are not substantially biased for English-speaking children born and raised in the United States. For assessing children and youth from other cultural and linguistic backgrounds, the best practice is to use a nonverbal intelligence test.

References

Achenbach, T. M., McConaughy, S. H., & Howell, C. T. (1987). Child/adolescent behavioral and emotional problems: Implications of cross-informant correlations for situational specificity. *Psychological Bulletin, 101*, 213–232.

Alfonso, V. C., Flanagan, D. P., & Radwan, S. (2005). The impact of the Cattell–Horn–Carroll theory on test development and interpretation of cognitive and academic abilities. In D. P. Flanagan & P. L. Harrison (Eds.), *Contemporary intellectual assessment: Theories, tests, and issues* (2nd ed., pp. 185–202). New York: Guilford Press.

Allport, G. W. (1937). *Personality: A psychological interpretation.* New York: Wiley.

American Association on Intellectual and Developmental Disabilities (AAIDD). (2010). *Intellectual disability: Definition, classification, and systems of supports* (11th ed.). Washington, DC: Author.

American Association on Mental Retardation. (1992). *Mental retardation: Definition, classification, and systems of supports* (9th ed.). Washington, DC: Author.

American Educational Research Association (AERA), American Psychological Association (APA), & National Council on Measurement in Education (NCME). (1999). *Standards for educational and psychological testing.* Washington, DC: American Educational Research Association.

American Psychiatric Association. (2000). *Diagnostic and statistical manual of mental disorders* (4th ed., text rev.). Washington, DC: Author.

American Psychiatric Association. (2013). *Diagnostic and statistical manual of mental disorders* (5th ed.). Arlington, VA: Author.

American Psychological Association (APA). (2002). Ethical principles of psychologists and code of conduct. *American Psychologist, 57*, 1060–1073.

American Psychological Association (APA). (2010a). Amendments to the 2002 ethical principles of psychologists and code of conduct. *American Psychologist, 65*, 493.

American Psychological Association (APA). (2010b). *Publication manual of the American Psychological Association* (6th ed.). Washington, DC: Author.

American Speech–Language–Hearing Association. (n.d.). *Self-test for hearing loss.* Retrieved from *www. asha.org/public/hearing/Self-Test-for-Hearing-Loss.*

Assouline, S. G., & Whiteman, C. S. (2011). Twice-exceptionality: Implications for school psychologists in the post-IDEA 2004 era. *Journal of Applied School Psychology, 27*, 380–402.

Bandura, A. (1978). The self system in reciprocal determinism. *American Psychologist, 33*, 344–358.

Barron, F. (1968). *Creativity and personal freedom.* New York: Van Nostrand.

Baum, S., & Owen, S. V. (1988). High ability/learning disabled students: How are they different? *Gifted Child Quarterly, 32*, 321–326.

Bender, L. (1938). A Visual Motor Gestalt Test and its clinical use. *American Orthopsychiatric Association Research Monograph*, No. 3.

Benson, J. (1998). Developing a strong program of construct validation: A test anxiety example. *Educational Measurement: Issues and Practices, 17*, 10–17.

Benson, N., Hulac, D., & Kranzler, J. (2010). Independent examination of the Wechsler Adult Intelligence Scale—Fourth Edition (WAIS-IV): What does the WAIS-IV measure? *Psychological Assessment, 22*, 121–130.

Berg, C. A., & Sternberg, R. J. (1992). Adults' conceptions of intelligence across the adult life span. *Psychology and Aging, 7*, 221–231.

Bergeron, R., & Floyd, R. G. (2006). Broad cognitive abilities of children with mental retardation: An analysis of group and individual profiles. *American Journal of Mental Retardation, 111*, 417–432.

Bergeron, R., & Floyd, R. G. (2013). Individual part score profiles of children with intellectual disability: A descriptive analysis across three intelligence tests. *School Psychology Review, 42*, 22–38.

Bergeron, R., Floyd, R. G., & Shands, E. I. (2008). States' eligibility guidelines for mental retardation: An update and consideration of part scores and unreliability of IQs. *Education and Training in Developmental Disabilities, 41*, 123–131.

Berninger, V. W. (2008). Defining and differentiating dysgraphia, dyslexia, and language learning disability within a working memory model. In M. Mody & E. R. Silliman (Eds.), *Brain, behavior, and learning in language and reading disorders: Challenges in language and literacy* (pp. 103–134). New York: Guilford Press.

Borland, J. (2009). The gifted constitute 3% to 5% of the population. Moreover, giftedness equals high IQ, which is a stable measure of aptitude: Spinal tap psychometrics in gifted education. *Gifted Child Quarterly, 53*, 236–238.

Bouchard, T. J. (2009). Strong inference: A strategy for advancing psychological science. In K. McCartney & R. A. Weinberg (Eds.), *Experience and development: A festschrift in honor of Sandra Wood Scarr. Modern pioneers in psychological science: An APS-Psychology Press series* (pp. 39–59). New York: Psychology Press.

Bouchard, T. J., Jr., & McGue, M. (1981). Familial studies of intelligence: A review. *Science, 250*, 223–238.

Bowen, C. (1998). *Developmental phonological disorders: A practical guide for families and teachers.* Melbourne: Australian Council for Educational Research.

Bracken, B. A. (1987). Limitations of preschool instruments and standards for minimal levels of technical adequacy. *Journal of Psychoeducational Assessment, 5*, 313–326.

Bracken, B. A. (2000). Maximizing construct relevant assessment: The optimal preschool testing situation. In B. A. Bracken (Ed.), *The psychoeducational assessment of preschool children* (pp. 33–44). Boston: Allyn & Bacon.

Bracken, B. A., Keith, L. K., & Walker, K. C. (1998). Assessment of preschool behavior and social-emotional functioning: A review of thirteen third-party instruments. *Journal of Psychoeducational Assessment, 16*, 153–169.

Bracken, B. A., & McCallum, R. S. (1998). *Universal Nonverbal Intelligence Test.* Chicago: Riverside.

Braden, J. P. (1997). The practical impact of intellectual assessment issues. *School Psychology Review, 26*, 242–248.

Braden, J. P., & Athanasiou, M. S. (2005). A comparative review of nonverbal measures of intelligence. In D. P. Flanagan & P. L. Harrison (Eds.), *Contemporary intellectual assessment: Theories, tests, and issues* (pp. 557–577). New York: Guilford Press.

Braden, J. P., & Elliott, S. N. (2003). *Accommodations on the Stanford–Binet Intelligence Scales, Fifth Edition* (Stanford–Binet Intelligence Scales, Fifth Edition, Assessment Service Bulletin No. 2). Itasca, IL: Riverside.

Braden, J. P., & Kratochwill, T. R. (1997). Treatment utility of assessment: Myths and realities. *School Psychology Review, 26*, 467–474.

Braden, J. P., & Shaw, S. R. (2009). Intervention validity of cognitive assessment: Knowns, unknowables, and unknowns. *Assessment for Effective Intervention, 34*, 106–115.

Bradley-Johnson, S., & Durmusoglu, G. (2005). Evaluation of floors and item gradients for reading and math tests for young children. *Journal of Psychoeducational Assessment, 23*, 262–278.

Breiger, D., & Majovski, L. V. (2009). Neuropsychological assessment and RTI in the assessment of learning disabilities: Are they mutually exclusive? In E. Fletcher-Janzen & C. R. Reynolds (Eds.), *Neuropsychological perspectives on learning disabilities in the era of RTI: Recommendations for diagnosis and intervention* (pp. 141–157). Hoboken, NJ: Wiley.

Brody, L. E., & Stanley, J. C. (2005). Youths who reason exceptionally well mathematically and/or verbally: Using the MVT:D4 model to develop their talents. In R. J. Sternberg & J. E. Davidson (Eds.), *Conceptions of giftedness* (2nd ed., pp. 20–37). New York: Cambridge University Press.

Brody, N. (1994). Cognitive abilities. *Psychological Science, 5*, 63–68.

Brown, E. F. (2012). Is response to intervention and gifted assessment compatible? *Journal of Psychoeducational Assessment, 30*, 103–116.

Brown, R. T., Daly, B. P., & Stefanatos, G. A (2009). Learning disabilities: Complementary views from neuroscience, neuropsychology, and public health. In E. Fletcher-Janzen & C. R. Reynolds (Eds.), *Neuropsychological perspectives on learning disabilities in the era of RTI: Recommendations for diagnosis and intervention* (pp. 159–178). Hoboken, NJ: Wiley.

Brown, R. T., Reynolds, C. R., & Whitaker, J. W. (1999). Bias in mental testing since "Bias in mental testing." *School Psychology Quarterly, 14,* 208–238.

Brown, W. (1910). Some experimental results in the correlation of mental abilities. *British Journal of Psychology, 3,* 296–322.

Brown-Chidsey, R. (2005). The role of published norm-referenced tests in problem-solving-based assessment. In R. Brown-Chidsey (Ed.), *Assessment for intervention: A problem-solving approach* (pp. 247–266). New York: Guilford Press.

Brown Waesche, J. S., Schatschneider, C., Maner, J. K., Ahmed, Y., & Wagner, R. K. (2011). Examining agreement and longitudinal stability among traditional and RTI-based definitions of reading disability using the affected-status agreement statistic. *Journal of Learning Disabilities, 44,* 296–307.

Browne-Miller, A. (1995). *Intelligence policy: Its impact on college admissions and other social policies.* New York: Plenum Press.

Buck, J. N., & Warren, W. L. (1992). *H-T-P manual and interpretive guide.* Torrance, CA: Western Psychological Services.

Buckingham, B. R. (1921). Intelligence and its measurement: A symposium—XIV. *Journal of Educational Psychology, 12,* 271–275.

Campbell, D. T., & Stanley, J. C. (1963). *Experimental and quasi-experimental designs for research.* Boston: Houghton Mifflin.

Campbell, J. M. (2006a). Autism spectrum disorders. In R. W. Kamphaus & J. M. Campbell (Eds.), *Psychodiagnostic assessment of children: Dimensional and categorical approaches* (pp. 119–168). Hoboken, NJ: Wiley.

Campbell, J. M. (2006b). Mental retardation/intellectual disability. In R. W. Kamphaus & J. M. Campbell (Eds.), *Psychodiagnostic assessment of children: Dimensional and categorical approaches* (pp. 45–85). New York: Wiley.

Canivez, G. L. (2008). Orthogonal higher–order factor structure of the Stanford–Binet Intelligence Scales for children and adolescents. *School Psychology Quarterly, 23,* 533–541.

Canivez, G. L. (2011). Hierarchical factor structure of the Cognitive Assessment System: Variance partitions from the Schmid–Leiman (1957) procedure. *School Psychology Quarterly, 26,* 305–317.

Canivez, G. L., & Watkins, M. W. (2010a). Exploratory and higher-order factor analyses of the Wechsler Adult Intelligence Scale—Fourth Edition (WAIS-IV) adolescent subsample. *School Psychology Quarterly, 25,* 223–235.

Canivez, G. L., & Watkins, M. W. (2010b). Investigation of the factor structure of the Wechsler Adult Intelligence Scale—Fourth Edition (WAIS-IV): Exploratory and higher-order factor analyses. *Psychological Assessment, 22,* 827–836.

Canter, A., Paige, L., & Shaw, S. (2010). *Helping children at home and school III.* Bethesda, MD: National Association of School Psychologists.

Carpenter, P. A., Just, M. A., & Shell, P. (1990). What one intelligence test measures: A theoretical account of the processing in the Raven Progressive Matrices Test. *Psychological Review, 97,* 404–431.

Carroll, J. B. (1982). The measurement of intelligence. In R. J. Sternberg (Ed.), *Handbook of human intelligence* (pp. 29–122). Cambridge, UK: Cambridge University Press.

Carroll, J. B. (1993). *Human cognitive abilities: A survey of factor-analytic studies.* New York: Cambridge University Press.

Carroll, J. B. (2005). The three-stratum theory of cognitive abilities. In D. P. Flanagan & P. L. Harrison (Eds.), *Contemporary intellectual assessment: Theories, tests, and issues* (pp. 69–75). New York: Guilford Press.

Cassidy, J., & Hossler, A. (1992). State and federal definitions of the gifted: An update. *Gifted Child Quarterly, 15,* 46–53.

Cattell, R. B. (1971). *Abilities: Their structure, growth, and action.* Boston: Houghton Mifflin.

Ceci, S. J. (1990). *On intelligence . . . more or less: A bio-ecological treatise on intellectual development.* Englewood Cliffs, NJ: Prentice-Hall.

Centers for Disease Control and Prevention. (n.d.). *Vision loss fact sheet.* Retrieved from *www.cdc.gov/ncbddd/actearly/pdf/parents_pdfs/VisionLossFactSheet.pdf.*

Chafouleas, S., Riley-Tillman, T. C., & Sugai, G. (2007). *School-based behavioral assessment: Informing intervention and instruction.* New York: Guilford Press.

Chapman, P. D. (1988). *Schools as sorters: Lewis M. Terman, applied psychology, and the intelligence testing movement, 1890–1930.* New York: New York University Press.

Chipeur, H. M., Rovine, M., & Plomin, R. (1990). LISREL modeling: Genetic and environmental influences on IQ revisited. *Intelligence, 14,* 11–29.

Christ, T. J., Zopluoglu, C., Long, J. D., & Monaghen, B. D. (2012). Curriculum-based measurement of oral reading: Quality of progress monitoring outcomes. *Council for Exceptional Children, 78,* 356–373.

Cizek, G. J., Bowen, D., & Church, K. (2010). Sources of validity evidence for educational and psychological tests: A follow up. *Educational and Psychological Measurement, 70,* 732–743.

Clarke, A. M., & Clarke, A. D. B. (1989). The later cognitive effects of early intervention. *Intelligence, 13,* 289–297.

Colom, R., & Thompson, P. M. (2011). Understanding human intelligence by imaging the brain. In T. Chamorro-Premuzic, S. von Stumm, & A. Furnham (Eds.), *The Wiley–Blackwell handbook of individual differences* (pp. 330–352). Malden, MA: Wiley–Blackwell.

Colour Blind Awareness. (n.d.). *Early symptoms.* Retrieved from *www.colourblindawareness.org/parents/early-symptoms.*

Cormier, D. C., McGrew, K. S., & Evans, J. J. (2011). Quantifying the "degree of linguistic demand" in spoken intelligence test directions. *Journal of Psychoeducational Assessment, 29,* 1–19.

Cox, C. M. (1926). *Genetic studies of genius: Vol. 2. The early mental traits of three hundred geniuses.* Stanford, CA: Stanford University Press.

Crawford, J. (2009). *Making sense of Census 2009.* Retrieved from *www.language-policy.org/content/features/article5.htm.*

Cronbach, L. J. (1975). Five decades of public controversy over mental testing. *American Psychologist, 30,* 1–14.

Cronbach, L. J. (1990). *Essentials of psychological testing* (5th ed.). New York: Harper & Row.

Cronbach, L. J., & Meehl, P. (1955). Construct validity of psychological tests. *Psychological Bulletin, 52,* 281–302.

Cronbach, L. J., & Snow, R. E. (1977). *Aptitudes and instructional methods: A handbook for research on interactions.* Oxford, UK: Irvington.

Cummins, J. (1984). *Bilingual and special education: Issues in assessment and pedagogy.* San Diego, CA: College-Hill Press.

Daniel, M. H. (2007). "Scatter" and the construct validity of the FSIQ: Comment on Fiorello et al. (2007). *Applied Neuropsychology, 14,* 291–295.

Das, J. P. (1999). *PASS Reading Enhancement Program (PREP).* Edmonton: Developmental Disabilities Centre, University of Alberta.

Das, J. P. (2004). *The Cognitive Enhancement Training program (COGENT).* New York: Springer.

Das, J. P., Naglieri, J. A., & Kirby, J. R. (1994). *Assessment of cognitive processes: The PASS theory of intelligence.* Boston: Allyn & Bacon.

Deary, I. J. (2001). *Intelligence: A very short introduction.* Oxford, UK: Oxford University Press.

Deary, I. J., Penke, L., & Johnson, W. (2010). Genetic foundations of human intelligence. *Human Genetics, 126,* 215–232.

DeFries, J. C., & Gillis, J. J. (1993). Genetics of reading disability. In R. Plomin & G. E. McClearn (Eds.), *Nature, nurture, and psychology* (pp. 121–145).

Washington, DC: American Psychological Association.

Delisle, J. R. (2003). To be or to do: Is a gifted child born or developed? *Roeper Review, 26,* 12–13.

Delisle, J. R., & Galbraith, J. (2002). *When gifted kids don't have all the answers: How to meet their social and emotional needs.* Minneapolis, MN: Free Spirit.

Derr-Minneci, T. F., & Shapiro, E. S. (1992). Validating curriculum-based measurement in reading from a behavioral perspective. *School Psychology Quarterly, 7,* 2–16.

Deno, S. L. (1989). Curriculum-based measurement and alternative special education services: A fundamental and direct relationship. In M. R. Shinn (Ed.), *Curriculum-based measurement: Assessing special children* (pp. 1–17). New York: Guilford Press.

Deno, S. L. (2002). Problem solving as "best practice." In A. Thomas & J. Grimes (Eds.), *Best practices in school psychology IV* (Vol. 1; pp. 37–55). Washington, DC: National Association of School Psychologists.

De Los Reyes, A., & Kazdin, A. E. (2005). Informant discrepancies in the assessment of childhood psychopathology: A critical review, theoretical framework, and recommendations for further study. *Psychological Bulletin, 131,* 483–509.

Detterman, D. K., & Sternberg, R. J. (Eds.). (1993). *Transfer on trial: Intelligence, cognition, and instruction.* Norwood, NJ: Ablex.

Dhaniram-Beharry, E. (2008). *Cultural and linguistic influences on test performance: Evaluation of alternate variables* (Doctoral dissertation). Retrieved from ProQuest (Accession No. 3336081).

DiStefano, C., & Dombrowski, S. C. (2006). Investigating the theoretical structure of the Stanford–Binet, Fifth Edition. *Journal of Psychoeducational Assessment, 24,* 123–136.

Dombrowski, S. C. (2003, September). Ethical standards and best practices in using newly revised intelligence tests. *Communiqué, 32,* pp. 1, 12.

Education for All Handicapped Children Act of 1975, Pub. L. No. 94-142 (1975).

Elliott, C. D. (2007). *Differential Ability Scales—Second Edition.* San Antonio, TX: Harcourt Assessment.

Embretson, S. E., & Reise, S. P. (2000). *Item response theory for psychologists.* Mahwah, NJ: Erlbaum.

Emmons, M. R., & Alfonso, V. (2005). Critical review of the technical characteristics of current preschool screening batteries. *Journal of Psychoeducational Assessment, 23,* 111–127.

Ericsson, K. A., & Simon, H. A. (1993). *Protocol analysis: Verbal reports as data* (rev. ed.). Cambridge, MA: MIT Press.

Esters, I. G., Ittenbach, R. F., & Han, K. (1997). Today's

IQ tests: Are they really better than their historical predecessors? *School Psychology Review, 26,* 211–244.

Eysenck, H. J. (1973). *The measurement of intelligence.* Baltimore: Williams & Wilkins.

Eysenck, H. J. (1979). *The structure and measurement of intelligence.* New York: Springer-Verlag.

Eysenck, H. J. (1994). Review of *Human cognitive abilities: A survey of factor-analytic studies. Personality and Individual Differences, 16,* 199.

Eysenck, H. J. (1998). *Intelligence: A new look.* New Brunswick, NJ: Transaction.

Fagan, T. K., & Wise, P. S. (2007). *School psychology: Past, present, and future* (3rd ed.). Bethesda, MD: National Association of School Psychologists.

Feuerstein, R., Rand, Y., & Hoffman, M. B. (1979). *The dynamic assessment of retarded performers: The Learning Potential Assessment Device theory, instruments, and techniques.* Baltimore: University Park Press.

Fiorello, C. A., Hale, J. B., & Snyder, L. (2006). Cognitive hypothesis testing and response to intervention for children with reading problems. *Psychology in the Schools, 8,* 835–853.

Fiorello, C. A., Hale, J. B., Holdnack, J. A., Kavanagh, J. A., Terrell, J., & Long, L. (2007). Interpreting intelligence test results for children with disabilities: Is global intelligence relevant? *Applied Neuropsychology, 14,* 2–12.

Fish, J. M. (1988). Reinforcement in testing: Research with children and adolescents. *Professional School Psychology, 3,* 203–218.

Flanagan, D. P., & Alfonso, A. C. (1995). A critical review of the technical characteristics of new and recently revised intelligence tests for preschool children. *Journal of Psychoeducational Assessment, 13,* 66–90.

Flanagan, D. P., Alfonso, V. C., & Ortiz, S. O. (2013). The cross-battery approach: An overview, historical perspective, and current directions. In D. P. Flanagan & P. L. Harrison (Eds.), *Contemporary intellectual assessment: Theories, tests, and issues* (pp. 459–484). New York: Guilford Press.

Flanagan, D. P., & Harrison, P. L. (Eds.). (2012). *Contemporary intellectual assessment: Theories, tests, and issues* (3rd ed.). New York: Guilford Press.

Flanagan, D. P., & Kaufman, A. S. (2009). *Essentials of WISC-IV assessment* (2nd ed.). Hoboken, NJ: Wiley.

Flanagan, D. P., Ortiz, S. O., & Alfonso, V. C. (2013). *Essentials of cross-battery assessment* (3rd ed.). Hoboken, NJ: Wiley.

Flanagan, D. P., Ortiz, S. O., Alfonso, V. C., & Mascolo, J. (2006). *Achievement test desk reference: A guide to learning disability identification* (2nd ed.). New York: Wiley.

Flesch, R. (1948). A new readability yardstick. *Journal of Applied Psychology, 32,* 221–233.

Flesch, R. (1949). *The art of readable writing.* New York: Harper.

Fletcher, J. M., Lyons, R. L., Fuchs, L. S., & Barnes, M. A. (2006). *Learning disabilities: From identification to intervention.* New York: Guilford Press.

Fletcher, J. M., Stuebing, K. K., Barth, A. E., Denton, C. A., Cirino, P. T., Francis, D. J., et al. (2011). Cognitive correlates of inadequate response to reading intervention. *School Psychology Review, 40,* 3–22.

Fletcher-Janzen, E., & Reynolds, C. R. (Eds.). (2009). *Neuropsychological perspectives on learning disabilities in the era of RTI: Recommendations for diagnosis and intervention.* Hoboken, NJ: Wiley.

Flipsen, P., Jr. (2006). Measuring the intelligibility of conversational speech in children. *Clinical Linguistics and Phonetics, 20,* 202–312.

Florida Department of Education. (2009). *Florida statutes and State Board of Education rules.* Retrieved from *www.fldoe.org/ese/pdf/1b-stats.pdf.*

Florida Department of Education. (2011). *Florida statutes and state board of education rules.* Tallahassee, FL: Bureau of Exceptional Education and Student Services.

Floyd, R. G. (2010). Cognitive abilities and cognitive processes: Issues, applications, and fit within a problem-solving model. In G. Gimpel Peacock, R. A. Ervin, E. J. Daly III, & K. W. Merrell (Eds.), *Practical handbook of school psychology: Effective practices for the 21st century* (pp. 48–66). New York: Guilford Press.

Floyd, R. G., & Bose, J. E. (2003). A critical review of rating scales assessing emotional disturbance. *Journal of Psychoeducational Assessment, 21,* 43–78.

Floyd, R. G., Clark, M. H., & Shadish, W. R. (2008). The exchangeability of intelligent quotients: Implications for professional psychology. *Professional Psychology: Research and Practice, 39,* 414–423.

Floyd, R. G., & Kranzler, J. H. (2012). Processing approaches to interpretation of information from cognitive ability tests: A critical review. In D. P. Flanagan & P. L. Harrison (Eds.), *Contemporary intellectual assessment: Theories, tests, and issues* (3rd ed., pp. 497–523). New York: Guilford Press.

Floyd, R. G., & Kranzler, J. H. (2013). The role of intelligence testing in understanding students' academic problems. In R. Brown-Chidsey & K. J. Andren (Eds.), *Assessment for intervention: A problem-solving approach* (2nd ed., pp. 229–249). New York: Guilford Press.

Floyd, R. G., McGrew, K. S., Barry, A., Rafael, F. A., & Rogers, J. (2009). General and specific effects on Cattell–Horn–Carroll broad ability composites: Analysis of the Woodcock–Johnson III Normative Update CHC factor clusters across development. *School Psychology Review, 38,* 249–265.

Floyd, R. G., Shaver, R. B., & McGrew, K. S. (2003). Interpretation of the Woodcock–Johnson III Tests of Cognitive Abilities: Acting on evidence. In F. A. Schrank & D. P. Flanagan (Eds.), *WJ III clinical use and interpretation* (pp. 1–46, 403–408). Boston: Academic Press.

Flynn, J. R. (1984). The mean IQ of Americans: Massive gains 1932 to 1978. *Psychological Bulletin, 95,* 29–51.

Flynn, J. R. (1987). Massive IQ gains in 14 nations: What IQ tests really measure. *Psychological Bulletin, 101,* 171–191.

Flynn, J. R. (1999). Searching for justice: The discovery of IQ gains over time. *American Psychologist, 54,* 5–20.

Flynn, J. R. (2007). *What is intelligence?* New York: Cambridge University Press.

Fox, L. H., Brody, L., & Tobin, D. (1983). *Learning-disabled/gifted children: Identification and programming.* Baltimore: University Park Press.

Francis, D. J., Fletcher, J. M., Stuebing, K. K., Lyon, R. L., Shaywitz, B. A., & Shaywitz, S. E. (2005). Psychometric approaches to the identification of LD: IQ and achievement scores are not sufficient. *Journal of Learning Disabilities, 38,* 98–108.

Freberg, M. E., Vandiver, B. J., Watkins, M. W., & Canivez, G. L. (2008). Significant factor score variability and the validity of the WISC-III Full Scale IQ in predicting later academic achievement. *Applied Neuropsychology, 15,* 131–139.

Frick, P. J., Barry, C. T., & Kamphaus, R. K. (2009). *Clinical assessment of child and adolescent personality and behavior* (3rd ed.). New York: Springer.

Frisby, C. L., & Braden, J. P. (1992). Feuerstein's dynamic assessment approach: A semantic, logical, and empirical critique. *Journal of Special Education, 26,* 281–301.

Frisby, C. L., & Braden, J. P. (Eds.). (1999). Bias in mental testing [Special issue]. *School Psychology Quarterly, 14*(4).

Fuchs, D., & Deshler, D. D. (2007). What we need to know about responsiveness to intervention (and shouldn't be afraid to ask). *Learning Disabilities Research and Practice, 22,* 129–136.

Fuchs, D., Fuchs, L. S., & Compton, D. L. (2004). Identifying reading disabilities by responsiveness-to-instruction: Specifying measures and criteria. *Learning Disability Quarterly, 27,* 216–227.

Fuchs, D., Mock, D., Morgan, P. L., & Young, C. L. (2003). Responsiveness-to-intervention: Definitions, evidence, and implications for the learning disabili-

ties construct. *Learning Disabilities Research and Practice, 18,* 157–171.

Fuchs, D., & Young, C. L. (2006). On the irrelevance of intelligence in predicting responsiveness to reading instruction. *Exceptional Children, 73,* 8–30.

Fuchs, L. S. (1995). Best practices in defining student goals and outcomes. In A. Thomas & J. Grimes (Eds.), *Best practices in school psychology III* (pp. 539–546). Washington, DC: National Association of School Psychologists.

Fuchs, L. S., & Fuchs, D. (1998). Treatment validity: A unifying concept for reconceptualizing the identification of learning disabilities. *Learning Disabilities Research and Practice, 13,* 204–219.

Galton, F. (1865). Hereditary talent and character. *Macmillan's Magazine, 12,* 318–327.

Galton, F. (1869). *Hereditary genius: An inquiry into its laws and consequences.* London: Macmillan.

Garber, H. L. (1988). *The Milwaukee project.* Washington, DC: American Association on Mental Retardation.

Gardner, H. (1983). *Frames of mind: The theory of multiple intelligences.* New York: Basic Books.

Gardner, H. (1993). *Multiple intelligences.* New York: Basic Books.

Gardner, H. (1999). *Intelligences reframed: Multiple intelligences for the 21st century.* New York: Basic Books.

Gardner, H. (2006). *Multiple intelligences: New horizons.* New York: Basic Books.

Gifford, B. R. (1989). Introduction. In B. R. Gifford (Ed.), *Testing policy and test performance: Education, language, and culture* (p. ix). Boston: Kluwer Academic.

Glutting, J. J., Adams, W., & Sheslow, D. (2000). *Wide Range Intelligence Test.* Wilmington, DE: Wide Range.

Glutting, J. J., McDermott, P. A., & Stanley, J. C. (1987). Resolving differences among methods of establishing confidence limits for test scores. *Educational and Psychological Measurement, 47,* 607–614.

Glutting, J. J., & Oakland, T. (1993). *Manual for the guide to the assessment of test session behavior.* San Antonio, TX: Psychological Corporation.

Good, R. H., III, Vollmer, M., Katz, L., Creek, R. J., & Chowdhri, S. (1993). Treatment utility of the Kaufman Assessment Battery for Children: Effects of matching instruction and student processing strength. *School Psychology Review, 22,* 8–26.

Goodman, J. F. (1990). Infant intelligence: Do we, can we, should we assess it? In C. R. Reynolds & R. W. Kamphaus (Eds.), *Handbook of psychological and educational assessment of children: Intelligence and achievement* (pp. 183–208). New York: Guilford Press.

Gordon, R. A. (1987). Jensen's contributions concerning test bias: A contextual view. In S. Modgil & C. Modgil (Eds.), *Arthur Jensen: Consensus and controversy* (pp. 77–154). Philadelphia: Falmer.

Gordon-Brannan, M. (1994). Assessing intelligibility: Children's expressive phonologies. *Topics in Language Disorders, 14*, 17–25.

Gottfredson, L. S. (1997). Why *g* matters: The complexity of everyday life. *Intelligence, 24*, 79–132.

Gottfredson, L. S. (2000). Pretending intelligence doesn't matter. *Cerebrum, 2*, 75–96.

Gottfredson, L. S. (2002). *g*: Highly general and highly practical. In R. J. Sternberg & E. L. Grigorenko (Eds.), *The general factor of intelligence: How general is it?* (pp. 331–380). Mahwah, NJ: Erlbaum.

Gottfredson, L. S. (2008). Of what value is intelligence? In A. Prifitera, D. Saklofske, & L. G. Weiss (Eds.), *WISC-IV applications for clinical assessment and intervention* (2nd ed., pp. 545–563). Amsterdam: Elsevier.

Gottfredson, L. S. (2011). Intelligence and social inequality: Why the biological link? In T. Chamorro-Preuzic, S. von Stumm, & A. Furnham (Eds.), *The Wiley–Blackwell handbook of individual differences* (pp. 538–575). Malden, MA: Wiley–Blackwell.

Gould, S. J. (1994, November 28). Curveball: Review of *The bell curve*. *The New Yorker, 70*, pp. 139–149.

Gould, S. J. (1996). *The mismeasure of man* (rev. ed.). New York: Norton.

Graesser, A. C., McNamara, D. S., Louwerse, M. M., & Cai, Z. (2004). Coh-Metrix: Analysis of text on cohesion and language. *Behavior Research Methods, Instruments, and Computers, 36*, 193–202.

Gresham, F. M., & Vellutino, F. R. (2010). What is the role of intelligence in the identification of specific learning disabilities?: Issues and clarifications. *Learning Disabilities Research and Practice, 25*, 194–206.

Gresham, F. M., & Witt, J. C. (1997). Utility of intelligence tests for treatment planning, classification, and placement decisions: Recent empirical findings and future directions. *School Psychology Quarterly, 12*, 249–267.

Gustafsson, J. (1984). A unifying model for the structure of intellectual abilities. *Intelligence, 8*, 179–203.

Gustafsson, J.-E. (2002). Measurement from a hierarchical point of view. In H. I. Braun, D. N. Jackson, & D. E. Wiley (Eds.), *The role of constructs in psychological and educational measurement* (pp. 73–96). Mahwah, NJ: Erlbaum.

Haier, R. J. (2011). Biological basis of intelligence. In R. J. Sternberg & S. B. Kaufman (Eds.), *The Cambridge handbook of intelligence* (pp. 351–370). Cambridge, UK: Cambridge University Press.

Hale, J. B., & Fiorello, C. A. (2001). Beyond the academic rhetoric of "*g*": Intelligence testing guidelines for practitioners. *The School Psychologist, 55*, 113–139.

Hambleton, R. K., & Li, S. (2005). Translaterion and adaptation issues and methods for educational and psychological tests. In C. L. Frisby & C. R. Reynolds (Eds.), *Comprehensive handbook of multicultural school psychology* (pp. 882–903). Hoboken, NJ: Wiley.

Hammill, D. D., Brown, L., & Bryant, B. R. (1992). *A consumer's guide to test in print* (2nd ed.). Austin, TX: PRO-ED.

Harrison, P. L., & Oakland, T. (2003). *Adaptive Behavior Assessment System—Second Edition*. San Antonio, TX: Psychological Corporation.

Harvey, V. S. (1997). Improving readability of psychological reports. *Professional Psychology: Research and Practice, 28*, 271–274.

Hayes, S. C., Nelson, R. O., & Jarrett, R. B. (1987). The treatment utility of assessment: A functional approach to evaluating assessment quality. *American Psychologist, 42*, 963–503.

Haynes, S. N., Smith, G. T., & Hunsley, J. D. (2012). *Scientific foundations of clinical assessment*. New York: Routledge.

Herrnstein, R. J., & Murray, C. (1994). *The bell curve: Intelligence and class structure in American life*. New York: Free Press.

Hintze, J. M., & Matthews, W. J. (2004). The generalizability of systematic direct observations across time and setting: A preliminary investigation of the psychometrics of behavioral assessment. *School Psychology Review, 33*, 258–270.

Holdnack, J. A., Dozdick, L. W., Weiss, L. G., & Iverson, G. (2013). *WAIS-IV/WMS-IV advanced clinical solutions*. San Diego, CA: Academic Press.

Horn, J. L. (1991). Measurement of intellectual capabilities: A review of theory. In K. S. McGrew, J. K. Werder, & R. W. Woodcock, *WJ-R technical manual* (pp. 197–232). Itasca, IL: Riverside.

Horn, J. L. (1994). Theory of fluid and crystallized intelligence. In R. J. Sternberg (Ed.), *Encyclopedia of intelligence* (pp. 443–451). New York: Macmillan.

Horn, J. L., & Noll, J. (1997). Human cognitive capabilities: Gf-Gc theory. In D. P. Flanagan, J. L. Genshaft, & P. L. Harrison (Eds.), *Contemporary intellectual assessment: Theories, tests, and issues* (pp. 53–91). New York: Guilford Press.

Howard, D. (1992). Knowing who may have a hearing loss: A simple speech reception game for use by teachers and parents. *The Aboriginal Child at School, 19*(1), 33–51.

Howell, K. W., Hosp, J. L., & Kurns, S. (2008). Best practices in curriculum-based evaluation. In A.

Thomas & J. Grimes (Eds.), *Best practices in school psychology V* (Vol. 2, pp. 349–362). Bethesda, MD: National Association of School Psychologists.

Humphreys, L. G. (1985). A conceptualization of intellectual giftedness. In F. D. Horowitz & M. O'Brien (Eds.), *The gifted and talented: Developmental perspectives* (pp. 331–360). Washington, DC: American Psychological Association.

Humphreys, L. G. (1989). Intelligence: Three kinds of instability and their consequences for policy. In R. L. Linn (Ed.), *Intelligence: Measurement, theory, and public policy* (pp. 193–216). Urbana: University of Illinois Press.

Hunsley, J., & Mash, E. J. (2008). Developing criteria for evidence-based assessment: An introduction to assessments that work. In J. Hunsley & E. J. Mash (Eds.), *A guide to assessments that work* (pp. 3–14). New York: Oxford University Press.

Hunter, J. E. (1986). Cognitive ability, cognitive aptitude, job knowledge, and job performance. *Journal of Vocational Behavior, 29,* 340–362.

Individuals with Disabilities Education Improvement Act of 2004, Pub. L. No. 108-446 (2004).

Institute of Education Sciences. (2008, December). *1.5 million homeschooled students in the United States in 2007.* National Center for Education Statistics, IES Issue Brief. Retrieved August 14, 2011, from *http://nces.ed.gov/pubs2009/2009030.pdf.*

Irby, S. M., & Floyd, R. G. (in press). Review the test Wechsler Abbreviated Scales of Intelligence, Second Edition. *Canadian Journal of School Psychology.*

Jacob, S., Decker, D. M., & Hartshorne, T. (2011). *Ethics and law for school psychologists* (6th ed.). Hoboken, NJ: Wiley.

Jacob K. Javits Gifted and Talented Students Education Act of 1988, 20 U.S.C. 3061 *et seq.* (1988).

Jensen, A. R. (1980). *Bias in mental testing.* New York: Free Press.

Jensen, A. R. (1981). *Straight talk about mental tests.* New York: Free Press.

Jensen, A. R. (1987). Mental chronometry in the study of learning disabilities. *Mental Retardation & Learning Disability Bulletin, 15,* 67–88.

Jensen, A. R. (1989a). Raising IQ without raising g?: A review of "The Milwaukee Project: Preventing mental retardation in children at risk." *Developmental Review, 9,* 234–258.

Jensen, A. R. (1989b). The relationship between learning and intelligence. *Learning and Individual Differences, 1,* 37–62.

Jensen, A. R. (1998). *The g factor: The science of mental ability.* Westport, CT: Preager.

Jensen, A. R. (2002). Galton's legacy to research on intelligence. *Journal of Biosocial Sciences, 34,* 145–172.

Jensen, A. R. (2006). *Clocking the mind: Mental chronometry and individual differences.* Oxford, UK: Elsevier.

Jimerson, S. R., Burns, M. K., & VanDerHeyden, A. M. (Eds.). (2007). *Handbook of response to intervention: The science and practice of assessment and intervention.* New York: Springer.

Johnson, te Nijenhuis, H., & Bouchard, T. J., Jr. (2008). Still one g: Consistent results from five test batteries. *Intelligence, 36,* 81–95.

Kamphaus, R. K. (2001). *Clinical assessment of child and adolescent intelligence* (2nd ed.). Boston: Allyn & Bacon.

Kamphaus, R. K. (2009). Assessment of intelligence and achievement. In T. B. Gutkin & C. R. Reynolds (Eds.), *The handbook of school psychology* (4th ed., pp. 230–246). New York: Wiley.

Kamphaus, R. W., & Campbell, J. M. (Eds.). (2006). *Psychodiagnostic assessment of children: Dimensional and categorical approaches.* Hoboken, NJ: Wiley.

Kamphaus, R. W., Winsor, A. P., Rowe, E. W., & Kim, S. (2012). A history of intelligence test interpretation. In D. P. Flanagan & P. Harrison (Eds.), *Contemporary intellectual assessment* (3rd ed., pp. 56–70). New York: Guilford Press.

Kaplan, E., Delis, D., Fein, D., Maerlender, A., Morris, R., & Kramer, J. (2004). *WISC-IV Integrated.* San Antonio, TX: Harcourt Assessment.

Kaufman, A. S. (1979). *Intelligent testing with the WISC-R.* New York: Wiley.

Kaufman, A. S. (1994). *Intelligent testing with the WISC-III.* New York: Wiley.

Kaufman, A. S., & Kaufman, N. L. (2004a). *Kaufman Assessment Battery for Children, Second Edition.* Circle Pines, MN: American Guidance Service.

Kaufman, A. S., & Kaufman, N. L. (2004b). *Kaufman Brief Intelligence Test, Second Edition.* Circle Pines, MN: American Guidance Service.

Kaufman, S. B., Reynolds, M. R., Liu, X., Kaufman, A. S., & McGrew, K. S. (2012). Are cognitive g and academic achievement g one and the same g?: An exploration on the Woodcock–Johnson and Kaufman tests. *Intelligence, 40,* 123–138.

Kaufman, S. B., & Sternberg, R. J. (2008). Conceptions of giftedness. In S. I. Pfeiffer (Ed.), *Handbook of giftedness in children: Psychoeducational theory, research, and best practices* (pp. 71–91). New York: Springer.

Kazdin, A. (2010). *Single-case research designs: Methods for clinical and applied settings* (2nd ed.). New York: Oxford University Press.

Keith, T. Z., Fine, J. G., Taub, G. E., Reynolds, M. R., & Kranzler, J. H. (2006). Hierarchical, multi-sample, confirmatory factor analysis of the Wechsler Intelligence Scale for Children—Fourth Edition: What does it measure? *School Psychology Review, 35,* 108–127.

Keith, T. Z., Kranzler, J. H., & Flanagan, D. P. (2001). What does the Cognitive Assessment System (CAS) measure?: Conjoint confirmatory factor analysis of the CAS and the Woodcock–Johnson Tests of Cognitive Ability (3rd ed.). *School Psychology Review, 30,* 89–117.

Keith, T. Z., Low, J. A., Reynolds, M. R., Patel, P. G., & Ridley, K. P. (2010). Higher-order factor structure of the Differential Ability Scales—II: Consistency across ages 4 to 17. *Psychology in the Schools, 47,* 676–697.

Keith, T. Z., & Reynolds, M. R. (2010). Cattell–Horn–Carroll theory and cognitive abilities: What we've learned from 20 years of research. *Psychology in the Schools, 47,* 635–650.

Keith, T. Z., & Reynolds, M. R. (2012). Using confirmatory factor analysis to aid in understanding the constructs measured by intelligence tests. In D. P. Flanagan & P. L. Harrison (Eds.), *Contemporary intellectual assessment: Theories, tests, and issues* (3rd ed., pp. 758–799). New York: Guilford Press.

Kelley, T. E. (1927). *Interpretation of educational measurements.* Yonkers-on-Hudson, NY: World Book.

Kirk, S. A. (1962). *Educating exceptional children.* Boston: Houghton-Mifflin.

Kirk, S. A., & Kirk, W. D. (1983). On defining learning disabilities. *Journal of Learning Disabilities, 16,* 20–21.

Kirschenbaum, R. J. (1998). Dynamic assessment and its use with underserved gifted and talented populations. *Gifted Child Quarterly, 42,* 140–147.

Kotz, K. M., Watkins, M. W., & McDermott, P. A. (2008). Validity of the general conceptual ability score from the Differential Ability Scales as a function of significant and rare interfactor variability. *School Psychology Review, 37,* 261–278.

Kranzler, J. H., Flores, C. G., & Coady, M. (2010). Examination of the cross-battery approach for the cognitive assessment of children and youth from diverse linguistic and cultural backgrounds. *School Psychology Review, 39,* 431–446.

Kranzler, J. H., & Keith, T. Z. (1999). Independent confirmatory factor analysis of the Cognitive Assessment System (CAS): What does the CAS measure? *School Psychology Review, 28,* 117–144.

Kranzler, J. H., & Weng, L. (1995). The factor structure of the PASS cognitive tasks: A reexamination of Naglieri et al. (1991). *Journal of School Psychology, 33,* 143–157.

Krasa, N. (2007). Is the Woodcock–Johnson III a test for all seasons?: Ceiling and item gradient considerations in its use with older students. *Journal of Psychoeducational Assessment, 25,* 3–16.

LaBuda, M. C., Vogler, G. P., DeFries, J. C., & Fulker, D. W. (1985). Multivariate familial analysis of cognitive measures in the Colorado Family Reading Study. Multivariate *Behavioral Research, 20,* 357–368.

Lichtenberger, E. O., & Kaufman, A. S. (2009). *Essentials of WAIS-IV assessment.* Hoboken, NJ: Wiley.

Lichtenberger, E. O., Mather, N., Kaufman, N. L., & Kaufman, A. S. (2004). *Essentials of assessment report writing.* New York: Wiley.

Lichtenstein, R. (2010, June). How soon must you switch to the new version of a test? *Communiqué, 38*(8), pp. 1, 12, 14–15.

Lilienfeld, S. O., Ammirati, R., & David, M. (2012). Distinguishing science from pseudoscience in school psychology: Science and scientific thinking as safeguard against human error. *Journal of School Psychology, 50,* 7–36.

Locurto, C. (1990). The malleability of IQ as judged from adoption studies. *Intelligence, 14,* 275–292.

Locurto, C. (1991). *Sense and nonsense about IQ: The case for uniqueness.* New York: Praeger.

Loehlin, J. C. (2007). The strange case of $c2 = 0$: What does it imply for views of human development? *Research in Human Development, 4,* 151–162.

Lohman, D. F., Korb, K., & Lakin, J. (2008). Identifying academically gifted English language learners using nonverbal tests: A comparison of the Raven, NNAT, and CogAT. *Gifted Child Quarterly, 52,* 275–296.

Lohman, D. F., & Lakin, J. (2008). Nonverbal test scores as one component of an identification system: Integrating ability, achievement, and teacher ratings. In J. L. VanTassel-Baska (Ed.), *Alternative assessments of identifying gifted and talented students* (pp. 41–66). Austin, TX: Prufrock Press.

Marín, G. (1992). Issues in the measurement of acculturation among Hispanics. In K. F. Geisinger (Ed.), *Psychological testing of Hispanics* (pp. 235–251). Washington, DC: American Psychological Association.

Marland, S. P., Jr. (1972). *Education of the gifted and talented: Report to the Congress of the United States by the U.S. Commissioner of Education.* Washington, DC: U.S. Government Printing Office.

Mash, E. J., & Barkley, R. A. (2007). *Assessment of childhood disorders* (4th ed.). New York: Guilford Press.

Mather, N., & Jaffe, L. E. (2002). *Woodcock–Johnson III: Reports, recommendations, and strategies.* New York: Wiley.

Mathers, M., Keyes, M., & Wright, M. (2010). A review of the evidence on the effectiveness of children's vision screening. *Child: Care, Health and Development, 36,* 756–780.

Maynard, J. L., Floyd, R. G., Acklie, T. J., & Houston, L. (2011). General factor loadings and specific effects of the Differential Ability Scales, Second Edition composites. *School Psychology Quarterly, 26,* 108–118.

McCallum, R. S., Bracken, B. A., & Wasserman, J. (2001). *Essentials of nonverbal assessment.* New York: Wiley.

McClain, M., & Pfeiffer, S. (2012). Identification of gifted students in the United States today: A look at state definitions, policies, and practices. *Journal of Applied School Psychology, 28,* 59–88.

McCoach, D. B., Kehle, T. J., Bray, M. A., & Siegle, D. (2001). Best practices in the identification of gifted students with disabilities. *Psychology in the Schools, 38,* 403–411.

McConaughy, S. H. (2005). Direct observational assessment during test sessions and child clinical interviews. *School Psychology Review, 34,* 490–506.

McConaughy, S. H., & Achenbach, T. M. (2004). *Manual for the Test Observation Form for Ages 2–18.* Burlington: University of Vermont, Research Center for Children, Youth, & Families.

McCrimmon, A. W., & Smith, A. D. (2013). Review of the Wechsler Abbreviated Scale of Intelligence, Second Edition (WASI-II). *Journal of Psychoeducational Assessment, 31,* 337–341.

McDermott, P. A., Fantuzzo, J. W., & Glutting, J. J. (1990). Just say no to subtest analysis: A critique on Wechsler theory and practice. *Journal of Psychoeducational Assessment, 8,* 290–302.

McDermott, P. A., & Glutting, J. J. (1997). Informing stylistic learning behavior, disposition, and achievement through ability subtests: Or more illusions of meaning? *School Psychology Review, 26,* 163–175.

McGrew, K. S., & Flanagan, D. P. (1998). *The intelligence test desk reference (ITDR): Gf-Gc cross-battery assessment.* Boston: Allyn & Bacon.

McGue, M., Bouchard, T. J., Jr., Iacono, W. G., & Lykken, D. T. (1993). Behavioral genetics of cognitive ability: A life-span perspective. In R. Plomin & G. E. McClearn (Eds.), *Nature, nurture, and psychology* (pp. 59–76). Washington, DC: American Psychological Association.

McNamara, J. K., Willoughby, T., & Chalmers, H. (2005). Psychosocial status of adolescents with learning disabilities with and without comorbid attention deficit hyperactivity disorder. *Learning Disabilities Research and Practice, 20,* 234–244.

Mercer, C. D., Jordan, L., Allsopp, D. H., & Mercer, A. R. (1996). Learning disabilities definitions and criteria used by state education departments. *Learning Disability Quarterly, 19,* 217–232.

Merrell, K. W. (2008). *Behavioral, social, and emotional assessment of children and adolescents* (3rd ed.). Mahwah, NJ: Erlbaum.

Merrell, K. W., Ervin, R. A., & Gimpel Peacock, G. (2012). *School psychology for the 21st century: Foundations and practices* (2nd ed.). New York: Guilford Press.

Mervis, C. B., & John, A. E. (2010). Intellectual disability syndromes. In K. O. Yeates, M. D. Ris, H. G. Taylor, & B. F. Pennington (Eds.), *Pediatric neuropsychology: Research, theory, and practice* (2nd ed., pp. 447–470) New York: Guilford Press.

Messick, S. (1995). Validity of psychological assessment: Validity of inferences from persons' responses and performances as scientific inquiry into score meaning. *American Psychologist, 50,* 741–749.

Naglieri, J. A., Booth, A. L., & Winsler, A. (2004). Comparison of Hispanic children with and without limited English proficiency on the Naglieri Nonverbal Ability Test. *Psychological Assessment, 16,* 81–84.

Naglieri, J. A., & Das, J. P. (1997). *Cognitive Assessment System.* Itasca, IL: Riverside.

Naglieri, J. A., & Kaufman, A. S. (2008). IDEIA and specific learning disabilities: What role does intelligence play? In E. L. Grigorenko (Ed.), *Educating individuals with disabilities: IDEIA 2004 and beyond* (pp. 165–195). New York: Springer.

Naglieri, J. A., & Otero, T. M. (2012). The Cognitive Assessment System: From theory to practice. In D. P. Flanagan & P. L. Harrison (Eds.), *Contemporary intellectual assessment: Theories, tests, and issues* (pp. 376–399). New York: Guilford Press.

National Association for Gifted Children (NAGC). (2009). *State of the states in gifted education.* Washington, DC: Author.

National Association of School Psychologists (NASP). (2010a). *Principles for professional ethics.* Bethesda, MD: Author. Retrieved from *www.nasponline.org/ standards/2010standards.aspx.*

National Association of School Psychologists (NASP). (2010b). *Position statement on identification of students with specific learning disabilities.* Bethesda, MD: Author. Retrieved from *www.nasponline.org/ profdevel/online-learning.aspx.*

National Center for Education Statistics (NCES). (2007). Status and trends in the education of racial and ethnic minorities. Retrieved from *http://nces. ed.gov/pubs2007/minoritytrends/ind_2_7.asp.*

National Center for Education Statistics (NCES). (2009). Number and percentage of elementary and secondary school students who spoke a language other than English at home and percentage who spoke English with difficulty, by grade level and race/ethnicity: 2005. Retrieved from *http://nces. ed.gov/pubs2007/minoritytrends/tables/table_8_2a. asp?referrer=report.*

National Center for Education Statistics (NCES).

(2011). *Digest of education statistics: 2010.* Washington, DC: U.S. Department of Education.

National Joint Committee on Learning Disabilities (NJCLD). (1994). *Collective perspectives on issues affecting learning disabilities: Position papers and statements.* Austin, TX: PRO-ED.

National Joint Committee on Learning Disabilities (NJCLD). (2010, June). Comprehensive assessment and evaluation of students with learning disabilities. Retrieved from *www.ldanatl.org/pdf/NJCLD%2520 Comp%2520Assess%2520Paper%2520.*

National Research Center on Learning Disabilities (NRCLD). (2007). *National SEA Conference on SLD Determination: Integrating RTI within the SLD determination process.* Retrieved from *www.nrcld. org/sea.*

Neisser, U., Boodoo, G., Bouchard, T. J., Jr., Boykin, A. W., Brody, N., Ceci, S. J., et al. (1996). Intelligence: Knowns and unknowns. *American Psychologist, 51,* 77–101.

Nelson, J. M., & Canivez, G. L. (2012). Examination of the structural, convergent, and incremental validity of the Reynolds Intellectual Assessment Scales (RIAS) with a clinical sample. *Psychological Assessment, 24,* 129–140.

Nelson, J. M., Canivez, G. L., Lindstrom, W., & Hatt, C. V. (2007). Higher-order exploratory factor analysis of the Reynolds Intellectual Assessment Scales with a referred sample. *Journal of School Psychology, 45,* 439–456.

Nelson-Gray, R. O. (2003). Treatment utility of psychological assessment. *Psychological Assessment, 15,* 521–531.

Nese, J. F. T., Biancarosa, G., Anderson, D., Lai, C.-F., Alonzo, J., & Tindal, G. (2012). Within-year oral reading fluency with CBM: A comparison of models. *Reading and Writing, 25,* 887–915.

Nesselroade, J. R, Stigler, S. M., & Baltes, P. B. (1980). Regression toward the mean and the study of change. *Psychological Bulletin, 88,* 622–637.

Nettelbeck, T. (2011). Basic processes of intelligence. In R. J. Sternberg & S. B. Kaufman (Eds.), *The Cambridge handbook of intelligence* (pp. 371–393). Cambridge, UK: Cambridge University Press.

Newton, J. H., & McGrew, K. S. (2010). Introduction to the special issue: Current research in Cattell–Horn–Carroll-based assessment. *Psychology in the Schools, 47,* 621–634.

Nicpon, M. F., & Pfeiffer, S. (2011). High-ability students: New ways to conceptualize giftedness and provide psychological services in the schools. *Journal of Applied School Psychology, 27,* 293–305.

Nieves-Brull, A. I. (2006). *Evaluation of the culture–language matrix: A validation study of test performance in monolingual English speaking and bilingual English/Spanish speaking populations* (Doctoral dissertation). Retrieved from ProQuest (Accession No. 3286026).

Nisbett, R., E., Aronson, J., Blair, C., Dickens, W., Flynn, J., Halpern, D. F., et al. (2012). Intelligence: New findings and theoretical developments. *American Psychologist, 67,* 130–159.

No Child Left Behind (NCLB) Act of 2001, Pub. L. 107-110 (2002).

Nunnally, J. C., & Bernstein, I. H. (1994). *Psychometric theory* (3rd ed.). New York: McGraw-Hill.

O'Connor, E., Pasternak, R., Bush, K., Paczak, H., Deri, J., Gibbons, K., et al. (2012, February). *Identifying SLD using RtI: Comparing state rules and best practices.* Paper presented at the annual conference of the National Association of School Psychologists, Philadelphia.

Oades-Sese, G. V., Esquivel, G. B., & Añon, C. (2007). Identifying gifted and talented culturally and linguistically diverse children and adolescents. In G. B. Esquivel & E. C. Lopez (Eds.), *Handbook of multicultural school psychology: An interdisciplinary perspective* (pp. 453–478). Mahwah, NJ: Erlbaum.

Oakland, T. (2003, November). Standards for using revised tests: A different opinion. *Communiqué, 32*(3), pp. 10–11.

Oh, H.-J., Glutting, J. J., Watkins, M. W., Youngstrom, E. A., & McDermott, P. A. (2004). Correct interpretation of latent versus observed abilities: Implications from structural equation modeling applied to the WISC-III and WIAT linking sample. *Journal of Special Education, 38,* 159–173.

Ownby, R. L. (1997). *Psychological reports: A guide to report writing in professional psychology* (3rd ed.). New York: Wiley.

Ortiz, S. O., Ochoa, S. H., & Dynda, A. M. (2012). Testing with culturally and linguistically diverse populations. In D. P. Flanagan & P. L. Harrison (Eds.), *Contemporary intellectual assessment: Theories, tests, and issues* (3rd ed., pp. 526–552). New York: Guilford Press.

Pagel, L. G. (2011). *Proofreading and editing precision.* Mason, OH: South-Western Cengage Learning.

Park, G., Lubinski, D., & Benow, C. P. (2007). Contrasting intellectual patterns predict creativity in the arts and sciences: Tracking intellectually precocious youth over 25 years. *Psychological Science, 18,* 948–952.

Park, G., Lubinski, D., & Benow, C. P. (2008). Ability differences among people who have commensurate degrees matter for scientific creativity. *Psychological Science, 19,* 957–961.

Percy, M. (2007). Factors that cause or contribute to intellectual and developmental disabilities. In I.

Brown & M. Percy (Eds.), *A comprehensive guide to intellectual and developmental disabilities* (pp. 125–148). Baltimore: Brookes.

Pfeiffer, S. I. (2003). Challenges and opportunities for students who are gifted: What the experts say. *Gifted Child Quarterly, 47*, 161–169.

Pfeiffer, S. I., & Blei, S. (2008). Gifted identification beyond the IQ test: Rating scales and other assessment procedures. In S. I. Pfeiffer (Ed.), *Handbook of giftedness in children: Psychoeducational theory, research, and best practices* (pp. 177–198). New York: Springer.

Pfeiffer, S. I., Reddy, L. A., Kletzel, J. E., Schmelzer, E. R., & Boyer, L. M. (2000). The practitioner's view of IQ testing and profile analysis. *School Psychology Quarterly, 15*, 376–385.

Phillips, S. E. (1994). High stakes testing accommodations: Validity versus disabled rights. *Applied Measurement in Education, 7*, 93–120.

Platt, S. A., & Sanislow, C. A. (1988). Norm-of-reaction: Definition and misinterpretation of animal research. *Journal of Comparative Psychology, 102*, 254–261.

Plomin, R., & Kovas, Y. (2005). Generalist genes and learning disabilities. *Psychological Bulletin, 131*, 592–617.

Plomin, R., & Spinath, F. M. (2004). Intelligence: Genetics, genes, and genomics. *Journal of Personality and Social Psychology, 86*, 112–129.

Pope, K. S. (2010). *Responsibilities in providing psychological test feedback to clients.* Retrieved from *www.kspope.com/kpope/index.php on 10/5/2010.*

Popper, K. (1968). *Conjectures and refutations: The growth of scientific knowledge.* New York: Harper.

President's Committee on Mental Retardation. (1969). *The six-hour retarded child.* Washington, DC: U.S. Government Printing Office.

Prifitera, A., Saklofske, D. H., & Weiss, L. G. (2005). *WISC-IV clinical use and interpretation: Scientist-practitioner perspectives.* New York: Elsevier.

Purcell, C. (1978). *Gifted and Talented Children's Education Act of 1978.* Congressional Record. Washington, DC: U.S. Government Printing Office.

Raiford, S. E., Weiss, L. G., Rolfhus, E., & Coalson, D. (2005). *WISC-IV General Ability Index* (Technical Report No. 4). San Antonio, TX: Psychological Corporation.

Raiford, S. E., Weiss, L. G., Rolfhus, E., & Coalson, D. (2010). *GAI utility* [Computer software]. San Antonio, TX: Pearson Education.

Ramey, C. T. (1992). High-risk children and IQ: Altering intergenerational patterns. *Intelligence, 16*, 239–256.

Ramey, C. T. (1994). Abecedarian project. In R. J. Sternberg (Ed.), *Encyclopedia of human intelligence* (Vol. 1, pp. 1–2). New York: Macmillan.

Rasch, G. (1960). *Probabilistic models for some intelligence and attainment tests.* Copenhagen: Danmarks Paedagogiske Institut.

Redfield, R., Linton, R., & Herskovitz, M. J. (1936). Memorandum for the study of acculturation. *American Anthropologist, 38*, 149–152.

Ree, M., & Earles, J. A. (1991). The stability of convergent estimates of *g. Intelligence, 15*, 86–89.

Ree, M., & Earles, J. A. (1992). Intelligence is the best predictor of job performance. *Psychological Science, 3*, 86–89.

Reis, S. M., & Renzulli, J. S. (2011). Intellectual giftedness. In R. J. Sternberg & S. B. Kaufman (Eds.), *The Cambridge handbook of intelligence* (pp. 235–252). Cambridge, UK: Cambridge University Press.

Renzulli, J. S. (1978). What makes giftedness?: Reexamining a definition. *Phi Delta Kappan, 60*, 180–184, 261.

Renzulli, J. S. (1986). The three ring conceptualization of giftedness: A developmental model for creative productivity. In R. J. Sternberg & J. E. Davidson (Eds.), *Conceptions of giftedness* (pp. 246–279). New York: Cambridge University Press.

Reschly, D. J. (1997). Diagnostic and treatment utility of intelligence tests. In D. P. Flanagan, J. L. Genshaft, & P. L. Harrison (Eds.), *Contemporary intellectual assessment: Theories, tests, and issues* (pp. 437–456). New York: Guilford Press.

Reschly, D. J., & Grimes, J. P. (1990). Intellectual assessment. In A. Thomas & J. Grimes (Eds.), *Best practices in school psychology II* (pp. 425–439). Washington, DC: National Association of School Psychologists.

Reschly, D. J., & Grimes, J. P. (1995). Best practices in intellectual assessment. In A. Thomas & J. Grimes (Eds.), *Best practices in school psychology III* (pp. 763–773). Bethesda, MD: National Association of School Psychologists.

Reschly, D. J., & Grimes, J. P. (2002). Best practices in intellectual assessment. In A. Thomas & J. Grimes (Eds.), *Best practices in school psychology IV* (Vol. 2, pp. 1337–1351). Bethesda, MD: National Association of School Psychologists.

Reschly, D. J., & Hosp, J. L. (2007). State SLD identification policies and practices. *Learning Disability Quarterly, 27*, 197–213.

Revelle, W., Wilt, J., & Condon, D. M. (2011). Individual differences and differential psychology: A brief history and prospect. In T. Chamorro-Premuzic, S. von Stumm, & A. Furnham (Eds.), *The Wiley–Blackwell handbook of personality and individual differences* (pp. 3–38). Malden, MA: Wiley–Blackwell.

Reynolds, C. R. (1984–1985). Critical measurement issues in learning disabilities. *The Journal of Special Education, 18*, 451–476.

Reynolds, C. R. (2009). RTI, neuroscience, and sense: Chaos in the diagnosis and treatment of learning disabilities. In E. Fletcher-Janzen & C. R. Reynolds (Eds.), *Neuropsychological perspectives on learning disabilities in the era of RTI: Recommendations for diagnosis and intervention* (pp. 14–27). Hoboken, NJ: Wiley.

Reynolds, C. R., & Carson, A. D. (2005). Methods for assessing cultural bias in tests. In C. L. Frisby & C. R. Reynolds (Eds.), *Comprehensive handbook of multicultural school psychology* (pp. 795–823). Hoboken, NJ: Wiley.

Reynolds, C. R., & Kaiser, S. (1992). Test bias in psychological assessment. In T. B. Gutkin & C. R. Reynolds (Eds.), *The handbook of school psychology* (2nd ed., pp. 487–525). New York: Wiley.

Reynolds, C. R., & Kamphaus, R. W. (2003). *Reynolds Intellectual Assessment Scales*. Lutz, FL: Psychological Assessment Resources.

Reynolds, C. R., & Kamphaus, R. W. (2004). *Behavior Assessment System for Children, Second Edition (BASC-2)*. Circle Pines, MN: American Guidance Service.

Reynolds, C. R., Lowe, P. A., & Saenz, A. (1999). The problem of bias in psychological assessment. In C. R. Reynolds & T. B. Gutkin (Eds.), *The handbook of school psychology* (3rd ed., pp. 549–595). New York: Wiley.

Reynolds, C. R., & Shaywitz, S. E. (2009). Response to intervention: Ready or not? Or, from wait-to-fail to watch-them-fail. *School Psychology Quarterly, 24*, 130–145.

Reynolds, M. R., Keith, T. Z., Fine, J. G., Fisher, M. E., & Low, J. (2007). Confirmatory factor structure of the Kaufman Assessment Battery for Children— Second Edition: Consistency with Cattell–Horn– Carroll theory. *School Psychology Quarterly, 22*, 511–539.

Rhodes, R. L., Ochoa, S. H., & Ortiz, S. O. (2005). *Assessing culturally and linguistically diverse students: A practical guide*. New York: Guilford Press.

Robertson, K. G., Smeets, S., Lubinski, D., & Benbow, C. P. (2010). Beyond the threshold hypothesis: Even among the gifted and top math/science graduate students, cognitive abilities, vocational interests, and lifestyle preferences matter for career choice, performance, and persistence. *Current Directions in Psychological Science, 19*, 346–351.

Roid, G. H. (2003). *Stanford–Binet Intelligence Scales, Fifth Edition*. Itasca, IL: Riverside.

Roid, G. H., & Miller, L. J. (1997). *Leiter International Performance Scale—Revised*. Wood Dale, IL: Stoelting.

Roid, G. H., Miller, L. J., Pomplun, M., & Koch, C.

(2013). *Leiter International Performance Scale, Third Edition*. Wood Dale, IL: Stoelting.

Rosa's law, Pub. L. No. 111-256 (2010).

Rowe, D. C. (1994). *The limits of family influence: Genes, experience, and behavior*. New York: Guilford Press.

Rugg, H. O. (1921). Intelligence and its measurement: A symposium. *Journal of Educational Psychology, 12*, 123–147.

Rushton, P. J. (1995). *Race, evolution and behavior: A life history perspective*. New Brunswick, NJ: Transaction.

Ryan-Arredondo, K., & Sandoval, J. (2005). Psychometric issues in the measurement of acculturation. In C. L. Frisby & C. R. Reynolds (Eds.), *Comprehensive handbook of multicultural school psychology* (pp. 861–880). Hoboken, NJ: Wiley.

Salthouse, T. A. (1996). The processing-speed theory of adult age differences in cognition. *Psychological Review, 103*, 403–428.

Salthouse, T. A. (2010). *Major issues in cognitive aging*. New York: Oxford University Press.

Saklofske, D. H., Prifitera, A., Weiss, L. G., Rolfhus, E., & Zhu, J. (2005). Clinical interpretation of the WISC-IV FSIQ and GAI. In A. Prifitera & D. Saklofske (Eds.), *WISC-IV clinical use and interpretation* (pp. 36–71). San Diego, CA: Academic Press.

Sattler, J. M. (2008). *Assessment of children: Cognitive foundations* (5th ed.). San Diego, CA: Author.

Sattler, J. M., & Hoge, R. D. (2006). *Assessment of children: Behavioral, social, and clinical foundations* (5th ed.). San Diego, CA: Author.

Schaie, K. (1996). Intellectual development in adulthood. In J. E. Birren, K. Schaie, R. P. Abeles, M. Gatz, & T. A. Salthouse (Eds.), *Handbook of the psychology of aging* (4th ed., pp. 266–286). San Diego, CA: Academic Press.

Scheuneman, J. D. (1987). An argument opposing Jensen on test bias: The psychological aspects. In S. Modgil & C. Modgil (Eds.), *Arthur Jensen: Consensus and controversy* (pp. 155–170). Philadelphia: Falmer Press.

Schneider, W. J. (2011a, March 29). A geometric representation of composite scores [Video file]. Retrieved from *http://assessingpsyche.wordpress. com/2011/03/29/a-geometric-representation-of-composite-scores*.

Schneider, W. J. (2011b, October 7). Re: Cathy Fiorello's table [Electronic mailing list message]. Retrieved from *http://groups.yahoo.com/group/NASP-Listserv*.

Schneider, W. J. (2013). What if we took our models seriously? Estimating latent scores in individuals. *Journal of Psychoeducational Assessment, 31*, 186–201.

Schneider, W. J., & McGrew, K. S. (2012). The Cattell–Horn–Carroll model of intelligence. In D. P. Flanagan & P. Harrison (Eds.), *Contemporary intellectual assessment* (3rd ed., pp. 99–144). New York: Guilford Press.

Semrud-Clikeman, M., Wilkinson, A., & Wellington, T. M. (2005). Evaluating and using qualitative approaches to neuropsychological assessment. In R. C. D'Amato, E. Fletcher-Janzen, & C. R. Reynolds (Eds.), *Handbook of school neuropsychology* (pp. 287–302). Hoboken, NJ: Wiley.

Shaw, S. R. (2010, February). Rescuing students from the slow learner trap. *Principal Leadership*, pp. 12–16.

Shaywitz, S. E., & Shaywitz, B. A. (2003). Neurobiological indices of dyslexia. In H. L. Swanson, K. R. Harris, & S. Graham (Eds.), *Handbook of learning disabilities* (pp. 514–531). New York: Guilford Press.

Shepard, L. A. (1989). Identification of mild handicaps. In R. L. Linn (Ed.), *Educational measurement* (3rd ed., pp. 545–572). New York: American Council on Education/Macmillan.

Shinn, M. R. (2005). Identifying and validating academic problems in a problem-solving model. In R. Brown-Chidsey (Ed.), *Assessment for intervention: A problem-solving approach* (pp. 219–246). New York: Guilford Press.

Shinn, M. R. (2007). Identifying students at risk, monitoring performance, and determining eligibility within response to intervention: Research on educational need and benefit from academic intervention. *School Psychology Review, 36,* 601–617.

Shinn, M. R., & Bamonto, S. (1998). Advanced applications of curriculum-based measurement: "Big ideas" and avoiding confusion. In M. R. Shinn (Ed.), *Advanced applications of curriculum-based measurement* (pp. 1–31). New York: Guilford Press.

Shinn, M. R., & Habedank, L. (1992). Curriculum-based measurement in special education problem identification and certification decisions. *Preventing School Failure, 36,* 11–15.

Shinn, M. R., & Walker, H. M. (2010). *Interventions for achievement and behavior problems in a three-tier model including RTI.* Bethesda, MD: National Association of School Psychologists.

Shriberg, L. D. (1993). Four new speech and prosody voice measures for genetics research and other studies in developmental phonological disorders. *Journal of Speech and Hearing Research, 36,* 105–140.

Siegel, L. S. (1989). I.Q. is irrelevant to the definition of learning disabilities. *Journal of Learning Disabilities, 22,* 469–478.

Siegel, L. S. (1992). An evaluation of the discrepancy definition of dyslexia. *Journal of Learning Disabilities, 25,* 618–629.

Simonton, D. K. (1999). Creativity and genius. In L. A. Pervin & O. P. John (Eds.), *Handbook of personality: Theory and research* (2nd ed., pp. 629–652). New York: Guilford Press.

Simonton, D. K. (2001). Talent development as a multidimensional, multiplicative, and dynamic process. *Current Directions in Psychological Science, 10,* 39–43.

Skibbe, L. E., Grimm, K. J., Bowles, R. P., & Morrison, F. J. (2012). Literacy growth in the academic year versus summer from preschool through second grade: Differential effects of schooling across four skills. *Scientific Studies of Reading, 16,* 141–165.

Snow, R. E. (1977). Research on aptitudes: A progress report. In L. S. Shulman (Ed.), *Review of research in education* (Vol. 4, pp. 50–105). Itasca, IL: Peacock.

Snow, R. E., & Yalow, R. (1982). Education and intelligence. In R. J. Sternberg (Ed.), *Handbook of human intelligence* (pp. 493–583). Cambridge, UK: Cambridge University Press.

Snyderman, M., & Rothman, S. (1987). Survey of expert opinion on intelligence and aptitude testing. *American Psychologist, 42,* 137–144.

Snyderman, M., & Rothman, S. (1988). *The IQ controversy, the media and public policy.* New Brunswick, NJ: Transaction.

Sparrow, S. S., Cicchetti, D. V., & Balla, D. A. (2005). *Vineland Adaptive Behavior Scales, Second Edition: Survey Forms manual.* Circles Pines, MN: American Guidance Service.

Spearman, C. E. (1904). "General intelligence" objectively determined and measured. *American Journal of Psychology, 15,* 201–293.

Spearman, C. E. (1910). Correlation calculated from faulty data. *British Journal of Psychology, 3,* 271–295.

Spearman, C. E. (1927). *The abilities of man.* London: Macmillan.

Spearman, C. E., & Jones, L. (1950). *Human ability.* London: Macmillan.

Spitz, H. H. (1986). *The raising of intelligence: A selected history of attempts to raise retarded intelligence.* Hillsdale, NJ: Erlbaum.

Spitz, H. H. (1999). *Attempts to raise intelligence.* Hove, UK: Psychology Press/Taylor & Francis.

Stanovich, K. E., & Siegel, L. S. (1994). Phenotypic performance profile of children with reading disabilities: A regression-based test of the phonological-core variable-difference model. *Journal of Educational Psychology, 86,* 24–53.

Steege, M. W., & Watson, T. S. (2009). *Conducting school-based functional behavioral assessments: A practitioner's guide* (2nd ed.). New York: Guilford Press.

Stephens, K. R. (2011). Federal and state response to the gifted and talented. *Journal of Applied School Psychology, 27*, 306–318.

Stephens, K. R., & Karnes, F. A. (2000). State definitions for the gifted and talented revisited. *Exceptional Children, 66*, 219–238.

Stern, W. (1912). *The psychological methods of intelligence testing*. Baltimore: Warwick & York.

Sternberg, R. J. (1985). *Beyond IQ: A triarchic theory of human intelligence*. New York: Cambridge University Press.

Sternberg, R. J. (1988a). A triarchic view of intelligence in cross-cultural perspective. In S. H. Irvine & J. W. Berry (Eds.), *Human abilities in cultural context* (pp. 60–85). New York: Cambridge University Press.

Sternberg, R. J. (1988b). *The triarchic mind: A new theory of human intelligence*. New York: Viking Press.

Sternberg, R. J. (1994). 468 factor-analyzed data sets: What they tell us and don't tell us about human intelligence. *Psychological Science, 5*, 63–65.

Sternberg, R. L. (1996). Myths, countermyths, and truths about intelligence. *Educational Researcher, 25*, 11–16.

Sternberg, R. J., & Davidson, J. E. (Eds.). (1986). *Conceptions of giftedness*. New York: Cambridge University Press.

Sternberg, R. J., & Davidson, J. E. (Eds.). (2005). *Conceptions of giftedness* (2nd ed.). New York: Cambridge University Press.

Sternberg, R. J., & Detterman, D. K. (1986). *What is intelligence?: Contemporary viewpoints on its nature and definition*. Norwood, NJ: Ablex.

Sternberg, R. J., & Kaufman, S. B. (Eds.). (2011). *The Cambridge handbook of intelligence*. Cambridge, UK: Cambridge University Press.

Stevenson, J., Graham, P., Fredman, G., & McLoughlin, V. (1987). A twin study of genetic influences on reading and spelling ability and disability. *Journal of Child Psychology and Psychiatry, 28*, 229–247.

Stuebing, K. K., Barth, A. E., Molfese, P. J., Weiss, B., & Fletcher, J. M. (2009). IQ is not strongly related to response to reading instruction: A meta-analytic interpretation. *Exceptional Children, 76*, 31–51.

Subotnik, R. F., Olszewski-Kubilius, & Worrell, F. C. (2011). Rethinking giftedness and gifted education: A proposed direction forward based on psychological science. *Psychological Science in the Public Interest, 12*, 3–54.

Suttle, C. M. (2001). Visual acuity assessment in infants and young children. *Clinical and Experimental Optometry, 84*, 337–345.

Suzuki, L. A., Short, E. L., & Lee, C. S. (2011). Racial and ethnic group differences in intelligence in the United States. In R. J. Sternberg & S. B. Kaufman (Eds.), *The Cambridge handbook of intelligence* (pp. 273–292). Cambridge, UK: Cambridge University Press.

Swanson, H. L. (2009). Neuroscience and RTI: A complementary role. In E. Fletcher-Janzen & C. R. Reynolds (Eds.), *Neuropsychological perspectives on learning disabilities in the era of RTI: Recommendations for diagnosis and intervention* (pp. 28–53). Hoboken, NJ: Wiley.

Tallent, N. (1993). *Psychological report writing* (4th ed.). Englewood Cliffs, NJ: Prentice-Hall.

Tannenbaum, A. J. (1986). Giftedness: A psychosocial approach. In R. J. Sternberg & J. E. Davidson (Eds.), *Conceptions of giftedness* (pp. 21–52). New York: Cambridge University Press.

Tannenbaum, A. J. (2003). Nature and nurture of giftedness. In N. Colangelo & G. A. Davis (Eds.), *Handbook of gifted education* (pp. 45–59). Boston: Allyn & Bacon.

Teller, D. Y., McDonald, M. A., Preston, K., Sebris, S. L., & Dobson, V. (2008). Assessment of visual acuity in infants and children: The acuity card procedure. *Developmental Medicine and Child Neurology, 28*, 779–789.

Terman, L. M. (1916). *The measurement of intelligence*. Boston: Houghton Mifflin.

Terman, L. M. (Ed.). (1925). *Genetic studies of genius: Vol. 1. Mental and physical traits of a thousand gifted children*. Stanford, CA: Stanford University Press.

Terman, L. M. (1954). The discovery and encouragement of exceptional talent. *American Psychologist, 9*, 221–230.

Terman, L. M., & Oden, M. H. (1947). *Genetic studies of genius: Vol. 4. The gifted child grows up: Twenty-five years' follow up of a superior group*. Stanford, CA: Stanford University Press.

Terman, L. M., & Oden, M. H. (1959). *Genetic studies of genius: Vol. 5. The gifted group at mid-life: Thirty-five years' follow up of the superior child*. Stanford. CA: Stanford University Press.

Therrien, W. J., Zaman, M., & Banda, D. (2011). How can meta-analyses guide practice?: A review of the learning disability research base. *Remedial and Special Education, 32*, 206–218.

Thorndike, R. L. (1985). The central role of general ability in prediction. *Multivariate Behavioral Research, 20*, 241–254.

Thorndike, R. L. (1986). The role of general ability in prediction. *Journal of Vocational Behavior, 29*, 332–339.

Thurstone, L. L. (1938). *Primary mental abilities*. Chicago: University of Chicago Press.

Torgesen, J. K., Alexander, A., Wagner, R., Rashotte, C., Voeller, K., & Conway, T. (2001). Intensive remedial instruction for children with severe reading disabilities: Immediate and long-term outcomes from two instructional approaches. *Journal of Learning Disabilities, 34,* 33–58.

Tychanska, J. (2009). *Evaluation of speech and language impairment using the culture–language test classifications and interpretive matrix.* (Doctoral dissertation). Retrieved from ProQuest (Accession No. 3365687).

U.S. Office of Education. (1977). Assistance to states for education of handicapped children: Procedures for evaluating specific learning disabilities. *Federal Register, 42,* 65082–65085.

U.S. Office of Education. (1978). Gifted and Talented Children's Education Act, passed in 1978 (PL 95-561, Title IX, sec. 902).

Valencia, R. R. (1988). The McCarthy scales and Hispanic children: A review of psychometric research. *Hispanic Journal of Behavioral Sciences, 10,* 81–104.

Valencia, R. R., & Lopez, R. (1992). Assessment of racial and ethnic minority students: Problems and prospects. In M. Zeidner & R. Most (Eds.), *Psychological testing: An inside view* (pp. 399–439). Palo Alto, CA: Consulting Psychologists Press.

VanTassel-Baska, J. (2005). Domain-specific giftedness: Applications in school and life. In R. J. Sternberg & J. E. Davidson (Eds.), *Conceptions of giftedness* (pp. 358–376). New York: Cambridge University Press.

Vaughn, S., & Fuchs, L. S. (2003). Redefining learning disabilities as inadequate response to instruction: The promise and potential problems. *Learning Disabilities Research and Practice, 18,* 137–146.

Vazquez-Nuttal, E., Li, C., Dynda, A. M., Ortiz, S. O., Armengol, C. G., Walton, J. W., et al. (2007). Cognitive assessment of culturally and linguistically diverse students. In G. B. Esquivel & E. C. Lopez (Eds.), *Handbook of multicultural school psychology: An interdisciplinary perspective* (pp. 265–288). Mahwah, NJ: Erlbaum.

Vellutino, F. R., Scanlon, D. M., Sipay, E. R., Small, S. G., Pratt, A., Chen, R., et al. (1996). Cognitive profiles of difficult-to-remediate and readily remediated poor readers: Early intervention as a vehicle for distinguishing between cognitive and experiential deficits as basic causes of specific reading disability. *Journal of Educational Psychology, 88,* 601–638.

Verderosa, F. A. (2007). *Examining the effects of language and culture on the differential ability scales with bilingual preschoolers.* (Doctoral dissertation). Retrieved from ProQuest (Accession No. 3286027).

Walters, J., & Gardner, H. (1986). The crystallizing experience: Discovery of an intellectual gift. In R.

Sternberg & J. E. Davidson (Eds.), *Conceptions of giftedness* (pp. 163–182). New York: Cambridge University Press.

Watkins, M. W. (2006). Orthogonal higher-order structure of the Wechsler Intelligence Scale for Children—Fourth Edition. *Psychological Assessment, 18,* 123–125.

Watkins, M. W. (2009). Errors in diagnostic decision making and clinical judgment. In T. B. Gutkin & C. R. Reynolds (Eds.), *The handbook of school psychology* (4th ed., pp. 210–229). Hoboken, NJ: Wiley.

Watkins, M. W., & Canivez, G. L. (2004). Temporal stability of WISC-III subtest composite: Strengths and weaknesses. *Psychological Assessment, 16,* 133–138.

Watkins, M. W., Glutting, J. J., & Lei, P. (2007). Validity of the Full-Scale IQ when there is significant variability among WISC-III and WISC-IV factor scores. *Applied Neuropsychology, 14,* 13–20.

Watkins, M. W., Glutting, J. J., & Youngstrom, E. A. (2005). Issues in subtest profile analysis. In D. P. Flanagan & P. L. Harrison (Eds.), *Contemporary intellectual assessment: Theories, tests, and issues* (2nd ed., pp. 251–268). New York: Guilford Press.

Wechsler, D. (2002). *Wechsler Preschool and Primary Scale of Intelligence—Third Edition.* San Antonio, TX: Psychological Corporation.

Wechsler, D. (2003). *Wechsler Intelligence Scale for Children—Fourth Edition.* San Antonio, TX: Psychological Corporation.

Wechsler, D. (2008). *Wechsler Adult Intelligence Scale—Fourth Edition.* San Antonio, TX: Pearson Assessments.

Wechsler, D. (2009). *Wechsler Individual Achievement Test—Third Edition.* San Antonio, TX: Pearson Assessments.

Wechsler, D. (2011). *Wechsler Abbreviated Scale of Intelligence—Second Edition.* San Antonio, TX: Pearson Assessments.

Wechsler, D. (2012). *Wechsler Preschool and Primary Scale of Intelligence—Fourth Edition.* San Antonio, TX: Pearson Assessments.

Wechsler, D., & Naglieri, J. A. (2006). *Wechsler Nonverbal Scale of Ability.* San Antonio, TX: Psychological Corporation.

Wharton-Michael, P. (2008). Print vs. computer screen: Effects of medium on proofreading accuracy. *Journalism and Mass Communication Educator, 63*(1), 28–41.

Whitmore, J. R., & Maker, C. J. (1985). *Intellectual giftedness in disabled persons.* Rockville, MD: Aspen Systems.

Whitcomb, S. A., & Merrell, K. W. (2012). *Behavioral, social, and emotional assessment of children and adolescents* (4th ed.). Mahwah, NJ: Erlbaum.

Wiener, J. (1985). Teachers' comprehension of psychological reports. *Psychology in the Schools, 22,* 60–64.

Wiener, J. (1987). Factors affecting educators' comprehension of psychological reports. *Psychology in the Schools, 24,* 116–126.

Wiener, J., & Constaris, L. (2011). Teaching psychological report writing: Content and process. *Canadian Journal of School Psychology, 27,* 119–135.

Wiener, J., & Kohler, S. (1986). Parents' comprehension of psychological reports. *Psychology in the Schools, 23,* 265–270.

Wigdor, A. K., & Garner, W. R. (Eds.). (1982). *Ability testing: Uses, consequences, and controversies.* Committee on Ability Testing, Assembly of Behavioral and Social Sciences. Washington, DC: National Academy Press.

Winner, E. (1996). *Gifted children: Myths and realities.* New York: Basic Books.

Wodrich, D. L., Spencer, M. L. S., & Daley, K. B. (2006). Combining RTI and psychoeducational assessment: what we must assume to do otherwise. *Psychology in the Schools, 43,* 797–806.

Woodcock, R. W., McGrew, K. S., & Mather, N. (2001). *Woodcock–Johnson III.* Itasca, IL: Riverside.

Woodcock, R. W., McGrew, K. S., Schrank, F. A., & Mather, N. (2007). *Woodcock–Johnson III Tests of Cognitive Abilities, Normative Update.* Itasca, IL: Riverside.

World Health Organization. (2007). *International statistical classification of diseases and related health problems* (10th rev.). Retrieved December 3, 2010, from *http://apps.who.int/classifications/apps/icd/icd10online.*

Worrell, F. C. (2009). What does gifted mean?: Personal and social identity perspectives on giftedness in adolescence. In F. D. Horowitz, R. F. Subotnik, & D. J. Matthews (Eds.), *The development of giftedness and talent across the lifespan* (pp. 131–152). Washington, DC: American Psychological Association.

Worrell, F. C., & Erwin, J. O. (2011). Best practices in identifying students for gifted and talented education programs. *Journal of Applied School Psychology, 27,* 319–340.

Ysseldyke, J., & Elliott, J. (1999). Effective instructional practices: Implications for assessing educational environments. In C. R. Reynolds & T. B. Gutkin (Eds.), *The handbook of school psychology* (3rd ed., pp. 497–518). New York: Wiley.

Zhu, J., Cayton, T., Weiss, L., & Gabel, A. (2008). Technical Report No. 7: WISC-IV extended norms. Retrieved from *www.pearsonassessments.com/NR/rdonlyres/C1C19227–BC79–46D9–B43C-8E4A114F7E1F/0/WISCIV_TechReport_7.pdf.*

Zigler, E., & Farber, E. A. (1985). Commonalities between the intellectual extremes: Giftedness and mental retardation. In F. D. Horowitz & M. O'Brien (Eds.), *The gifted and talented: Developmental perspectives* (pp. 387–408). Washington, DC: American Psychological Association.

Index

"f" following a page number indicates a figure; "t" following a page number indicates a table